ICD·9·CM

FOURTH EDITION

THE INTERNATIONAL CLASSIFICATION OF DISEASES

9TH REVISION

CLINICAL MODIFICATION

Volume 3

PROCEDURES: TABULAR LIST & ALPHABETIC INDEX

Context Software Systems, Inc.

McGraw–Hill Inc.

New York St. Louis San Francisco Auckland Bogatá Caracas
Lisbon London Madrid Mexico Milan Montreal New Delhi Paris
San Juan Singapore Sydney Tokyo Toronto

**THE INTERNATIONAL CLASSIFICATION OF DISEASES–9TH REVISION–
CLINICAL MODIFICATION (ICD•9•CM) FOURTH EDITION**

Copyright © 1995 by McGraw–Hill, Inc. All rights reserved. Printed in the United States of America. Except as permitted under the United States Copyright Act of 1976, no part of this publication may be reproduced or distributed in any form or by any means, electronic or mechanical, including photocpy, recording, or stored in a data base or retrieval system, without the prior written permission of the publisher.

1 2 3 4 5 6 7 8 9 0 VNH VNH 9 5

ISBN 0–07–600729–4

DISCLAIMER

This book contains the same information that is published by the U.S. Public Health Service and Health Care Financing Administration. All official authorized addenda through September 30, 1993 have been included. The publisher has added color coding to assist in identifying codes requiring fourth and fifth digits and to assist in identifying codes which should only be used with caution. The publisher has also annotated codes for patient age, sex, and maternity. All information is believed to be reliable, but accuracy is not guaranteed by the editor or the publisher. Neither the editor nor the publisher may be held responsible for any misuse or misinterpretation of the information in this manual.

TABLE OF CONTENTS

Volume 3

Disclaimer ii
Foreword iv
Preface v
Introduction vi
Conventions Used in the Tabular List viii
Publisher's Annotations x

Tabular List

    1. Operations on the Nervous System 3
    2. Operations on the Endocrine System 7
    3. Operations on the Eye 9
    4. Operations on the Ear 15
    5. Operations on the Nose, Mouth, and Pharynx 19
    6. Operations on the Respiratory System 25
    7. Operations on the Cardiovascular System 29
    8. Operations on the Hemic and Lymphatic System 39
    9. Operations on the Digestive System 41
  10. Operations on the Urinary System 55
  11. Operations on the Male Genital Organs 61
  12. Operations on the Female Genital Organs 65
  13. Obstetrical Procedures 71
  14. Operations on the Musculoskeletal System 73
  15. Operations on the Integumentary System 83
  16. Miscellaneous Diagnostic and Therapeutic Procedures 87

Alphabetic Index 101

FOREWORD

This color–coded and specially annotated version of *ICD–9–CM* Volume 3 was produced in response to the significant changes that have taken place related to the reporting of procedures and services. Not only must *ICD–9–CM* procedure codes be reported to HCFA, the coding needs to be accurate. In the hospital setting special knowledge is required to meet the demands of DRG coding and Medicare Code Edits.

Through the use of a straightforward color–coding system, this *ICD–9–CM* Volume 3 manual provides visual cautions and warnings designed to help eliminate the most common types of procedure coding errors. The color red is used to flag non-specific codes (i.e., unspecified, not otherwise specified); amber–orange signifies that the code is an operating room procedure as defined by the DRG system; blue is used to highlight procedures which are not covered by Medicare. You will also find notations regarding non-operating room procedures, bilateral procedures, and patient sex.

The production of this manual required the extraordinary efforts of several individuals. William Elliott and Leslie Garvey spent numerous hours color-coding and proofing this manual. Erin Poto–Dill, RRA, CCS, of Optimal Coding and Reimbursement Resources, provided insight into the workings of the DRG system, along with suggested notations. Finally, John Christoffersson with McGraw–Hill provided the insightful guidance which led to the simple and conceptually elegant color–coding scheme incorporated in this version of *ICD–9–CM*.

Every effort has been made to create an *ICD–9–CM* Volume 3 that meets the needs of today's hospitals. Any comments and suggestions for improvement are welcomed. All correspondence should be sent to Context at the address below.

Leslie Garvey, Project Coordinator
Context Software Systems, Inc.
241 S. Frontage Road, Suite 38
Burr Ridge, Illinois 60521

PREFACE

This fourth edition of the *International Classification of Diseases, 9th Revision, Clinical Modification (ICD–9–CM)* is originally published by the United States Government in recognition of its responsibility to promulgate this classification throughout the United States for morbidity coding. The *International Classification of Diseases, 9th Revision,* published by the World Health Organization (WHO) is the foundation of the *ICD–9–CM* and continues to be the classification employed in cause–of–death coding in the United States. The *ICD–9–CM* is completely comparable with *ICD–9*. The WHO Collaborating Center for Classification of Diseases in North America serves as liaison between the international obligations for comparable classifications and the national health data needs of the United States.

The *ICD–9–CM* is recommended for use in all clinical settings but is required for reporting diagnoses and diseases to all U.S. Public Health Service and Health Care Financing Administration programs.

This version faithfully follows and contains the same information found in the U.S. Public Health Service and Health Care Financing Administration version of *ICD–9–CM*. All extensions, interpretations, modifications, addenda, or errata other than those approved by the U.S. Public Health Service and the Health Care Financing Administration are not to be considered official and should not be utilized. Continuous maintenance of the *ICD–9–CM* is the responsibility of the Federal Government. However, because the *ICD–9–CM* represents the best in contemporary thinking of clinicians, nosologists, epidemiologists, and statisticians from both public and private sectors, no future modifications will be considered without extensive advice from the appropriate representatives of all major users.

All official authorized addenda through October 1, 1994, have been included in this fourth edition.

INTRODUCTION

Volume 3
Procedure Classification: Tabular List & Alphabetic Index

An important new development occurred with the publication of the 9th Revision of the *International Classification of Diseases*—a classification of procedures in medicine was added. Although some countries, notably the United States, had included classifications of surgical procedures in their adaptations of *ICD* since 1959, international accord in this area had never been obtained and the classifications of procedures had never been included in *ICD* itself.

The World Health Organization had recognized the growing need for a classification of procedures used in medicine and in 1971 sponsored an international working party which was convened by the American Hospital Association to coordinate the recommendations for a classification of procedures, with the primary emphasis on surgery. At the International Conference for the 9th Revision of the International Classification of Diseases, convened at WHO Headquarters in Geneva in 1975, a proposal for a classification of procedures was submitted. The report of that conference states:

> In response to the requests from a number of member states, the Organization has drafted a classification of therapeutic, diagnostic, and prophylactic procedures in medicine, covering surgery, radiology, laboratory and other procedures. Various national classifications of this kind had been studied and advice sought from hospital associations in a number of countries. The intention was to provide a tool for use in the analysis of health services provided to patients in hospitals, clinics, outpatient departments, etc.
>
> The conference congratulates the Secretariat on this important development and,
>
> *Recommends* that the provisional procedures classification should be published as a supplement to, and not as integral parts, of the Ninth Revision of the International Classification of Diseases. They should be published in some inexpensive form, and after two or three years' experience, revised in the light of users' comments.

Accordingly, the *ICD-9* Classification of Procedures in Medicine appears as a series of separate sections called fascicles. Each fascicle provides a classification of a different mode of therapy, e.g., surgery, radiology, and laboratory procedures. Significant input to Fascicle V, "Surgical Procedures," came from the United States.

The *ICD-9-CM* Procedure Classification draws heavily on WHO's Fascicle V, "Surgical Procedures." Selected detail from the remaining fascicles of *ICD-9* was added where appropriate, but compatibility with the *ICD-9* Classification of Procedures in Medicine was not maintained when a different axis was deemed more clinically useful. The specifications for the *ICD-9-CM* Procedure Classification are:

1. The *ICD-9-CM* Procedure Classification is published in its own volume containing both a Tabular List and an Alphabetic Index.
2. The classification is a modification of Fascicle V, "Surgical Procedures," of the *ICD-9* Classification of Procedures in Medicine, working from the draft dated Geneva, 30 September — 6 October 1975, and labeled WHO/ICD-9/Rev. Conf. 75.4.
3. All three digit rubrics in the range 01–86 are maintained as they appear in Fascicle V, whenever feasible.
4. Nonsurgical procedures are segregated from the surgical procedures and are confined to the rubrics 87–99, whenever feasible.
5. Selected detail contained in the remaining fascicles of *ICD-9* Classification of Procedures in Medicine is accommodated where possible.
6. The structure of the classification is based on anatomy rather than surgical specialty.

INTRODUCTION

7. The *ICD-9-CM* Procedure Classification is numeric only, i.e., no alphabetic characters are used.
8. The classification is based on a two-digit structure with two decimal digits where necessary.
9. Compatibility with the *ICD-9* Classification of Procedures in Medicine was not maintained when a different axis was deemed more clinically appropriate.

The need for more specific clinical detail necessitated the expansion from three digits in *ICD-9* to four digits in the *ICD-9-CM* Procedure Classifications. While the major emphasis on clinical specificity is found in the section dealing with operative procedures, the codes for diagnostic and therapeutic procedures are also considerably more detailed than those appearing in previous classifications. This latter expansion is in response to the need for a procedure classification which could be used with equal efficiency both in hospitals and other primary care settings.

The Procedure Classification is published as Volume 3 of *ICD-9-CM* and contains both a Tabular List and an Alphabetic Index. This fourth edition of the Procedure Classification (Volume 3) contains all official authorized addenda published as of October 1, 1994.

CONVENTIONS USED IN THE TABULAR LISTS

The *ICD–9–CM* Tabular List for both the Disease and Procedure Classification makes use of certain abbreviations, punctuation, symbols, and other conventions which need to be clearly understood.

Abbreviations

NEC   *Not elsewhere classifiable.* The category number for the term including NEC is to be used only when the coder lacks the information necessary to code the term to a more specific category.

NOS   *Not otherwise specified.* This abbreviation is the equivalent of "unspecified."

Punctuation

[ ]   Brackets are used to enclose synonyms, alternative wordings, or explanatory phrases.

( )   Parentheses are used to enclose supplementary words which may be present or absent in the statement of a disease or procedure without affecting the code number to which it is assigned.

:   Colons are used in the Tabular List after an incomplete term which needs one or more of the modifiers which follow in order to make it assignable to a given category.

}   Braces are used to enclose a series of terms, each of which is modified by the statement appearing at the right of the brace.

Symbols

□   The lozenge symbol printed in the left margin preceding the disease code denotes a four–digit rubric unique to *ICD–9–CM*. The contents of these rubrics in *ICD–9–CM* are not the same as those in *ICD–9*. This symbol is used only in Volume 1 Diseases: Tabular List.

§   The section mark symbol preceding a code denotes the placement of a footnote at the bottom of the page which is applicable to all subdivisions in that code.

Other Conventions

Type Face

     Bold: Bold type face is used for all codes and titles in the Tabular List.

     Italics: Italicized type face is used for all exclusion notes and to identify those rubrics which are not to be used for primary tabulations of disease.

Format

     ICD–9–CM uses an indented format for ease in reference.

CONVENTIONS USED IN THE TABULAR LISTS

Instructional Notations

Includes: This note appears immediately under a three–digit code title to further define, or give example of, the contents of the category.

Excludes: Terms following the word excludes are to be coded elsewhere as indicated in each case.

Use additional code if desired:

> This instruction is placed in the Tabular List in those categories where the user may wish to add further information (by using an additional code) to give a more complete picture of the diagnosis or procedure.

Code also underlying disease:

> This instruction is used in those categories not intended for primary tabulation of disease. In such cases, the code, its title, and instructions appear in italics. The note requires that the underlying disease (etiology) be recorded first and the particular manifestation recorded secondarily. This note appears only in Volume 1 Diseases: Tabular List.

PUBLISHER'S ANNOTATIONS

This version of *ICD–9–CM* has been annotated to facilitate proper procedure coding by hospitals. Colors have been added to code numbers or descriptions where coding errors are likely to be made. Patient sex notations have also been included where appropriate. These annotations are in addition to the standard symbols and formats included in the United States Government original, reference to which may be found on pages xvii through xviii. The following is an explanation of the publisher–added annotations.

Color Notations

You will note that the need for additional digits is not highlighted in Volume 3. It is felt this information would be redundant for this volume, since there are no two-digit codes, and very few three-digit codes which are acceptable for reporting purposes.

There are a few codes that have a fourth-digit subclassification list located just after the main code description. The subclassification codes that could be applicable are located in brackets under the third-digit code. You must take care to expand these codes to four digits when using them.

Example:

> **78 Other operations on bones, except facial bones**
>
> **78.2 Limb shortening procedures**
> **[0,2-5,7-9]**

In any situation, always code out to the most specific code available.

 A red code number signifies that the procedure is non-specific (i.e., unspecified, not otherwise specified). Before assigning a code marked in red, review the medical record documentation and/or consult with the physician for more detailed information in order to possibly assign a more specific code. Use of non-specific codes can adversely affect reimbursement.

If the specific information given about the procedure does not allow classification to one of the specified subcategories, then assign the procedure to the "other" subcategory.

Example:

> **35.2 Replacement of heart valve**
>
> > 35.20 Replacement of unspecified heart valve
> > 35.21 Replacement of aortic valve with tissue graft
> > 35.22 Other replacement of aortic valve

If an aortic valve replacement with tissue graft was performed you would not use code 35.20, since code 35.21 specifies the procedure actually performed. If some other type of aortic valve replacement was performed, you would use code 35.22. If no specific heart valve is mentioned it is recommended that you attempt to obtain further information.

PUBLISHER'S ANNOTATIONS

 Amber–orange signifies that a code is considered an operating room procedure as defined by the DRG system.

Example:

42 Operations on esophagus

   42.5 Intrathoracic anastomosis of esophagus
      42.51 Intrathoracic esophagoesophagostomy

 Blue signifes a procedure that is not covered by Medicare.

Example:

50 Operations on liver

   50.5 Liver transplant
      50.51 Auxilliary liver transplant

Patient Sex Notations

♀   The female symbol appears to the right of a code's description when the diagnosis is specific to female patients.

Example:

   68.5 Vaginal hysterectomy ♀

♂   Thie male symbol appears to the right of a code's description when the diagnoses is specific to male patients.

Example:

   60.0 Incision of prostate ♂

ICD–9–CM

Operating Room Notations

|BIL| Bilateral Procedure. Some codes do not accurately reflect procedures that are performed in one admission on two or more <u>different</u> bilateral joints of the lower extremities. These codes, when combined, show a bilateral procedure when, actually, they could be duplicate procedures (i.e., procedures performed on a single joint). These codes are identified by the MCE as "Bilateral Procedure" whenever two or more <u>different</u> joint procedures are coded, and the principal diagnois causes assignment to MDC 8.

<u>Example:</u>

81.54 Total knee replacement |BIL|

81.55 Revise knee replacement |BIL|

If both are coded on the claim, the edit "Bilateral Procedure" will appear next to each code. This edit instructs the fiscal intermediary to verify that these procedures were performed on two separate joints. However, if 81.54 is coded twice, the edit would not appear since this signifies a true bilateral procedure.

|NOR| Non-operating room procedure. Signifies a non-operating room procedure as defined by the DRG system. These codes can affect the choice of DRG.

<u>Example:</u>

37.21 Right heart cardiac catheterization |NOR|

Revision Notations

● The appearance of a darkened circle to the left of a code number in the Tabular List signifies that the code is new to the 1995 version of ICD–9–CM.

▲ A delta (or triangle) to the left of a code number in the Tabular List signifies that the code's description has changed.

▸ An arrow to the left of an entry in the Index signifies that new or revised material now appears in the entry.

Volume 3

PROCEDURES: TABULAR LIST & ALPHABETIC INDEX

1. OPERATIONS ON THE NERVOUS SYSTEM (01–05)

01 Incision and excision of skull, brain, and cerebral meninges

01.0 Cranial puncture

01.01 Cisternal puncture
Cisternal tap

Excludes: pneumocisternogram (87.02)

01.02 Ventriculopuncture through previously implanted catheter
Puncture of ventricular shunt tubing

01.09 Other cranial puncture
Aspiration of
 subarachnoid space
 subdural space
Cranial aspiration NOS
Puncture of anterior fontanel
Subdural tap (through fontanel)

01.1 Diagnostic procedures on skull, brain, and cerebral meninges

01.11 Closed [percutaneous] [needle] biopsy of cerebral meninges
Burr hole approach

01.12 Open biopsy of cerebral meninges

01.13 Closed [percutaneous] [needle] biopsy of brain
Burr hole approach
Stereotactic method

01.14 Open biopsy of brain

01.15 Biopsy of skull

01.18 Other diagnostic procedures on brain and cerebral meninges

Excludes: cerebral:
   arteriography (88.41)
   thermography (88.81)
 contrast radiogram of brain (87.01–87.02)
 echoencephalogram (88.71)
 electroencephalogram (89.14)
 microscopic examination of specimen from nervous system and of spinal fluid (90.01–90.09)
 neurologic examination (89.13)
 phlebography of head and neck (88.61)
 pneumoencephalogram (87.01)
 radioisotope scan:
   cerebral (92.11)
   head NEC (92.12)
 tomography of head:
   C.A.T. scan (87.03)
   other (87.04)

01.19 Other diagnostic procedures on skull

Excludes: transillumination of skull (89.16)
 x-ray of skull (87.17)

01.2 Craniotomy and craniectomy

Excludes: decompression of skull fracture (02.02)
 exploration of orbit (16.01–16.09)
 that as operative approach — omit code

01.21 Incision and drainage of cranial sinus

01.22 Removal of intracranial neurostimulator

Excludes: removal with synchronous replacement (02.93)

01.23 Reopening of craniotomy site

01.24 Other craniotomy
Cranial
 decompression
 exploration
 trephination
Craniotomy NOS
Craniotomy with removal of:
 epidural abscess
 extradural hematoma
 foreign body of skull

Excludes: removal of foreign body with incision into brain (01.39)

01.25 Other craniectomy
Debridement of skull NOS
Sequestrectomy of skull

Excludes: debridement of compound fracture of skull (02.02)
 strip craniectomy (02.01)

01.3 Incision of brain and cerebral meninges

01.31 Incision of cerebral meninges
Drainage of
 intracranial hygroma
 subarachnoid abscess (cerebral)
 subdural empyema

01.32 Lobotomy and tractotomy
Division of:
 brain tissue
 cerebral tracts
Percutaneous (radiofrequency) cingulotomy

01.39 Other incision of brain
Amygdalohippocampotomy
Drainage of intracerebral hematoma
Incision of brain NOS

Excludes: division of cortical adhesions (02.91)

01.4 Operations on thalamus and globus pallidus

01.41 Operations on thalamus
Chemothalamectomy
Thalamotomy

01.42 Operations on globus pallidus
Pallidoansectomy
Pallidotomy

01.5 Other excision or destruction of brain and meninges

01.51 Excision of lesion or tissue of cerebral meninges
Decortication ⎫
Resection ⎬ of (cerebral) meninges
Stripping of subdural membrane ⎭

Excludes: biopsy of cerebral meninges (01.11–01.12)

01.52 Hemispherectomy

01.53 Lobectomy of brain

01.59 Other excision or destruction of lesion or tissue of brain
Curettage of brain
Debridement of brain
Marsupialization of brain cyst
Transtemporal (mastoid) excision of brain tumor

Excludes: biopsy of brain (01.13–01.14)

01.6 Excision of lesion of skull
Removal of granulation tissue of cranium

Excludes: biopsy of skull (01.15)
 sequestrectomy (01.25)

02 Other operations on skull, brain, and cerebral meninges

02.0 Cranioplasty

> *Excludes:* that with synchronous repair of encephalocele (02.12)

02.01 Opening of cranial suture
Linear craniectomy
Strip craniectomy

02.02 Elevation of skull fracture fragments
Debridement of compound fracture of skull
Decompression of skull fracture
Reduction of skull fracture

Code also any synchronous debridement of brain (01.59)

> *Excludes:* debridement of skull NOS (01.25)
> removal of granulation tissue of cranium (01.6)

02.03 Formation of cranial bone flap
Repair of skull with flap

02.04 Bone graft to skull
Pericranial graft (autogenous) (heterogenous)

02.05 Insertion of skull plate
Replacement of skull plate

02.06 Other cranial osteoplasty
Repair of skull NOS
Revision of bone flap of skull

02.07 Removal of skull plate

> *Excludes:* removal with synchronous replacement (02.05)

02.1 Repair of cerebral meninges

> *Excludes:* marsupialization of cerebral lesion (01.59)

02.11 Simple suture of dura matter of brain

02.12 Other repair of cerebral meninges
Closure of fistula of cerebrospinal fluid
Dural graft
Repair of encephalocele including synchronous cranioplasty
Repair of meninges NOS
Subdural patch

02.13 Ligation of meningeal vessel
Ligation of:
  longitudinal sinus
  middle meningeal artery

02.14 Choroid plexectomy
Cauterization of choroid plexus

02.2 Ventriculostomy
Anastomosis of ventricle to:
  cervical subarachnoid space
  cisterna magna
Insertion of Holter valve
Ventriculocisternal intubation

02.3 Extracranial ventricular shunt
Includes: that with insertion of valve

02.31 Ventricular shunt to structure in head and neck
Ventricle to nasopharynx shunt
Ventriculomastoid anastomosis

02.32 Ventricular shunt to circulatory system
Ventriculoatrial anastomosis
Ventriculocaval shunt

02.33 Ventricular shunt to thoracic cavity
Ventriculopleural anastomosis

02.34 Ventricular shunt to abdominal cavity and organs
Ventriculocholecystostomy
Ventriculoperitoneostomy

02.35 Ventricular shunt to urinary system
Ventricle to ureter shunt

02.39 Other operations to establish drainage of ventricle
Ventricle to bone marrow shunt
Ventricular shunt to extracranial site NEC

02.4 Revision, removal, and irrigation or ventricular shunt

02.41 Irrigation of ventricular shunt

02.42 Replacement of ventricular shunt
Reinsertion of Holter valve
Replacement of ventricular catheter

02.43 Removal of ventricular shunt

02.9 Other operations on skull, brain, and cerebral meninges

> *Excludes:* operations on:
> pineal gland (07.17, 07.51–07.59)
> pituitary gland [hypophysis] (07.13–07.15, 07.61–07.79)

02.91 Lysis of cortical adhesions

02.92 Repair of brain

02.93 Implantation of intracranial neurostimulator
Implantation, insertion, placement, or replacement of intracranial:
  brain pacemaker [neuropacemaker]
  depth electrodes
  electroencephalographic receiver
  epidural pegs
    electroencephalographic receiver
  foramen ovale electrodes
    intracranial electrostimulator
  subdural grids
  subdural strips

02.94 Insertion or replacement of skull tongs or halo traction device

02.95 Removal of skull tongs or halo traction device

02.96 Insertion of sphenoidal electrodes

02.99 Other

> *Excludes:* chemical shock therapy (94.24)
> electroshock therapy:
>   subconvulsive (94.26)
>   other (94.27)

03 Operations on spinal cord and spinal canal structures

03.0 Exploration and decompression of spinal canal structures

03.01 Removal of foreign body from spinal canal

03.02 Reopening of laminectomy site

03.09 Other exploration and decompression of spinal canal
Decompression:
  laminectomy
  laminotomy
Exploration of spinal nerve root
Foraminotomy

> *Excludes:* drainage of spinal fluid by anastomosis (03.71–03.79)
> laminectomy with excision of intervertebral disc (80.51)
> spinal tap (03.31)
> that as operative approach — omit code

03.1 Division of intraspinal nerve root
Rhizotomy

OPERATIONS ON THE NERVOUS SYSTEM (01-05)

03.2 Chordotomy

03.21 Percutaneous chordotomy
Stereotactic chordotomy

03.29 Other chordotomy
Chordotomy NOS
Tractotomy (one-stage) (two-stage) of spinal cord
Transection of spinal cord tracts

03.3 Diagnostic procedures on spinal cord and spinal canal structures

03.31 Spinal tap
Lumbar puncture for removal of dye

> Excludes: lumbar puncture for injection of dye [myelogram] (87.21)

03.32 Biopsy of spinal cord or spinal meninges

03.39 Other diagnostic procedures on spinal cord and spinal canal structures

> Excludes: microscopic examination of specimen from system or of spinal fluid (90.01–90.09)
> x-ray of spine (87.21–87.29)

03.4 Excision or destruction of lesion of spinal cord or spinal meninges

Curettage
Debridement   } of spinal cord or spinal meninges
Marsupialization of cyst
Resection

> Excludes: biopsy of spinal cord or meninges (03.32)

03.5 Plastic operations on spinal cord structures

03.51 Repair of spinal meningocele
Repair of meningocele NOS

03.52 Repair of spinal myelomeningocele

03.53 Repair of vertebral fracture
Elevation of spinal bone fragments
Reduction of fracture of vertebrae
Removal of bony spicules from spinal canal

03.59 Other repair and plastic operations on spinal cord structures
Repair of:
  diastematomyelia
  spina bifida NOS
  spinal cord NOS
  spinal meninges NOS
  vertebral arch defect

03.6 Lysis of adhesions of spinal cord and nerve roots

03.7 Shunt of spinal theca
Includes: that with valve

03.71 Spinal subarachnoid-peritoneal shunt

03.72 Spinal subarachnoid-ureteral shunt

03.79 Other shunt of spinal theca
Lumbar-subarachnoid shunt NOS
Pleurothecal anastomosis
Salpingothecal anastomosis

03.8 Injection of destructive agent into spinal canal

03.9 Other operations on spinal cord and spinal canal structures

03.90 Insertion of catheter into spinal canal for infusion of therapeutic or palliative substances
Insertion of catheter into epidural, subarachnoid, or subdural space of spine with intermittent or continuous infusion of drug (with creation of any reservoir)

Code also any implantation of infusion pump (86.06)

03.91 Injection of anesthetic into spinal canal for analgesia

> Excludes: that for operative anesthesia—omit code

03.92 Injection of other agent into spinal canal
Intrathecal injection of steroid
Subarachnoid perfusion of refrigerated saline

> Excludes: injection of:
>   contrast material for myelogram (87.21)
>   destructive agent into spinal canal (03.8)

03.93 Insertion or replacement of spinal neurostimulator

03.94 Removal of spinal neurostimulator

03.95 Spinal blood patch

03.96 Percutaneous denervation of facet

03.97 Revision of spinal thecal shunt

03.98 Removal of spinal thecal shunt

03.99 Other

04 Operations on cranial and peripheral nerves

04.0 Incision, division, and excision of cranial and peripheral nerves

> Excludes: opticociliary neurectomy (12.79)
> sympathetic ganglionectomy (05.21–05.29)

04.01 Excision of acoustic neuroma
That by craniotomy

> Excludes: that by radiosurgery (04.07)

04.02 Division of trigeminal nerve
Retrogasserian neurotomy

04.03 Division or crushing of other cranial and peripheral nerves

> Excludes: that of:
>   glossopharyngeal nerve (29.92)
>   laryngeal nerve (31.91)
>   nerves to adrenal glands (07.42)
>   phrenic nerve for collapse of lung (33.31)
>   vagus nerve (44.00–44.03)

04.04 Other incision of cranial and peripheral nerves

04.05 Gasserian ganglionectomy

04.06 Other cranial or peripheral ganglionectomy

> Excludes: sympathetic ganglionectomy (05.21–05.29)

04.07 Other excision or avulsion of cranial and peripheral nerves
Curettage
Debridement } of peripheral nerve
Resection
Excision of peripheral neuroma [Morton's]

> Excludes: biopsy of cranial or peripheral nerve (04.11–04.12)

04.1 Diagnostic procedures on peripheral nervous system

04.11 Closed [percutaneous] [needle] biopsy of cranial or peripheral nerve or ganglion

04.12 Open biopsy of cranial or peripheral nerve or ganglion

04.19 Other diagnostic procedures on cranial and peripheral nerves and ganglia

> Excludes: microscopic examination of specimen from nervous system (90.01–90.09)
> neurologic examination (89.13)

04.2 Destruction of cranial and peripheral nerves

Destruction of cranial or peripheral nerves by:
injection of neurolytic agent
radiofrequency

04.3 Suture of cranial and peripheral nerves

04.4 Lysis of adhesions and decompression of cranial and peripheral nerves

04.41 Decompression of trigeminal nerve root

04.42 Other cranial nerve decompression

04.43 Release of carpal tunnel

04.44 Release of tarsal tunnel

04.49 Other peripheral nerve or ganglion decompression or lysis of adhesions

Peripheral nerve neurolysis NOS

04.5 Cranial or peripheral nerve graft

04.6 Transposition of cranial and peripheral nerves

Nerve transplantation

04.7 Other cranial or peripheral neuroplasty

04.71 Hypoglossal-facial anastomosis

04.72 Accessory-facial anastomosis

04.73 Accessory-hypoglossal anastomosis

04.74 Other anastomosis of cranial or peripheral nerve

04.75 Revision of previous repair of cranial and peripheral nerves

04.76 Repair of old traumatic injury of cranial and peripheral nerves

04.79 Other neuroplasty

04.8 Injection into peripheral nerve

> Excludes: destruction of nerve (by injection of neurolytic agent) (04.2)

Peripheral nerve injection, not otherwise specified

04.81 Injection of anesthetic into peripheral nerve for analgesia

> Excludes: that for operative anesthesia — omit code

04.89 Injection of other agent, except neurolytic

> Excludes: injection of neurolytic agent (04.2)

04.9 Other operations on cranial and peripheral nerves

04.91 Neurectasis

04.92 Implantation or replacement of peripheral neurostimulator

04.93 Removal of peripheral neurostimulator

04.99 Other

05 Operations on sympathetic nerves or ganglia

> Excludes: paracervical uterine denervation (69.3)

05.0 Division of sympathetic nerve or ganglion

> Excludes: that of nerves to adrenal glands (07.42)

05.1 Diagnostic procedures on sympathetic nerves or ganglia

05.11 Biopsy of sympathetic nerve or ganglion

05.19 Other diagnostic procedures on sympathetic nerves or ganglia

05.2 Sympathectomy

05.21 Sphenopalatine ganglionectomy

05.22 Cervical sympathectomy

05.23 Lumbar sympathectomy

05.24 Presacral sympathectomy

05.29 Other sympathectomy and ganglionectomy

Excision or avulsion of sympathetic nerve NOS
Sympathetic ganglionectomy NOS

> Excludes: biopsy of sympathetic nerve or ganglion (05.11)
> opticociliary neurectomy (12.79)
> periarterial sympathectomy (39.7)
> tympanosympathectomy (20.91)

05.3 Injection into sympathetic nerve or ganglion

> Excludes: injection of ciliary sympathetic ganglion (12.79)

05.31 Injection of anesthetic into sympathetic nerve for analgesia

05.32 Injection of neurolytic agent into sympathetic nerve

05.39 Other injection into sympathetic nerve or ganglion

05.8 Other operations on sympathetic nerves or ganglia

05.81 Repair of sympathetic nerve or ganglion

05.89 Other

05.9 Other operations on nervous system

2. OPERATIONS ON THE ENDOCRINE SYSTEM (06–07)

06 Operations on thyroid and parathyroid glands
Includes: incidental resection of hyoid bone

06.0 Incision of thyroid field

> Excludes: division of isthmus (06.91)

06.01 Aspiration of thyroid field
Percutaneous or needle drainage of thyroid field

> Excludes: aspiration biopsy of thyroid (06.11)
> drainage by incision (06.09)
> postoperative aspiration of field (06.02)

06.02 Reopening of wound of thyroid field
Reopening of wound of thyroid field for:
  control of (postoperative) hemorrhage
  examination
  exploration
  removal of hematoma

06.09 Other incision of thyroid field
Drainage of hematoma
Drainage of thyroglossal tract
Exploration:
  neck
  thyroid (field)
Removal of foreign body
} by incision
Thyroidotomy NOS

> Excludes: postoperative exploration (06.02)
> removal of hematoma by aspiration (06.01)

06.1 Diagnostic procedures on thyroid and parathyroid glands

06.11 Closed [percutaneous] [needle] biopsy of thyroid gland
Aspiration biopsy of thyroid

06.12 Open biopsy of thyroid gland

06.13 Biopsy of parathyroid gland

06.19 Other diagnostic procedures on thyroid and parathyroid glands

> Excludes: radioisotope scan of:
> parathyroid (92.13)
> thyroid (92.01)
> soft tissue x-ray of thyroid field (87.09)

06.2 Unilateral thyroid lobectomy
Complete removal of one lobe of thyroid (with removal of isthmus or portion of other lobe)
Hemithyroidectomy

> Excludes: partial substernal thyroidectomy (06.51)

06.3 Other partial thyroidectomy

06.31 Excision of lesion of thyroid

> Excludes: biopsy of thyroid (06.11–06.12)

06.39 Other
Isthmectomy
Partial thyroidectomy NOS

> Excludes: partial substernal thyroidectomy (06.51)

06.4 Complete thyroidectomy

> Excludes: complete substernal thyroidectomy (06.52)
> that with laryngectomy (30.3–30.4)

06.5 Substernal thyroidectomy

06.50 Substernal thyroidectomy, not otherwise specified

06.51 Partial substernal thyroidectomy

06.52 Complete substernal thyroidectomy

06.6 Excision of lingual thyroid
Excision of thyroid by:
  submental route
  transoral route

06.7 Excision of thyroglossal duct or tract

06.8 Parathyroidectomy

06.81 Complete parathyroidectomy

06.89 Other parathyroidectomy
Parathyroidectomy NOS
Partial parathyroidectomy

> Excludes: biopsy of parathyroid (06.13)

06.9 Other operations on thyroid (region) and parathyroid

06.91 Division of thyroid isthmus
Transection of thyroid isthmus

06.92 Ligation of thyroid vessels

06.93 Suture of thyroid gland

06.94 Thyroid tissue reimplantation
Autotransplantation of thyroid tissue

06.95 Parathyroid tissue reimplantation
Autotransplantation of parathyroid tissue

06.98 Other operations on thyroid glands

06.99 Other operations on parathyroid glands

07 Operations on other endocrine glands
Includes: operations on:
  adrenal glands
  pineal gland
  pituitary gland
  thymus

> cludes: operations on:
> aortic and carotid bodies (39.8)
> ovaries (65.0–65.99)
> pancreas (52.01–52.99)
> testes (62.0–62.99)

07.0 Exploration of adrenal field

> Excludes: incision of adrenal (gland) (07.41)

07.00 Exploration of adrenal field, not otherwise specified

07.01 Unilateral exploration of adrenal field

07.02 Bilateral exploration of adrenal field

07.1 Diagnostic procedures on adrenal glands, pituitary gland, pineal gland, and thymus

07.11 Closed [percutaneous] [needle] biopsy of adrenal gland

07.12 Open biopsy of adrenal gland

07.13 Biopsy of pituitary gland, transfrontal approach

07.14 Biopsy of pituitary gland, transsphenoidal approach

07.15 Biopsy of pituitary gland, unspecified approach

07.16 Biopsy of thymus

07.17 Biopsy of pineal gland

07.19 Other diagnostic procedures on adrenal glands, pituitary gland, pineal gland, and thymus

> Excludes: microscopic examination of specimen from endocrine gland (90.11–90.19)
> radioisotope scan of pituitary gland (92.11)

07.2 Partial adrenalectomy

07.21 Excision of lesion of adrenal gland
> Excludes: biopsy of adrenal gland (07.11–07.12)

07.22 Unilateral adrenalectomy
Adrenalectomy NOS
> Excludes: excision of remaining adrenal gland (07.3)

07.29 Other partial adrenalectomy
Partial adrenalectomy NOS

07.3 Bilateral adrenalectomy
Excision of remaining adrenal gland
> Excludes: bilateral partial adrenalectomy (07.29)

07.4 Other operations on adrenal glands, nerves, and vessels

07.41 Incision of adrenal gland
Adrenalotomy (with drainage)

07.42 Division of nerves to adrenal glands

07.43 Ligation of adrenal vessels

07.44 Repair of adrenal gland

07.45 Reimplantation of adrenal tissue
Autotransplantation of adrenal tissue

07.49 Other

07.5 Operations on pineal gland

07.51 Exploration of pineal field
> Excludes: that with incision of pineal gland (07.52)

07.52 Incision of pineal gland

07.53 Partial excision of pineal gland
> Excludes: biopsy of pineal gland (07.17)

07.54 Total excision of pineal gland
Pinealectomy (complete) (total)

07.59 Other operations on pineal gland

07.6 Hypophysectomy

07.61 Partial excision of pituitary gland, transfrontal approach
Cryohypophysectomy, partial
Division of hypophyseal stalk
Excision of lesion of pituitary [hypophysis] } transfrontal approach
Hypophysectomy, subtotal
Infundibulectomy, hypophyseal
> Excludes: biopsy of pituitary gland, transfrontal approach (07.13)

07.62 Partial excision of pituitary gland, transsphenoidal approach
> Excludes: biopsy of pituitary gland, transsphenoidal approach (07.14)

07.63 Partial excision of pituitary gland, unspecified approach
> Excludes: biopsy of pituitary gland NOS (07.15)

07.64 Total excision of pituitary gland, transfrontal approach
Ablation of pituitary by implantation (strontium-yttrium) (Y) } transfrontal approach
Cryohypophysectomy, complete

07.65 Total excision of pituitary gland, transsphenoidal approach

07.68 Total excision of pituitary gland, other specified approach
Ablation of pituitary:
  Bragg peak proton beam
  Cobalt-60

07.69 Total excision of pituitary gland, unspecified approach
Hypophysectomy NOS
Pituitectomy NOS

07.7 Other operations on hypophysis

07.71 Exploration of pituitary fossa
> Excludes: exploration with incision of pituitary gland (07.72)

07.72 Incision of pituitary gland
Aspiration of:
  craniobuccal pouch
  craniopharyngioma
  hypophysis
  pituitary gland
  Rathke's pouch

07.79 Other
Insertion of pack into sella turcica

07.8 Thymectomy

07.80 Thymectomy, not otherwise specified

07.81 Partial excision of thymus
> Excludes: biopsy of thymus (07.16)

07.82 Total excision of thymus

07.9 Other operations on thymus

07.91 Exploration of thymus field
> Excludes: exploration with incision of thymus (07.92)

07.92 Incision of thymus

07.93 Repair of thymus

07.94 Transplantation of thymus

07.99 Other
Thymopexy

3. OPERATIONS ON THE EYE (08–16)

08 Operations on eyelids

Includes: operations on the eyebrow

08.0 Incision of eyelid

08.01 Incision of lid margin

08.02 Severing of blepharorrhaphy

08.09 Other incision of eyelid

08.1 Diagnostic procedures on eyelid

08.11 Biopsy of eyelid

08.19 Other diagnostic procedures on eyelid

08.2 Excision or destruction of lesion or tissue of eyelid

Code also any synchronous reconstruction (08.61–08.74)

Excludes: biopsy of eyelid (08.11)

08.20 Removal of lesion of eyelid, not otherwise specified
Removal of meibomian gland NOS

08.21 Excision of chalazion

08.22 Excision of other minor lesion of eyelid
Excision of:
 verucca
 wart

08.23 Excision of major lesion of eyelid, partial-thickness
Excision involving one-fourth or more of lid margin, partial-thickness

08.24 Excision of major lesion of eyelid, full-thickness
Excision involving one-fourth or more of lid margin, full-thickness
Wedge resection of eyelid

08.25 Destruction of lesion of eyelid

08.3 Repair of blepharoptosis and lid retraction

08.31 Repair of blepharoptosis by frontalis muscle technique with suture

08.32 Repair of blepharoptosis by frontalis muscle technique with fascial sling

08.33 Repair of blepharoptosis by resection or advancement of levator muscle or aponeurosis

08.34 Repair of blepharoptosis by other levator muscle techniques

08.35 Repair of blepharoptosis by tarsal technique

08.36 Repair of blepharoptosis by other techniques
Correction of eyelid ptosis NOS
Orbicularis oculi muscle sling for correction of blepharoptosis

08.37 Reduction of overcorrection of ptosis

08.38 Correction of lid retraction

08.4 Repair of entropion or ectropion

08.41 Repair of entropion or ectropion by thermocauterization

08.42 Repair of entropion or ectropion by suture technique

08.43 Repair of entropion or ectropion with wedge resection

08.44 Repair of entropion or ectropion with lid reconstruction

08.49 Other repair of entropion or ectropion

08.5 Other adjustment of lid position

08.51 Canthotomy
Enlargement of palpebral fissure

08.52 Blepharorrhaphy
Canthorrhaphy
Tarsorrhaphy

08.59 Other
Canthoplasty NOS
Repair of epicanthal fold

08.6 Reconstruction of eyelid with flaps or grafts

Excludes: that associated with repair of entropion and ectropion (08.44)

08.61 Reconstruction of eyelid with skin flap or graft

08.62 Reconstruction of eyelid with mucous membrane flap or graft

08.63 Reconstruction of eyelid with hair follicle graft

08.64 Reconstruction of eyelid with tarsoconjunctival flap
Transfer of tarsoconjunctival flap from opposing lid

08.69 Other reconstruction of eyelid with flaps or grafts

08.7 Other reconstruction of eyelid

Excludes: that associated with repair of entropion and ectropion (08.44)

08.70 Reconstruction of eyelid, not otherwise specified

08.71 Reconstruction of eyelid involving lid margin, partial-thickness

08.72 Other reconstruction of eyelid, partial-thickness

08.73 Reconstruction of eyelid involving lid margin, full-thickness

08.74 Other reconstruction of eyelid, full-thickness

08.8 Other repair of eyelid

08.81 Linear repair of laceration of eyelid or eyebrow

08.82 Repair of laceration involving lid margin, partial-thickness

08.83 Other repair of laceration of eyelid, partial-thickness

08.84 Repair of laceration involving lid margin, full-thickness

08.85 Other repair of laceration of eyelid, full-thickness

08.86 Lower eyelid rhytidectomy

08.87 Upper eyelid rhytidectomy

08.89 Other eyelid repair

08.9 Other operations on eyelids

08.91 Electrosurgical epilation of eyelid

08.92 Cryosurgical epilation of eyelid

08.93 Other epilation of eyelid

08.99 Other

09 Operations on lacrimal system

09.0 Incision of lacrimal gland

Incision of lacrimal cyst (with drainage)

09.1 Diagnostic procedures on lacrimal system

09.11 Biopsy of lacrimal gland

09.12 Biopsy of lacrimal sac

09.19 Other diagnostic procedures on lacrimal system

Excludes: contrast dacryocystogram (87.05)
soft tissue x-ray of nasolacrimal duct (87.09)

09.2 Excision of lesion or tissue of lacrimal gland

09.20 Excision of lacrimal gland, not otherwise specified

09.21 Excision of lesion of lacrimal gland

> Excludes: biopsy of lacrimal gland (09.11)

09.22 Other partial dacryoadenectomy

> Excludes: biopsy of lacrimal gland (09.11)

09.23 Total dacryoadenectomy

09.3 Other operations on lacrimal gland

09.4 Manipulation of lacrimal passage
Includes: removal of calculus
that with dilation

> Excludes: contrast dacryocystogram (87.05)

09.41 Probing of lacrimal punctum

09.42 Probing of lacrimal canaliculi

09.43 Probing of nasolacrimal duct

> Excludes: that with insertion of tube or stent (09.44)

09.44 Intubation of nasolacrimal duct
Insertion of stent into nasolacrimal duct

09.49 Other manipulation of lacrimal passage

09.5 Incision of lacrimal sac and passages

09.51 Incision of lacrimal punctum

09.52 Incision of lacrimal canaliculi

09.53 Incision of lacrimal sac

09.59 Other incision of lacrimal passages
Incision (and drainage) of nasolacrimal duct NOS

09.6 Excision of lacrimal sac and passage

> Excludes: biopsy of lacrimal sac (09.12)

09.7 Repair of canaliculus and punctum

> Excludes: repair of eyelid (08.81–08.89)

09.71 Correction of everted punctum

09.72 Other repair of punctum

09.73 Repair of canaliculus

09.8 Fistulization of lacrimal tract to nasal cavity

09.81 Dacryocystorhinostomy [DCR]

09.82 Conjunctivocystorhinostomy
Conjunctivodacryocystorhinostomy [CDCR]

> Excludes: that with insertion of tube or stent (09.83)

09.83 Conjunctivorhinostomy with insertion of tube or stent

09.9 Other operations on lacrimal system

09.91 Obliteration of lacrimal punctum

09.99 Other

10 Operations on conjunctiva

10.0 Removal of embedded foreign body from conjunctiva by incision

> Excludes: removal of:
> embedded foreign body without incision (98.22)
> superficial foreign body (98.21)

10.1 Other incision of conjunctiva

10.2 Diagnostic procedures on conjunctiva

10.21 Biopsy of conjunctiva

10.29 Other diagnostic procedures on conjunctiva

10.3 Excision or destruction of lesion or tissue of conjunctiva

10.31 Excision of lesion or tissue of conjunctiva
Excision of ring of conjunctiva around cornea

> Excludes: biopsy of conjunctiva (10.21)

10.32 Destruction of lesion of conjunctiva

> Excludes: excision of lesion (10.31)
> thermocauterization for entropion (08.41)

10.33 Other destructive procedures on conjunctiva
Removal of trachoma follicles

10.4 Conjunctivoplasty

10.41 Repair of symblepharon with free graft

10.42 Reconstruction of conjunctival cul-de-sac with free graft

> Excludes: revision of enucleation socket with graft (16.63)

10.43 Other reconstruction of conjunctival cul-de-sac

> Excludes: revision of enucleation socket (16.64)

10.44 Other free graft to conjunctiva

10.49 Other conjunctivoplasty

> Excludes: repair of cornea with conjunctival flap (11.53)

10.5 Lysis of adhesions of conjunctiva and eyelid
Division of symblepharon (with insertion of conformer)

10.6 Repair of laceration of conjunctiva

> Excludes: that with repair of sclera (12.81)

10.9 Other operations on conjunctiva

10.91 Subconjunctival injection

10.99 Other

11 Operations on cornea

11.0 Magnetic removal of embedded foreign body from cornea

> Excludes: that with incision (11.1)

11.1 Incision of cornea
Incision of cornea for removal of foreign body

11.2 Diagnostic procedures on cornea

11.21 Scraping of cornea for smear or culture

11.22 Biopsy of cornea

11.29 Other diagnostic procedures on cornea

11.3 Excision of pterygium

11.31 Transposition of pterygium

11.32 Excision of pterygium with corneal graft

11.39 Other excision of pterygium

11.4 Excision or destruction of tissue or other lesion of cornea

11.41 Mechanical removal of corneal epithelium
That by chemocauterization

> Excludes: that for smear or culture (11.21)

11.42 Thermocauterization of corneal lesion

11.43 Cryotherapy of corneal lesion

11.49 Other removal or destruction of corneal lesion
Excision of cornea NOS

> Excludes: biopsy of cornea (11.22)

OPERATIONS ON THE EYE (08-16)

11.5 Repair of cornea

    11.51 Suture of corneal laceration

    11.52 Repair of postoperative wound dehiscence of cornea

    11.53 Repair of corneal laceration or wound with conjunctival flap

    11.59 Other repair of cornea

11.6 Corneal transplant

    Excludes: excision of pterygium with corneal graft (11.32)

    11.60 Corneal transplant, not otherwise specified
        Keratoplasty NOS

    11.61 Lamellar keratoplasty with autograft

    11.62 Other lamellar keratoplasty

    11.63 Penetrating keratoplasty with autograft
        Perforating keratoplasty with autograft

    11.64 Other penetrating keratoplasty
        Perforating keratoplasty (with homograft)

    11.69 Other corneal transplant

11.7 Other reconstructive and refractive surgery on cornea

    11.71 Keratomeleusis

    11.72 Keratophakia

    11.73 Keratoprosthesis

    11.74 Thermokeratoplasty

    11.75 Radial keratotomy

    11.76 Epikeratophakia

    11.79 Other

11.9 Other operations on cornea

    11.91 Tattooing of cornea

    11.92 Removal of artificial implant from cornea

    11.99 Other

12 Operations on iris, ciliary body, sclera, and anterior chamber

Excludes: operations on cornea (11.0–11.99)

12.0 Removal of intraocular foreign body from anterior segment of eye

    12.00 Removal of intraocular foreign body from anterior segment of eye, not otherwise specified

    12.01 Removal of intraocular foreign body from anterior segment of eye with use of magnet

    12.02 Removal of intraocular foreign body from anterior segment of eye without use of magnet

12.1 Iridotomy and simple iridectomy

    Excludes: iridectomy associated with:
            cataract extraction (13.11–13.69)
            removal of lesion (12.41–12.42)
            scleral fistulization (12.61–12.69)

    12.11 Iridotomy with transfixion

    12.12 Other iridotomy
        Corectomy
        Discission of iris
        Iridotomy NOS

    12.13 Excision of prolapsed iris

    12.14 Other iridectomy
        Iridectomy (basal) (peripheral) (total)

12.2 Diagnostic procedures on iris, ciliary body, sclera, and anterior chamber

    12.21 Diagnostic aspiration of anterior chamber of eye

    12.22 Biopsy of iris

    12.29 Other diagnostic procedures on iris, ciliary body, sclera, and anterior chamber

12.3 Iridoplasty and coreoplasty

    12.31 Lysis of goniosynechiae
        Lysis of goniosynechiae by injection of air or liquid

    12.32 Lysis of other anterior synechiae
        Lysis of anterior synechiae:
            NOS
            by injection of air or liquid

    12.33 Lysis of posterior synechiae
        Lysis of iris adhesions NOS

    12.34 Lysis of corneovitreal adhesions

    12.35 Coreoplasty
        Needling of pupillary membrane

    12.39 Other iridoplasty

12.4 Excision or destruction of lesion of iris and ciliary body

    12.40 Removal of lesion of anterior segment of eye, not otherwise specified

    12.41 Destruction of lesion of iris, nonexcisional
        Destruction of lesion of iris by:
            cauterization
            cryotherapy
            photocoagulation

    12.42 Excision of lesion of iris
        Excludes: biopsy of iris (12.22)

    12.43 Destruction of lesion of ciliary body, nonexcisional

    12.44 Excision of lesion of ciliary body

12.5 Facilitation of intraocular circulation

    12.51 Goniopuncture without goniotomy

    12.52 Goniotomy without goniopuncture

    12.53 Goniotomy with goniopuncture

    12.54 Trabeculotomy ab externo

    12.55 Cyclodialysis

    12.59 Other facilitation of intraocular circulation

12.6 Scleral fistulization

    Excludes: exploratory sclerotomy (12.89)

    12.61 Trephination of sclera with iridectomy

    12.62 Thermocauterization of sclera with iridectomy

    12.63 Iridencleisis and iridotasis

    12.64 Trabeculectomy ab externo

    12.65 Other scleral fistulization with iridectomy

    12.66 Postoperative revision of scleral fistulization procedure
        Revision of filtering bleb

        Excludes: repair of fistula (12.82)

    12.69 Other fistulizing procedure

12.7 Other procedures for relief of elevated intraocular pressure

    12.71 Cyclodiathermy

    12.72 Cyclocryotherapy

    12.73 Cyclophotocoagulation

12.74 Diminution of ciliary body, not otherwise specified

12.79 Other glaucoma procedures

12.8 Operations on sclera

> Excludes: those associated with:
> retinal reattachment (14.41–14.59)
> scleral fistulization (12.61–12.69)

12.81 Suture of laceration of sclera
Suture of sclera with synchronous repair of conjunctiva

12.82 Repair of scleral fistula

> Excludes: postoperative revision of scleral fistulization procedure (12.66)

12.83 Revision of operative wound of anterior segment, not elsewhere classified

> Excludes: postoperative revision of scleral fistulization procedure (12.66)

12.84 Excision or destruction of lesion of sclera

12.85 Repair of scleral staphyloma with graft

12.86 Other repair of scleral staphyloma

12.87 Scleral reinforcement with graft

12.88 Other scleral reinforcement

12.89 Other operations on sclera
Exploratory sclerotomy

12.9 Other operations on iris, ciliary body, and anterior chamber

12.91 Therapeutic evacuation of anterior chamber
Paracentesis of anterior chamber

> Excludes: diagnostic aspiration (12.21)

12.92 Injection into anterior chamber
Injection of:
air
liquid } into anterior chamber
medication

12.93 Removal or destruction of epithelial downgrowth from anterior chamber

> Excludes: that with iridectomy (12.41–12.42)

12.97 Other operations on iris

12.98 Other operations on ciliary body

12.99 Other operations on anterior chamber

13 Operations on lens

13.0 Removal of foreign body from lens

> Excludes: removal of pseudophakos (13.8)

13.00 Removal of foreign body from lens, not otherwise specified

13.01 Removal of foreign body from lens with use of magnet

13.02 Removal of foreign body from lens without use of magnet

13.1 Intracapsular extraction of lens

Code also any synchronous insertion of pseudophakos (13.71)

13.11 Intracapsular extraction of lens by temporal inferior route

13.19 Other intracapsular extraction of lens
Cataract extraction NOS
Cryoextraction of lens
Erysiphake extraction of cataract
Extraction of lens NOS

13.2 Extracapsular extraction of lens by linear extraction technique

13.3 Extracapsular extraction of lens by simple aspiration (and irrigation) technique
Irrigation of traumatic cataract

13.4 Extracapsular extraction of lens by fragmentation and aspiration technique

13.41 Phacoemulsification and aspiration of cataract

13.42 Mechanical phacofragmentation and aspiration of cataract by posterior route

Code also any synchronous vitrectomy (14.74)

13.43 Mechanical phacofragmentation and other aspiration of cataract

13.5 Other extracapsular extraction of lens

Code also any synchronous insertion of pseudophakos (13.71)

13.51 Extracapsular extraction of lens by temporal inferior route

13.59 Other extracapsular extraction of lens

13.6 Other cataract extraction

Code also any synchronous insertion of pseudophakos (13.71)

13.64 Discission of secondary membrane [after cataract]

13.65 Excision of secondary membrane [after cataract]
Capsulectomy

13.66 Mechanical fragmentation of secondary membrane [after cataract]

13.69 Other cataract extraction

13.7 Insertion of prosthetic lens [pseudophakos]

13.70 Insertion of pseudophakos, not otherwise specified

13.71 Insertion of intraocular lens prosthesis at time of cataract extraction, one-stage

Code also synchronous extraction of cataract (13.11–13.69)

13.72 Secondary insertion of intraocular lens prosthesis

13.8 Removal of implanted lens
Removal of pseudophakos

13.9 Other operations on lens

14 Operations on retina, choroid, vitreous, and posterior chamber

14.0 Removal of foreign body from posterior segment of eye

> Excludes: removal of surgically implanted material (14.6)

14.00 Removal of foreign body from posterior segment of eye, not otherwise specified

14.01 Removal of foreign body from posterior segment of eye with use of magnet

14.02 Removal of foreign body from posterior segment of eye without use of magnet

14.1 Diagnostic procedures on retina, choroid, vitreous, and posterior chamber

14.11 Diagnostic aspiration of vitreous

14.19 Other diagnostic procedures on retina, choroid, vitreous, and posterior chamber

OPERATIONS ON THE EYE (08-16)

14.2 Destruction of lesion of retina and choroid
Includes: destruction of chorioretinopathy or isolated chorioretinal lesion

Excludes: that for repair of retina (14.31–14.59)

14.21 Destruction of chorioretinal lesion by diathermy

14.22 Destruction of chorioretinal lesion by cryotherapy

14.23 Destruction of chorioretinal lesion by xenon arc photocoagulation

14.24 Destruction of chorioretinal lesion by laser photocoagulation

14.25 Destruction of chorioretinal lesion by photocoagulation of unspecified type

14.26 Destruction of chorioretinal lesion by radiation therapy

14.27 Destruction of chorioretinal lesion by implantation of radiation source

14.29 Other destruction of chorioretinal lesion
Destruction of lesion of retina and choroid NOS

14.3 Repair of retinal tear
Includes: repair of retinal defect

Excludes: repair of retinal detachment (14.41–14.59)

14.31 Repair of retinal tear by diathermy

14.32 Repair of retinal tear by cryotherapy

14.33 Repair of retinal tear by xenon arc photocoagulation

14.34 Repair of retinal tear by laser photocoagulation

14.35 Repair of retinal tear by photocoagulation of unspecified type

14.39 Other repair of retinal tear

14.4 Repair of retinal detachment with scleral buckling and implant

14.41 Scleral buckling with implant

14.49 Other scleral buckling
Scleral buckling with:
 air tamponade
 resection of sclera
 vitrectomy

14.5 Other repair of retinal detachment
Includes: that with drainage

14.51 Repair of retinal detachment with diathermy

14.52 Repair of retinal detachment with cryotherapy

14.53 Repair of retinal detachment with xenon arc photocoagulation

14.54 Repair of retinal detachment with laser photocoagulation

14.55 Repair of retinal detachment with photocoagulation of unspecified type

14.59 Other

14.6 Removal of surgically implanted material from posterior segment of eye

14.7 Operations on vitreous

14.71 Removal of vitreous, anterior approach
Open sky technique
Removal of vitreous, anterior approach (with replacement)

14.72 Other removal of vitreous
Aspiration of vitreous by posterior sclerotomy

14.73 Mechanical vitrectomy by anterior approach

14.74 Other mechanical vitrectomy

14.75 Injection of vitreous substitute

Excludes: that associated with removal (14.71–14.72)

14.79 Other operations on vitreous

14.9 Other operations on retina, choroid, and posterior chamber

15 Operations on extraocular muscles

15.0 Diagnostic procedures on extraocular muscles or tendons

15.01 Biopsy of extraocular muscle or tendon

15.09 Other diagnostic procedures on extraocular muscles and tendons

15.1 Operations on one extraocular muscle involving temporary detachment from globe

15.11 Recession of one extraocular muscle

15.12 Advancement of one extraocular muscle

15.13 Resection of one extraocular muscle

15.19 Other operations on one extraocular muscle involving temporary detachment from globe

Excludes: transposition of muscle (15.5)

15.2 Other operations on one extraocular muscle

15.21 Lengthening procedure on one extraocular muscle

15.22 Shortening procedure on one extraocular muscle

15.29 Other

15.3 Operations on two or more extraocular muscles involving temporary detachment from globe, one or both eyes

15.4 Other operations on two or more extraocular muscles, one or both eyes

15.5 Transposition of extraocular muscles

Excludes: that for correction of ptosis (08.31–08.36)

15.6 Revision of extraocular muscle surgery

15.7 Repair of injury of extraocular muscle
Freeing of entrapped extraocular muscle
Lysis of adhesions of extraocular muscle
Repair of laceration of extraocular muscle, tendon, or Tenon's capsule

15.9 Other operations on extraocular muscles and tendons

16 Operations on orbit and eyeball

Excludes: reduction of fracture of orbit (76.78–76.79)

16.0 Orbitotomy

16.01 Orbitotomy with bone flap
Orbitotomy with lateral approach

16.02 Orbitotomy with insertion of orbital implant

Excludes: that with bone flap (16.01)

16.09 Other orbitotomy

16.1 Removal of penetrating foreign body from eye, not otherwise specified

Excludes: removal of nonpenetrating foreign body (98.21)

16.2 Diagnostic procedures on orbit and eyeball

16.21 Ophthalmoscopy

16.22 Diagnostic aspiration of orbit

16.23 Biopsy of eyeball and orbit

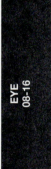

16.29 Other diagnostic procedures on orbit and eyeball

> Excludes: examination of form and structure of eye (95.11–95.16)
> general and subjective eye examination (95.01–95.09)
> microscopic examination of specimen from eye (90.21–90.29)
> objective functional tests of eye (95.21–95.26)
> ocular thermography (88.82)
> tonometry (89.11)
> x-ray of orbit (87.14, 87.16)

16.3 Evisceration of eyeball

16.31 Removal of ocular contents with synchronous implant into scleral shell

16.39 Other evisceration of eyeball

16.4 Enucleation of eyeball

16.41 Enucleation of eyeball with synchronous implant into tenon's capsule with attachment of muscles
Integrated implant of eyeball

16.42 Enucleation of eyeball with other synchronous implant

16.49 Other enucleation of eyeball
Removal of eyeball NOS

16.5 Exenteration of orbital contents

16.51 Exenteration of orbit with removal of adjacent structures
Radical orbitomaxillectomy

16.52 Exenteration of orbit with therapeutic removal of orbital bone

16.59 Other exenteration of orbit
Evisceration of orbit NOS
Exenteration of orbit with temporalis muscle transplant

16.6 Secondary procedures after removal of eyeball

> Excludes: that with synchronous:
> enucleation of eyeball (16.41–16.42)
> evisceration of eyeball (16.31)

16.61 Secondary insertion of ocular implant

16.62 Revision and reinsertion of ocular implant

16.63 Revision of enucleation socket with graft

16.64 Other revision of enucleation socket

16.65 Secondary graft to exenteration cavity

16.66 Other revision of exenteration cavity

16.69 Other secondary procedures after removal of eyeball

16.7 Removal of ocular or orbital implant

16.71 Removal of ocular implant

16.72 Removal of orbital implant

16.8 Repair of injury of eyeball and orbit

16.81 Repair of wound of orbit

> Excludes: reduction of orbital fracture (76.78–76.79)
> repair of extraocular muscles (15.7)

16.82 Repair of rupture of eyeball
Repair of multiple structures of eye

> Excludes: repair of laceration of:
> cornea (11.51–11.59)
> sclera (12.81)

16.89 Other repair of injury of eyeball or orbit

16.9 Other operations on orbit and eyeball

> Excludes: irrigation of eye (96.51)
> prescription and fitting of low vision aids (95.31–95.33)
> removal of:
> eye prosthesis NEC (97.31)
> nonpenetrating foreign body from eye without incision (98.21)

16.91 Retrobulbar injection of therapeutic agent

> Excludes: injection of radiographic contrast material (87.14)
> opticociliary injection (12.79)

16.92 Excision of lesion of orbit

> Excludes: biopsy of orbit (16.23)

16.93 Excision of lesion of eye, unspecified structure

> Excludes: biopsy of eye NOS (16.23)

16.98 Other operations on orbit

16.99 Other operations on eyeball

4. OPERATIONS ON THE EAR (18–20)

18 Operations on external ear

Includes: operations on:
external auditory canal
skin and cartilage of:
auricle
meatus

18.0 Incision of external ear

Excludes: removal of intraluminal foreign body (98.11)

18.01 Piercing of ear lobe
Piercing of pinna

18.02 Incision of external auditory canal

18.09 Other incision of external ear

18.1 Diagnostic procedures on external ear

18.11 Otoscopy

18.12 Biopsy of external ear

18.19 Other diagnostic procedures on external ear

Excludes: microscopic examination of specimen from ear (90.31–90.39)

18.2 Excision or destruction of lesion of external ear

18.21 Excision of preauricular sinus
Radical excision of preauricular sinus or cyst

Excludes: excision of preauricular remnant [appendage] (18.29)

18.29 Excision or destruction of other lesion of external ear
Cauterization
Coagulation
Cryosurgery   } of external ear
Curettage
Electrocoagulation
Enucleation
Excision of:
exostosis of external auditory canal
preauricular remnant [appendage]
Partial excision of ear

Excludes: biopsy of external ear (18.12)
radical excision of lesion (18.31)
removal of cerumen (96.52)

18.3 Other excision of external ear

Excludes: biopsy of external ear (18.12)

18.31 Radical excision of lesion of external ear

Excludes: radical excision of preauricular sinus (18.21)

18.39 Other
Amputation of external ear

Excludes: excision of lesion (18.21–18.29, 18.31)

18.4 Suture of laceration of external ear

18.5 Surgical correction of prominent ear
Ear:
pinning
setback

18.6 Reconstruction of external auditory canal
Canaloplasty of external auditory meatus
Construction [reconstruction] of external meatus of ear:
osseous portion
skin-lined portion (with skin graft)

18.7 Other plastic repair of external ear

18.71 Construction of auricle of ear
Prosthetic appliance for absent ear
Reconstruction:
auricle
ear

18.72 Reattachment of amputated ear

18.79 Other plastic repair of external ear
Otoplasty NOS
Postauricular skin graft
Repair of lop ear

18.9 Other operations on external ear

Excludes: irrigation of ear (96.52)
packing of external auditory canal (96.11)
removal of:
cerumen (96.52)
foreign body (without incision) (98.11)

19 Reconstructive operations on middle ear

19.0 Stapes mobilization
Division otosclerotic: Remobilization of stapes
material   Stapediolysis
process   Transcrural stapes mobilization

Excludes: that with synchronous stapedectomy (19.11–19.19)

19.1 Stapedectomy

Excludes: revision of previous stapedectomy (19.21–19.29)
stapes mobilization only (19.0)

19.11 Stapedectomy with incus replacement
Stapedectomy with incus:
homograft
prosthesis

19.19 Other stapedectomy

19.2 Revision of stapedectomy

19.21 Revision of stapedectomy with incus replacement

19.29 Other revision of stapedectomy

19.3 Other operations on ossicular chain
Incudectomy NOS
Ossiculectomy NOS
Reconstruction of ossicles, second stage

19.4 Myringoplasty
Epitympanic, type I
Myringoplasty by:
cauterization
graft
Tympanoplasty (type I)

19.5 Other tympanoplasty

19.52 Type II tympanoplasty
Closure of perforation with graft against incus or malleus

19.53 Type III tympanoplasty
Graft placed in contact with mobile and intact stapes

19.54 Type IV tympanoplasty
Mobile footplate left exposed with air pocket between round window and graft

19.55 Type V tympanoplasty
Fenestra in horizontal semicircular canal covered by graft

19.6 Revision of tympanoplasty

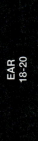

19.9 Other repair of middle ear
Closure of mastoid fistula
Mastoid myoplasty
Obliteration of tympanomastoid cavity

20 Other operations on middle and inner ear

20.0 Myringotomy

20.01 Myringotomy with insertion of tube
Myringostomy

20.09 Other myringotomy
Aspiration of middle ear NOS

20.1 Removal of tympanostomy tube

20.2 Incision of mastoid and middle ear

20.21 Incision of mastoid

20.22 Incision of petrous pyramid air cells

20.23 Incision of middle ear
Atticotomy
Division of tympanum
Lysis of adhesions of middle ear

> Excludes: division of otosclerotic process (19.0)
> stapediolysis (19.0)
> that with stapedectomy (19.11–19.19)

20.3 Diagnostic procedures on middle and inner ear

20.31 Electrocochleography

20.32 Biopsy of middle and inner ear

20.39 Other diagnostic procedures on middle and inner ear

> Excludes: auditory and vestibular function tests (89.13, 95.41–95.49)
> microscopic examination of specimen from ear (90.31–90.39)

20.4 Mastoidectomy

Code also any:
skin graft (18.79)
tympanoplasty (19.4–19.55)

> Excludes: that with implantation of cochlear prosthetic device (20.96–20.98)

20.41 Simple mastoidectomy

20.42 Radical mastoidectomy

20.49 Other mastoidectomy
Atticoantrostomy
Mastoidectomy:
NOS
modified radical

20.5 Other excision of middle ear

> Excludes: that with synchronous mastoidectomy (20.41–20.49)

20.51 Excision of lesion of middle ear

> Excludes: biopsy of middle ear (20.32)

20.59 Other
Apicectomy of petrous pyramid
Tympanectomy

20.6 Fenestration of inner ear

20.61 Fenestration of inner ear (initial)
Fenestration of:
labyrinth
semicircular canals } with graft (skin) (vein)
vestibule

> Excludes: that with tympanoplasty, type V (19.55)

20.62 Revision of fenestration of inner ear

20.7 Incision, excision, and destruction of inner ear

20.71 Endolymphatic shunt

20.72 Injection into inner ear
Destruction by injection (alcohol):
inner ear
semicircular canals
vestibule

20.79 Other incision, excision, and destruction of inner ear
Decompression of labyrinth
Drainage of inner ear
Fistulization:
endolymphatic sac
labyrinth
Incision of endolymphatic sac
Labyrinthectomy (transtympanic)
Opening of bony labyrinth
Perilymphatic tap

> Excludes: biopsy of inner ear (20.32)

20.8 Operations on eustachian tube

Catheterization
Inflation
Injection (Teflon paste)
Insufflation (boric acid-salicylic acid) } of Eustachian tube
Intubation
Politzerization

20.9 Other operations on inner and middle ear

20.91 Tympanosympathectomy

20.92 Revision of mastoidectomy

20.93 Repair of oval and round windows
Closure of fistula:
oval window
perilymph
round window

20.94 Injection of tympanum

20.95 Implantation of electromagnetic hearing device
Bone conduction hearing device

> Excludes: cochlear prosthetic device (20.96–20.98)

20.96 Implantation or replacement of cochlear prosthetic device, not otherwise specified
Implantation of receiver (within skull) and insertion of electrode(s) in cochlea
Includes: mastoidectomy

> Excludes: electromagnetic hearing device (20.95)

20.97 Implantation or replacement of cochlear prosthetic device, single channel
Implantation of receiver and insertion of electrode to cochlea
Includes: mastoidectomy

> Excludes: electromagnetic hearing device (20.95)

20.98 Implantation or replacement of cochlear prosthetic device, multiple channel
      Implantation of receiver (within skull) and insertion of electrode to cochlea
      Includes: mastoidectomy

      Excludes: electromagnetic hearing device (20.95)

20.99 Other operations on middle and inner ear
      Repair or removal of cochlear prosthetic device (receiver) (electrode)

      Excludes: adjustment (external components) of cochlear prosthetic device (95.49)
                 fitting of hearing aid (95.48)

OPERATIONS ON THE NOSE, MOUTH, AND PHARYNX (21-29)

5. OPERATIONS ON THE NOSE, MOUTH, AND PHARYNX (21-29)

21 Operations on nose

Includes: operations on:
- bone } of nose
- skin

21.0 Control of epistaxis

- **21.00** Control of epistaxis, not otherwise specified
- **21.01** Control of epistaxis by anterior nasal packing
- **21.02** Control of epistaxis by posterior (and anterior) packing
- **21.03** Control of epistaxis by cauterization (and packing)
- **21.04** Control of epistaxis by ligation of ethmoidal arteries
- **21.05** Control of epistaxis by (transantral) ligation of the maxillary artery
- **21.06** Control of epistaxis by ligation of the external carotid artery
- **21.07** Control of epistaxis by excision of nasal mucosa and skin grafting of septum and lateral nasal wall
- **21.09** Control of epistaxis by other means

21.1 Incision of nose
- Chrondrotomy
- Incision of skin of nose
- Nasal septotomy

21.2 Diagnostic procedures on nose

- **21.21** Rhinoscopy [NOR]
- **21.22** Biopsy of nose
- **21.29** Other diagnostic procedures on nose

  Excludes: microscopic examination of specimen from nose (90.31–90.39)
  nasal:
  function study (89.12)
  x-ray (87.16)
  rhinomanometry (89.12)

21.3 Local excision or destruction of lesion of nose

  Excludes: biopsy of nose (21.22)
  nasal fistulectomy (21.82)

- **21.30** Excision or destruction of lesion of nose, not otherwise specified
- **21.31** Local excision or destruction of intranasal lesion
  Nasal polypectomy
- **21.32** Local excision or destruction of other lesion of nose

21.4 Resection of nose
Amputation of nose

21.5 Submucous resection of nasal septum

21.6 Turbinectomy

- **21.61** Turbinectomy by diathermy or cryosurgery
- **21.62** Fracture of the turbinates
- **21.69** Other turbinectomy

  Excludes: turbinectomy associated with sinusectomy (22.31–22.39, 22.42, 22.60–22.64)

21.7 Reduction of nasal fracture

- **21.71** Closed reduction of nasal fracture
- **21.72** Open reduction of nasal fracture

21.8 Repair and plastic operations on the nose

- **21.81** Suture of laceration of nose
- **21.82** Closure of nasal fistula
  - Nasolabial
  - Nasopharyngeal } fistulectomy
  - Oronasal
- **21.83** Total nasal reconstruction
  Reconstruction of nose with:
  - arm flap
  - forehead flap
- **21.84** Revision rhinoplasty
  - Rhinoseptoplasty
  - Twisted nose rhinoplasty
- **21.85** Augmentation rhinoplasty
  Augmentation rhinoplasty with:
  - graft
  - synthetic implant
- **21.86** Limited rhinoplasty
  - Plastic repair of nasolabial flaps
  - Tip rhinoplasty
- **21.87** Other rhinoplasty
  - Rhinoplasty NOS
- **21.88** Other septoplasty
  - Crushing of nasal septum
  - Repair of septal perforation

  Excludes: septoplasty associated with submucous resection of septum (21.5)

- **21.89** Other repair and plastic operations on nose
  Reattachment of amputated nose

21.9 Other operations on nose

- **21.91** Lysis of adhesions of nose
  Posterior nasal scrub
- **21.99** Other

  Excludes: dilation of frontonasal duct (96.21)
  irrigation of nasal passages (96.53)
  removal of:
  intraluminal foreign body without incision (98.12)
  nasal packing (97.32)
  replacement of nasal packing (97.21)

22 Operations on nasal sinuses

22.0 Aspiration and lavage of nasal sinus

- **22.00** Aspiration and lavage of nasal sinus, not otherwise specified
- **22.01** Puncture of nasal sinus for aspiration or lavage
- **22.02** Aspiration or lavage of nasal sinus through natural ostium

22.1 Diagnostic procedures on nasal sinus

- **22.11** Closed [endoscopic] [needle] biopsy of nasal sinus
- **22.12** Open biopsy of nasal sinus
- **22.19** Other diagnostic procedures on sinuses
  Endoscopy without biopsy

  Excludes: transillumination of sinus (89.35)
  x-ray of sinus (87.15–87.16)

22.2 Intranasal antrotomy

  Excludes: antrotomy with external approach (22.31–22.39)

22.3 External maxillary antrotomy

- **22.31** Radical maxillary antrotomy
  Removal of lining membrane of maxillary sinus using Caldwell-Luc approach

22.39 Other external maxillary antrotomy
Exploration of maxillary antrum with Caldwell-Luc approach

22.4 Frontal sinusotomy and sinusectomy

22.41 Frontal sinusotomy

22.42 Frontal sinusectomy
Excision of lesion of frontal sinus
Obliteration of frontal sinus (with fat)

> Excludes: biopsy of nasal sinus (22.11–22.12)

22.5 Other nasal sinusotomy

22.50 Sinusotomy, not otherwise specified

22.51 Ethmoidotomy

22.52 Sphenoidotomy

22.53 Incision of multiple nasal sinuses

22.6 Other nasal sinusectomy
Includes: that with incidental turbinectomy

> Excludes: biopsy of nasal sinus (22.11–22.12)

22.60 Sinusectomy, not otherwise specified

22.61 Excision of lesion of maxillary sinus with Caldwell-Luc approach

22.62 Excision of lesion of maxillary sinus with other approach

22.63 Ethmoidectomy

22.64 Sphenoidectomy

22.7 Repair of nasal sinus

22.71 Closure of nasal sinus fistula
Repair of oro-antral fistula

22.79 Other repair of nasal sinus
Reconstruction of frontonasal duct
Repair of bone of accessory sinus

22.9 Other operations on nasal sinuses
Exteriorization of maxillary sinus
Fistulization of sinus

> Excludes: dilation of frontonasal duct (96.21)

23 Removal and restoration of teeth

23.0 Forceps extraction of tooth

23.01 Extraction of deciduous tooth [NOR]

23.09 Extraction of other tooth [NOR]
Extraction of tooth NOS

23.1 Surgical removal of tooth

23.11 Removal of residual root [NOR]

23.19 Other surgical extraction of tooth [NOR]
Odontectomy NOS
Removal of impacted tooth
Tooth extraction with elevation of mucoperiosteal flap

23.2 Restoration of tooth by filling [NOR]

23.3 Restoration of tooth by inlay [NOR]

23.4 Other dental restoration

23.41 Application of crown [NOR]

23.42 Insertion of fixed bridge [NOR]

23.43 Insertion of removable bridge

23.49 Other [NOR]

23.5 Implantation of tooth [NOR]

23.6 Prosthetic dental implant [NOR]
Endosseous dental implant

23.7 Apicoectomy and root canal therapy

23.70 Root canal, not otherwise specified [NOR]

23.71 Root canal therapy with irrigation [NOR]

23.72 Root canal therapy with apicoectomy [NOR]

23.73 Apicoectomy

24 Other operations on teeth, gums, and alveoli

24.0 Incision of gum or alveolar bone
Apical alveolotomy

24.1 Diagnostic procedures on teeth, gums, and alveoli

24.11 Biopsy of gum

24.12 Biopsy of alveolus

24.19 Other diagnostic procedures on teeth, gums, and alveoli

> Excludes: dental:
>   examination (89.31)
>   x-ray
>   full-mouth (87.11)
>   other (87.12)
>   microscopic examination of dental specimen (90.81–90.89)

24.2 Gingivoplasty
Gingivoplasty with bone or soft tissue graft

24.3 Other operations on gum

24.31 Excision of lesion or tissue of gum

> Excludes: biopsy of gum (24.11)
> excision of odontogenic lesion (24.4)

24.32 Suture of laceration of gum

24.39 Other

24.4 Excision of dental lesion of jaw
Excision of odontogenic lesion

24.5 Alveoloplasty
Alveolectomy (interradicular) (intraseptal) (radical) (simple) (with graft or implant)

> Excludes: biopsy of alveolus (24.12)
> en bloc resection of alveolar process and palate (27.32)

24.6 Exposure of tooth

24.7 Application of orthodontic appliance
Application, insertion, or fitting of:
  arch bars
  orthodontic obturator
  orthodontic wiring
  periodontal splint

> Excludes: nonorthodontic dental wiring (93.55)

24.8 Other orthodontic operation
Closure of diastema (alveolar) (dental)
Occlusal adjustment
Removal of arch bars
Repair of dental arch

> Excludes: removal of nonorthodontic wiring (97.33)

24.9 Other dental operations

24.91 Extension or deepening of buccolabial or lingual sulcus

OPERATIONS ON THE NOSE, MOUTH, AND PHARYNX (21-29)

24.99 Other

Excludes: *dental:*
debridement (96.54)
examination (89.31)
prophylaxis (96.54)
scaling and polishing (96.54)
wiring (93.55)
fitting of dental appliance [denture] (99.97)
microscopic examination of dental specimen (90.81–90.89)
removal of dental:
packing (97.34)
prosthesis (97.35)
wiring (97.33)
replacement of dental packing (97.22)

25 Operations on tongue

25.0 Diagnostic procedures on tongue

25.01 Closed [needle] biopsy of tongue

25.02 Open biopsy of tongue
Wedge biopsy

25.09 Other diagnostic procedures on tongue

25.1 Excision or destruction of lesion or tissue of tongue

Excludes: *biopsy of tongue (25.01–25.02)*
frenumectomy
labial (27.41)
lingual (25.92)

25.2 Partial glossectomy

25.3 Complete glossectomy
Glossectomy NOS

Code also any neck dissection (40.40–40.42)

25.4 Radical glossectomy

Code also any:
neck dissection (40.40–40.42)
tracheostomy (31.1–31.29)

25.5 Repair of tongue and glossoplasty

25.51 Suture of laceration of tongue

25.59 Other repair and plastic operations on tongue
Fascial sling of tongue
Fusion of tongue (to lip)
Graft of mucosa or skin to tongue

Excludes: *lysis of adhesions of tongue (25.93)*

25.9 Other operations on tongue

25.91 Lingual frenotomy

Excludes: *labial frenotomy (27.91)*

25.92 Lingual frenectomy

Excludes: *labial frenectomy (27.41)*

25.93 Lysis of adhesions of tongue

25.94 Other glossotomy

25.99 Other

26 Operations on salivary glands and ducts

Includes: operations on:
lesser salivary
parotid
sublingual
submaxillary
} gland and duct

Code also any neck dissection (40.40–40.42)

26.0 Incision of salivary gland or duct

26.1 Diagnostic procedures on salivary glands and ducts

26.11 Closed [needle] biopsy of salivary gland or duct

26.12 Open biopsy of salivary gland or duct

26.19 Other diagnostic procedures on salivary glands and ducts

Excludes: *x-ray of salivary gland (87.09)*

26.2 Excision of lesion of salivary gland

26.21 Marsupialization of salivary gland cyst

26.29 Other excision of salivary gland lesion

Excludes: *biopsy of salivary gland (26.11–26.12)*
salivary fistulectomy (26.42)

26.3 Sialoadenectomy

26.30 Sialoadenectomy, not otherwise specified

26.31 Partial sialoadenectomy

26.32 Complete sialoadenectomy
En bloc excision of salivary gland lesion
Radical sialoadenectomy

26.4 Repair of salivary gland or duct

26.41 Suture of laceration of salivary gland

26.42 Closure of salivary fistula

26.49 Other repair and plastic operations on salivary gland or duct
Fistulization of salivary gland
Plastic repair of salivary gland or duct NOS
Transplantation of salivary duct opening

26.9 Other operations on salivary gland or duct

26.91 Probing of salivary duct

26.99 Other

27 Other operations on mouth and face

Includes: operations on:
lips
palate
soft tissue of face and mouth, except tongue and gingiva

Excludes: *operations on:*
gingiva (24.0–24.99)
tongue (25.01–25.99)

27.0 Drainage of face and floor of mouth
Drainage of:
facial region (abscess)
fascial compartment of face
Ludwig's angina

Excludes: *drainage of thyroglossal tract (06.09)*

27.1 Incision of palate

27.2 Diagnostic procedures on oral cavity

27.21 Biopsy of bony palate

27.22 Biopsy of uvula and soft palate

27.23 Biopsy of lip

27.24 Biopsy of mouth, unspecified structure

27.29 Other diagnostic procedures on oral cavity

Excludes: *soft tissue x-ray (87.09)*

27.3 Excision of lesion or tissue of bony palate

27.31 Local excision or destruction of lesion or tissue of bony palate
Local excision or destruction of palate by:
- cautery
- chemotherapy
- cryotherapy

Excludes: biopsy of bony palate (27.21)

27.32 Wide excision or destruction of lesion or tissue of bony palate
En bloc resection of alveolar process and palate

27.4 Excision of other parts of mouth

27.41 Labial frenectomy

Excludes: division of labial frenum (27.91)

27.42 Wide excision of lesion of lip

27.43 Other excision of lesion or tissue of lip

27.49 Other excision of mouth

Excludes: biopsy of mouth NOS (27.24)
excision of lesion of:
  palate (27.31–27.32)
  tongue (25.1)
  uvula (27.72)
fistulectomy of mouth (27.53)
frenectomy of:
  lip (27.41)
  tongue (25.92)

27.5 Plastic repair of mouth

Excludes: palatoplasty (27.61–27.69)

27.51 Suture of laceration of lip

27.52 Suture of laceration of other part of mouth

27.53 Closure of fistula of mouth

Excludes: fistulectomy:
  nasolabial (21.82)
  oro-antral (22.71)
  oronasal (21.82)

27.54 Repair of cleft lip

27.55 Full-thickness skin graft to lip and mouth

27.56 Other skin graft to lip and mouth

27.57 Attachment of pedicle or flap graft to lip and mouth

27.59 Other plastic repair of mouth

27.6 Palatoplasty

27.61 Suture of laceration of palate

27.62 Correction of cleft palate
Correction of cleft palate by push-back operation

Excludes: revision of cleft palate repair (27.63)

27.63 Revision of cleft palate repair
Secondary:
  attachment of pharyngeal flap
  lengthening of palate

27.69 Other plastic repair of palate

Excludes: fistulectomy of mouth (27.53)

27.7 Operations on uvula

27.71 Incision of uvula

27.72 Excision of uvula

Excludes: biopsy of uvula (27.22)

27.73 Repair of uvula

Excludes: that with synchronous cleft palate repair (27.62)
uranostaphylorrhaphy (27.62)

27.79 Other operations on uvula

27.9 Other operations on mouth and face

27.91 Labial frenotomy
Division of labial frenum

Excludes: lingual frenotomy (25.91)

27.92 Incision of mouth, unspecified structure

Excludes: incision of:
  gum (24.0)
  palate (27.1)
  salivary gland or duct (26.0)
  tongue (25.94)
  uvula (27.71)

27.99 Other operations on oral cavity
Graft of buccal sulcus

Excludes: removal of:
  intraluminal foreign body (98.01)
  penetrating foreign body from mouth without incision (98.22)

28 Operations on tonsils and adenoids

28.0 Incision and drainage of tonsil and peritonsillar structures
Drainage (oral) (transcervical) of:
  parapharyngeal ⎫
  peritonsillar   ⎬ abscess
  retropharyngeal ⎪
  tonsillar   ⎭

28.1 Diagnostic procedures on tonsils and adenoids

28.11 Biopsy of tonsils and adenoids

28.19 Other diagnostic procedures on tonsils and adenoids

Excludes: soft tissue x-ray (87.09)

28.2 Tonsillectomy without adenoidectomy

28.3 Tonsillectomy with adenoidectomy

28.4 Excision of tonsil tag

28.5 Excision of lingual tonsil

28.6 Adenoidectomy without tonsillectomy
Excision of adenoid tag

28.7 Control of hemorrhage after tonsillectomy and adenoidectomy

28.9 Other operations on tonsils and adenoids

28.91 Removal of foreign body from tonsil and adenoid by incision

Excludes: that without incision (98.13)

28.92 Excision of lesion of tonsil and adenoid

Excludes: biopsy of tonsil and adenoid (28.11)

28.99 Other

29 Operations on pharynx

Includes: operations on:
  hypopharynx
  nasopharynx
  oropharynx
  pharyngeal pouch
  pyriform sinus

OPERATIONS ON THE NOSE, MOUTH, AND PHARYNX (21-29)

29.0 Pharyngotomy
Drainage of pharyngeal bursa

> Excludes: incision and drainage of retropharyngeal abscess (28.0)
> removal of foreign body (without incision) (98.13)

29.1 Diagnostic procedures on pharynx

29.11 Pharyngoscopy NOR

29.12 Pharyngeal biopsy
Biopsy of supraglottic mass

29.19 Other diagnostic procedures on pharynx

> Excludes: x-ray of nasopharynx:
> contrast (87.06)
> other (87.09)

29.2 Excision of branchial cleft cyst or vestige

> Excludes: branchial cleft fistulectomy (29.52)

29.3 Excision or destruction of lesion or tissue of pharynx

29.31 Cricopharyngeal myotomy

> Excludes: that with pharyngeal diverticulectomy (29.32)

29.32 Pharyngeal diverticulectomy

29.33 Pharyngectomy (partial)

> Excludes: laryngopharyngectomy (30.3)

29.39 Other excision or destruction of lesion or tissue of pharynx

29.4 Plastic operation on pharynx
Correction of nasopharyngeal atresia

> Excludes: pharyngoplasty associated with cleft palate repair (27.62–27.63)

29.5 Other repair of pharynx

29.51 Suture of laceration of pharynx

29.52 Closure of branchial cleft fistula

29.53 Closure of other fistula of pharynx
Pharyngoesophageal fistulectomy

29.54 Lysis of pharyngeal adhesions

29.59 Other

29.9 Other operations on pharynx

29.91 Dilation of pharynx
Dilation of nasopharynx

29.92 Division of glossopharyngeal nerve

29.99 Other

> Excludes: insertion of radium into pharynx and nasopharynx (92.27)
> removal of intraluminal foreign body (98.13)

6. OPERATIONS ON THE RESPIRATORY SYSTEM (30–34)

30 Excision of larynx

30.0 Excision or destruction of lesion or tissue of larynx

30.01 Marsupialization of laryngeal cyst

30.09 Other excision or destruction of lesion or tissue of larynx
Stripping of vocal cords

> Excludes: biopsy of larynx (31.43)
> laryngeal fistulectomy (31.62)
> laryngotracheal fistulectomy (31.62)

30.1 Hemilaryngectomy

30.2 Other partial laryngectomy

30.21 Epiglottidectomy

30.22 Vocal cordectomy
Excision of vocal cords

30.29 Other partial laryngectomy
Excision of laryngeal cartilage

30.3 Complete laryngectomy
Block dissection of larynx (with thyroidectomy) (with synchronous tracheostomy)
Laryngopharyngectomy

> Excludes: that with radical neck dissection (30.4)

30.4 Radical laryngectomy
Complete [total] laryngectomy with radical neck dissection (with thyroidectomy) (with synchronous tracheostomy)

31 Other operations on larynx and trachea

31.0 Injection of largnx
Injection of inert material into larynx or vocal cords

31.1 Temporary tracheostomy NOR
Tracheostomy for assistance in breathing

31.2 Permanent tracheostomy

31.21 Mediastinal tracheostomy

31.29 Other permanent tracheostomy

> Excludes: that with laryngectomy (30.3–30.4)

31.3 Other incision of larynx or trachea

> Excludes: that for assistance in breathing (31.1–31.29)

31.4 Diagnostic procedures on larynx and trachea

31.41 Tracheoscopy through artificial stoma NOR

> Excludes: that with biopsy (31.43–31.44)

31.42 Laryngoscopy and other tracheoscopy NOR

> Excludes: that with biopsy (31.43–31.44)

31.43 Closed [endoscopic] biopsy of larynx NOR

31.44 Closed [endoscopic] biopsy of trachea NOR

31.45 Open biopsy of larynx or trachea

31.48 Other diagnostic procedures on larynx

> Excludes: contrast laryngogram (87.07)
> microscopic examination of specimen from larynx (90.31–90.39)
> soft tissue x-ray of larynx NEC (87.09)

31.49 Other diagnostic procedures on trachea

> Excludes: microscopic examination of specimen from trachea (90.41–90.49)
> x-ray of trachea (87.49)

31.5 Local excision or destruction of lesion or tissue of trachea

> Excludes: biopsy of trachea (31.44–31.45)
> laryngotracheal fistulectomy (31.62)
> tracheoesophageal fistulectomy (31.73)

31.6 Repair of larynx

31.61 Suture of laceration of larynx

31.62 Closure of fistula of larynx
Laryngotracheal fistulectomy
Take-down of laryngostomy

31.63 Revision of laryngostomy

31.64 Repair of laryngeal fracture

31.69 Other repair of larynx
Arytenoidopexy
Graft of larynx
Transposition of vocal cords

> Excludes: construction of artificial larynx (31.75)

31.7 Repair and plastic operations on trachea

31.71 Suture of laceration of trachea

31.72 Closure of external fistula of trachea
Closure of tracheotomy

31.73 Closure of other fistula of trachea
Tracheoesophageal fistulectomy

> Excludes: laryngotracheal fistulectomy (31.62)

31.74 Revision of tracheostomy

31.75 Reconstruction of trachea and construction of artificial larynx
Tracheoplasty with artificial larynx

31.79 Other repair and plastic operations on trachea

31.9 Other operations on larynx and trachea

31.91 Division of laryngeal nerve

31.92 Lysis of adhesions of trachea or larynx

31.93 Replacement of laryngeal or tracheal stent

31.94 Injection of locally-acting therapeutic substance into trachea

31.95 Tracheoesophageal fistulization

31.98 Other operations on larynx
Dilation
Division of congenital web } of larynx
Removal of keel or stent

> Excludes: removal of intraluminal foreign body from larynx without incision (98.14)

31.99 Other operations on trachea

> Excludes: removal of:
> intraluminal foreign body from trachea without incision (98.15)
> tracheostomy tube (97.37)
> replacement of tracheostomy tube (97.23)
> tracheostomy toilette (96.55)

32 Excision of lung and bronchus

Includes: rib resection
sternotomy
sternum-splitting incision
thoracotomy } as operative approach

Code also any synchronous bronchoplasty (33.48)

32.0 Local excision or destruction of lesion or tissue of bronchus

> Excludes: biopsy of bronchus (33.24–33.25)
> bronchial fistulectomy (33.42)

32.01 Endoscopic excision or destruction of lesion or tissue of bronchus NOR

32.09 Other local excision or destruction of lesion or tissue of bronchus

> *Excludes:* that by endoscopic approach (32.01)

32.1 Other excision of bronchus

Resection (wide sleeve) of bronchus

> *Excludes:* radical dissection [excision] of bronchus (32.6)

32.2 Local excision or destruction of lesion or tissue of lung

32.21 Plication of emphysematous bleb

32.28 Endoscopic excision or destruction of lesion or tissue of lung

> *Excludes:* biopsy of lung (33.26–33.27)

32.29 Other local excision or destruction of lesion or tissue of lung

Resection of lung:
 NOS
 wedge

> *Excludes:* biopsy of lung (33.26–33.27)
> that by endoscopic approach (32.28)
> wide excision of lesion of lung (32.3)

32.3 Segmental resection of lung

Partial lobectomy

32.4 Lobectomy of lung

Lobectomy with segmental resection of adjacent lobes of lung

> *Excludes:* that with radical dissection [excision] of thoracic structures (32.6)

32.5 Complete pneumonectomy

Excision of lung NOS
Pneumonectomy (with mediastinal dissection)

32.6 Radical dissection of thoracic structures

Block [en bloc] dissection of bronchus, lobe of lung, brachial plexus, intercostal structure, ribs (transverse process), and sympathetic nerves

32.9 Other excision of lung

> *Excludes:* biopsy of lung and bronchus (33–24–33.27)
> pulmonary decortication (34.51)

33 Other operations on lung and bronchus

Includes: rib resection
 sternotomy
 sternum-splitting incision
 thoracotomy
 } as operative approach

33.0 Incision of bronchus

33.1 Incision of lung

> *Excludes:* puncture of lung (33.93)

33.2 Diagnostic procedures on lung and bronchus

33.21 Bronchoscopy through artificial stoma NOR

> *Excludes:* that with biopsy (33.24, 33.27)

33.22 Fiber-optic bronchoscopy NOR

> *Excludes:* that with biopsy (33.24, 33.27)

33.23 Other bronchoscopy NOR

> *Excludes:* that for:
> aspiration (96.05)
> biopsy 33.27)

33.24 Closed [endoscopic] biopsy of bronchus

Bronchoscopy (fiberoptic) (rigid) with:
 brush biopsy of "lung"
 brushing or washing for specimen collection
 excision (bite) biopsy

> *Excludes:* closed biopsy of lung, other than brush biopsy of "lung" (33.26, 33.27)

33.25 Open biopsy of bronchus

> *Excludes:* open biopsy of lung (33.28)

33.26 Closed [percutaneous] [needle] biopsy of lung

> *Excludes:* endoscopic biopsy of lung (33.27)

▲**33.27 Closed endoscopic biopsy of lung**

Fiber-optic (flexible) bronchoscopy with fluoroscopic guidance with biopsy
Transbronchial lung biopsy

> *Excludes:* brush biopsy of "lung" (33.24)
> percutaneous biopsy of lung (33.26)

33.28 Open biopsy of lung

33.29 Other diagnostic procedures on lung and bronchus

> *Excludes:* contrast bronchogram:
> endotracheal (87.31)
> other (87.32)
> lung scan (92.15)
> magnetic resonance imaging (88.92)
> microscopic examination of specimen from bronchus or lung (90.41–90.49)
> routine chest x-ray (87.44)
> ultrasonography of lung (88.73)
> vital capacity determination (89.37)
> x-ray of bronchus or lung NOS (87.49)

33.3 Surgical collapse of lung

33.31 Destruction of phrenic nerve for collapse of lung

33.32 Artificial pneumothorax for collapse of lung
Thoracotomy for collapse of lung

33.33 Pneumoperitoneum for collapse of lung

33.34 Thoracoplasty

33.39 Other surgical collapse of lung
Collapse of lung NOS

33.4 Repair and plastic operation on lung and bronchus

33.41 Suture of laceration of bronchus

33.42 Closure of bronchial fistula
Closure of bronchostomy
Fistulectomy:
 bronchocutaneous
 bronchoesophageal
 bronchovisceral

> *Excludes:* closure of fistula:
> bronchomediastinal (34.73)
> bronchopleural (34.73)
> bronchopleuromediastinal (34.73)

33.43 Closure of laceration of lung

33.48 Other repair and plastic operations on bronchus

33.49 Other repair and plastic operations on lung

> *Excludes:* closure of pleural fistula (34.73)

33.5 Lung transplant

> *Excludes:* combined heart-lung transplantation (33.6)

Combined heart-lung transplantation

Code also cardiopulmonary bypass [extracorporeal circulation] [heart-lung machine] (39.61)

OPERATIONS ON THE RESPIRATORY SYSTEM (30-34)

33.9 Other operations on lung and bronchus

33.91 Bronchial dilation

33.92 Ligation of bronchus

33.93 Puncture of lung

> Excludes: needle biopsy (33.26)

33.98 Other operations on bronchus

> Excludes: bronchial lavage (96.56)
> removal of intraluminal foreign body from bronchus without incision (98.15)

33.99 Other operations on lung

> Excludes: other continuous mechanical ventilation (96.70–96.72)
> respiratory therapy (93.90–93.99)

34 Operations on chest wall, pleura, mediastinum, and diaphragm

> Excludes: operations on breast (85.0–85.99)

34.0 Incision of chest wall and pleura

> Excludes: that as operative approach — omit code

34.01 Incision of chest wall
Extrapleural drainage

> Excludes: incision of pleura (34.09)

34.02 Exploratory thoracotomy

34.03 Reopening of recent thoracotomy site

34.04 Insertion of intercostal catheter for drainage
Closed chest drainage

●**34.05 Creation of pleuroperitoneal shunt** NOR

34.09 Other incision of pleura
Creation of pleural window for drainage
Intercostal stab
Open chest drainage

> Excludes: thoracoscopy (34.21)
> thoracotomy for collapse of lung (33.32)

34.1 Incision of mediastinum

> Excludes: mediastinoscopy (34.22)
> mediastinotomy associated with pneumonectomy (32.5)

34.2 Diagnostic procedures on chest wall, pleura, mediastinum, and diaphragm

34.21 Transpleural thoracoscopy

34.22 Mediastinoscopy

Code also any lymph node biopsy (40.11)

34.23 Biopsy of chest wall

34.24 Pleural biopsy

34.25 Closed [percutaneous] [needle] biopsy of mediastinum

34.26 Open biopsy of mediastinum

34.27 Biopsy of diaphragm

34.28 Other diagnostic procedures on chest wall, pleura, and diaphragm

> Excludes: angiocardiography (88.50–88.58)
> aortography (88.42)
> arteriography of:
>   intrathoracic vessels NEC (88.44)
>   pulmonary arteries (88.43)
> microscopic examination of specimen from chest wall, pleura, and diaphragm (90.41–90.49)
> phlebography of:
>   intrathoracic vessels NEC (88.63)
>   pulmonary veins (88.62)
> radiological examinations of thorax:
>   C.A.T. scan (87.41)
>   diaphragmatic x-ray (87.49)
>   intrathoracic lymphangiogram (87.34)
>   routine chest x-ray (87.44)
>   sinogram of chest wall (87.38)
>   soft tissue x-ray of chest wall NEC (87.39)
>   tomogram of thorax NEC (87.42)
>   ultrasonography of thorax (88.73)

34.29 Other diagnostic procedures on mediastinum

> Excludes: mediastinal:
>   pneumogram (87.33)
>   x-ray NEC (87.49)

34.3 Excision or destruction of lesion or tissue of mediastinum

> Excludes: biopsy of mediastinum (34.25–34.26)
> mediastinal fistulectomy (34.73)

34.4 Excision or destruction of lesion of chest wall
Excision of lesion of chest wall NOS (with excision of ribs)

> Excludes: biopsy of chest wall (34.23)
> costectomy not incidental to thoracic procedure (77.91)
> excision of lesion of:
>   breast (85.20–85.25)
>   cartilage (80.89)
>   skin (86.2–86.3)
> fistulectomy (34.73)

34.5 Pleurectomy

34.51 Decortication of lung

34.59 Other excision of pleura
Excision of pleural lesion

> Excludes: biopsy of pleura (34.24)
> pleural fistulectomy (34.73)

34.6 Scarification of pleura
Pleurosclerosis

> Excludes: injection of sclerosing agent (34.92)

34.7 Repair of chest wall

34.71 Suture of laceration of chest wall

> Excludes: suture of skin and subcutaneous tissue alone (86.59)

34.72 Closure of thoracostomy

34.73 Closure of other fistula of thorax
Closure of:
  bronchopleural
  bronchopleurocutaneous } fistula
  bronchopleuromediastinal

34.74 Repair of pectus deformity
Repair of:
  pectus carinatum } (with implant)
  pectus excavatum

34.79 Other repair of chest wall
Repair of chest wall NOS

34.8 Operations on diaphragm

    34.81 Excision of lesion or tissue of diaphragm

        Excludes: *biopsy of diaphragm (34.27)*

    34.82 Suture of laceration of diaphragm

    34.83 Closure of fistula of diaphragm
        Thoracicoabdominal ⎫
        Thoracicogastric   ⎬ fistulectomy
        Thoracicointestinal ⎭

    34.84 Other repair of diaphragm

        Excludes: *repair of diaphragmatic hernia (53.7–53.82)*

    34.85 Implantation of diaphragmatic pacemaker

    34.89 Other operations on diaphragm

34.9 Other operations on thorax

    34.91 Thoracentesis

    34.92 Injection into thoracic cavity
        Chemical pleurodesis
        Injection of cytotoxic agent or tetracycline
        Requires additional code for any cancer chemotherapeutic substance (99.25)

        Excludes: *that for collapse of lung (33.32)*

    34.93 Repair of pleura

    34.99 Other

        Excludes: *removal of:*
            mediastinal drain (97.42)
            sutures (97.43)
            thoracotomy tube (97.41)

7. OPERATIONS ON THE CARDIOVASCULAR SYSTEM (35–39)

35 Operations on valves and septa of heart

Includes: sternotomy (median) (transverse) thoracotomy } as operative approach

Code also cardiopulmonary bypass [extracorporeal circulation] [heart-lung machine] (39.61)

35.0 Closed heart valvotomy

Excludes: percutaneous (balloon) valvuloplasty (35.96)

35.00 Closed heart valvotomy, unspecified valve

35.01 Closed heart valvotomy, aortic valve

35.02 Closed heart valvotomy, mitral valve

35.03 Closed heart valvotomy, pulmonary valve

35.04 Closed heart valvotomy, tricuspid valve

35.1 Open heart valvuloplasty without replacement

Includes: open heart valvotomy

Excludes: percutaneous (balloon valvuloplasty (35.96)
that associated with repair of:
endocardial cushion defect (35.54, 35.63, 35.73)
valvular defect associated with atrial and ventricular septal defects (35.54, 35.63, 35.73)

Code also cardiopulmonary bypass, if performed [extracorporeal circulation] [heart-lung machine] (39.61)

35.10 Open heart valvuloplasty without replacement, unspecified valve

35.11 Open heart valvuloplasty of aortic valve without replacement

35.12 Open heart valvuloplasty of mitral valve without replacement

35.13 Open heart valvuloplasty of pulmonary valve without replacement

35.14 Open heart valvuloplasty of tricuspid valve without replacement

35.2 Replacement of heart valve

Includes: Excision of heart valve with replacement

Code also cardiopulmonary bypass [extracorporeal circulation] [heart-lung machine] (39.61)

Excludes: that associated with repair of:
endocardial cushion defect (35.54, 35.63, 35.73)
valvular defect associated with atrial and ventricular septal defects (35.54, 35.63, 35.73)

35.20 Replacement of unspecified heart valve
Repair of unspecified heart valve with tissue graft or prosthetic implant

35.21 Replacement of aortic valve with tissue graft
Repair of aortic valve with tissue graft (autograft) (heterograft) (homograft)

35.22 Other replacement of aortic valve
Repair of aortic valve with replacement:
NOS
prosthetic (partial) (synthetic) (total)

35.23 Replacement of mitral valve with tissue graft
Repair of mitral valve with tissue graft (autograft) (heterograft) (homograft)

35.24 Other replacement of mitral valve
Repair of mitral valve with replacement:
NOS
prosthetic (partial) (synthetic) (total)

35.25 Replacement of pulmonary valve with tissue graft
Repair of pulmonary valve with tissue graft (autograft) (heterograft) (homograft)

35.26 Other replacement of pulmonary valve
Repair of pulmonary valve with replacement:
NOS
prosthetic (partial) (synthetic) (total)

35.27 Replacement of tricuspid valve with tissue graft
Repair of tricuspid valve with tissue graft (autograft) (heterograft) (homograft)

35.28 Other replacement of tricuspid valve
Repair of tricuspid valve with replacement:
NOS
prosthetic (partial) (synthetic) (total)

35.3 Operations on structures adjacent to heart valves

Code also cardiopulmonary bypass [extracorporeal circulation] [heart-lung machine] (39.61)

35.31 Operations on papillary muscle
Division
Reattachment } of papillary muscle
Repair

35.32 Operations on chordae tendineae
Division } of chordae tendineae
Repair

35.33 Annuloplasty
Plication of annulus

35.34 Infundibulectomy
Right ventricular infundibulectomy

35.35 Operations on trabeculae carneae cordis
Division } of trabeculae carneae cordis
Excision
Excision of aortic subvalvular ring

35.39 Operations on other structures adjacent to valves of heart
Repair of sinus of Valsalva (aneurysm)

35.4 Production of septal defect in heart

35.41 Enlargement of existing atrial septal defect
Rashkind procedure
Septostomy (atrial) (balloon)

35.42 Creation of septal defect in heart
Blalock-Hanlon operation

35.5 Repair of atrial and ventricular septa with prosthesis

Includes: Repair of septa with synthetic implant or patch

Code also cardiopulmonary bypass [extracorporeal circulation] [heart-lung machine] (39.61)

35.50 Repair of unspecified septal defect of heart with prosthesis

Excludes: that associated with repair of:
endocardial cushion defect (35.54)
septal defect associated with valvular defect (35.54)

35.51 Repair of atrial septal defect with prosthesis, open technique
Atrioseptoplasty ⎫
Correction of atrial septal defect ⎬ with prosthesis
Repair: ⎪
   foramen ovale (patent) ⎪
   ostium secundum defect ⎭

Excludes: that associated with repair of:
   atrial septal defect associated with valvular and ventricular septal defects (35.54)
   endocardial cushion defect (35.54)

35.52 Repair of atrial septal defect with prosthesis, closed technique
Insertion of atrial septal umbrella [King-Mills]

35.53 Repair of ventricular septal defect with prosthesis
Correction of ventricular ⎫
   septal defect ⎬ with prosthesis
Repair of supracristal defect ⎭

Excludes: that associated with repair of:
   endocardial cushion defect (35.54)
   ventricular defect associated with valvular and atrial septal defects (35.54)

35.54 Repair of endocardial cushion defect with prosthesis
Repair:
   atrioventricular canal ⎫
   ostium primum defect ⎬ with prosthesis
   valvular defect associated ⎪ (grafted to septa)
     with atrial and ventricular ⎪
     defects ⎭

Excludes: repair of isolated:
   atrial septal defect (35.51–35.52)
   valvular defect (35.20, 35.22, 35.24, 35.26, 35.28)
   ventricular septal duct (35.53)

35.6 Repair of atrial and ventricular septa with tissue graft

Code also cardiopulmonary bypass [extracorporeal circulation] [heart-lung machine] (39.61)

35.60 Repair of unspecified septal defect of heart with tissue graft

Excludes: that associated with repair of:
   endocardial cushion defect (35.63)
   septal defect associated with valvular defect (35.63)

35.61 Repair of atrial septal defect with tissue graft
Atrioseptoplasty ⎫
Correction of atrial septal defect ⎬
Repair: ⎪ with tissue graft
   foramen ovale (patent) ⎪
   ostium secundum defect ⎭

Excludes: that associated with repair of:
   atrial septal defect associated with valvular and ventricular septal defects (35.63)
   endocardial cushion defect (35.63)

35.62 Repair of ventricular septal defect with tissue graft
Correction of ventricular ⎫
   septal defect ⎬ with tissue graft
Repair of supracristal defect ⎭

Excludes: that associated with repair of:
   endocardial cushion defect (35.63)
   ventricular defect associated with valvular and atrial septal defects (35.63)

35.63 Repair of endocardial cushion defect with tissue graft
Repair of:
   atrioventricular canal ⎫
   ostium primum defect ⎬
   valvular defect associated ⎪ with tissue graft
     with atrial and ⎪
     ventricular septal defects ⎭

Excludes: repair of isolated:
   atrial septal defect (35.61), Valvular defect (35.20–35.21, 35.23, 35.25, 35.27)
   ventricular septal defect (35.62)

35.7 Other and unspecified repair of atrial and ventricular septa

Code also cardiopulmonary bypass [extracorporeal circulation] [heart-lung machine] (39.61)

35.70 Other and unspecified repair of unspecified septal defect of heart
Repair of septal defect NOS

Excludes: that associated with repair of:
   endocardial cushion defect (35.73)
   septal defect associated with valvular defect (35.73)

35.71 Other and unspecified repair of atrial septal defect
Repair NOS:
   atrial septum
   foramen ovale (patent)
   ostium secundum defect

Excludes: that associated with repair of:
   atrial septal defect associated with valvular and ventricular septal defects (35.73)
   endocardial cushion defect (35.73)

35.72 Other and unspecified repair of ventricular septal defect
Repair NOS:
   supracristal defect
   ventricular septum

Excludes: that associated with repair of:
   endocardial cushion defect (35.73)
   ventricular septal defect associated with valvular and atrial septal defects (35.73)

35.73 Other and unspecified repair of endocardial cushion defect
Repair NOS:
   atrioventricular canal
   ostium primum defect
   valvular defect associated with atrial and ventricular septal defects

Excludes: repair of isolated:
   atrial septal defect (35.71), Valvular defect (35.20, 35.22, 35.24, 35.26, 35.28)
   ventricular septal duct (35.72)

35.8 Total repair of certain congenital cardiac anomalies
Note: For partial repair of defect [e.g. repair of atrial septal defect in tetralogy of Fallot] — code to specific procedure

35.81 Total repair of tetralogy of Fallot
One-stage total correction of tetralogy of Fallot with or without:
   commissurotomy of pulmonary valve
   infundibulectomy
   outflow tract prosthesis
   patch graft of outflow tract
   prosthetic tube for pulmonary artery
   repair of ventricular septal defect (with prosthesis)
   take-down of previous systemic-pulmonary artery anastomosis

OPERATIONS ON THE CARDIOVASCULAR SYSTEM (35-39)

35.82 Total repair of total anomalous pulmonary venous connection
One-stage total correction of total anomalous pulmonary venous connection with or without:
anastomosis between (horizontal) common pulmonary trunk and posterior wall of left atrium (side-to-side)
enlargement of foramen ovale
incision [excision] of common wall between posterior left atrium and coronary sinus and roofing of resultant defect with patch graft (synthetic)
ligation of venous connection (descending anomalous vein) (to left innominate vein) (to superior vena cava)
repair of atrial septal defect (with prosthesis)

35.83 Total repair of truncus arteriosus
One-stage total correction of truncus arteriosus with or without:
construction (with aortic homograft) (with prosthesis) of a pulmonary artery placed from right ventricle to arteries supplying the lung
ligation of connections between aorta and pulmonary artery
repair of ventricular septal defect (with prosthesis)

35.84 Total correction of transposition of great vessels, not elsewhere classified
Arterial switch operation [Jatene]
Total correction of transposition of great arteries at the arterial level by switching the great arteries, including the left or both coronary arteries, implanted in the wall of the pulmonary artery

Excludes: baffle operation [Mustard] [Senning] (35.91)
creation of shunt between right ventricle and pulmonary artery [Rastelli] (35.92)

35.9 Other operations on valves and septa of heart

Code also cardiopulmonary bypass, if performed [extracorporeal circulation] [heart-lung machine] (39.61)

35.91 Interatrial transposition of venous return
Baffle:
atrial
interatrial
Mustard's operation
Resection of atrial septum and insertion of patch to direct systemic venous return to tricuspid valve aid pulmonary venous return to mitral valve

35.92 Creation of conduit between right ventricle and pulmonary artery
Creation of shunt between right ventricle and (distal) pulmonary artery

Excludes: that associated with total repair of truncus arteriosus (35.83)

35.93 Creation of conduit between left ventricle and aorta
Creation of apicoaortic shunt
Shunt between apex of left ventricle and aorta

35.94 Creation of conduit between atrium and pulmonary artery
Fontan procedure

35.95 Revision of corrective procedure on heart
Replacement of prosthetic heart valve poppet
Resuture of prosthesis of:
septum
valve

Excludes: complete revision — code to specific procedure
replacement of prosthesis or graft of:
septum (35.50–35.63)
valve (35.20–35.28)

35.96 Percutaneous valvuloplasty
Percutaneous balloon valvuloplasty

35.98 Other operations on septa of heart

35.99 Other operations on valves of heart

36 Operations on vessels of heart

Includes: sternotomy (median) (transverse)
thoracotomy } as operative approach

Code also cardiopulmonary bypass, if performed [extracorporeal circulation] [heart-lung machine] (39.61)

36.0 Removal of coronary artery obstruction

▲ **36.01 Single vessel percutaneous transluminal coronary angioplasty [PTCA] or coronary atherectomy without mention of thrombolytic agent**
Balloon angioplasty of coronary artery
Coronary atherectomy
Percucaneous coronary angioplasty NOS
PTCA NOS

Excludes: multiple vessel percutaneous transluminal coronary angioplasty [PTCA] or coronary atherectomy performed during the same operation (36.05)

▲ **36.02 Single vessel percutaneous transluminal coronary angioplasty [PTCA] or coronary atherectomy with thrombolytic agent**
Balloon angioplasty of coronary artery with infusion of thrombolytic agent [streptokinase]
Coronary atherectomy

Excludes: multiple vessel percutaneous transluminal coronary angioplasty [PTCA] or coronary atherectomy performed during the same operation (36.05)
single vessel [PTCA] or coronary atherectomy without mention of thrombolytic agent (36.01)

36.03 Open chest coronary artery angioplasty
Coronary (artery):
endarterectomy (with patch graft)
thromboendarterectomy (with patch graft)
Open surgery for direct relief of coronary artery obstruction

Excludes: that with coronary artery bypass graft (36.10–36.19)

36.04 Intracoronary artery thrombolytic infusion
That by direct coronary artery injection, infusion, or catheterization

Excludes: that administered intravenously [IV infusion] (99.29)
that associated with any procedure in 36.02, 36.03

▲ **36.05 Multiple vessel percutaneous transluminal coronary angioplasty [PTCA] or coronary atherectomy performed during the same operation, with or without mention of thrombolytic agent**
Balloon angioplasty of multiple coronary arteries
Coronary atherectomy

Code also any intracoronary artery thrombolytic infusion (36.04)

Excludes: single vessel [PTCA] or coronary atherectomy without mention of thrombolytic agent (36.01)
with mention of thrombolytic agent (36.02)

▲**36.09 Other specified removal of coronary artery obstruction**
Coronary angioplasty NOS

> Excludes: that by open angioplasty (36.03)
> that by percutaneous transluminal coronary angioplasty [PTCA] or coronary atherectomy (36.01–36.02, 36.05)

36.1 Bypass anastomosis for heart revascularization

Code also cardiopulmonary bypass [extracorporeal circulation] [heart-lung machine] (39.61)

36.10 Aortocoronary bypass for heart revascularization, not otherwise specified
Direct revascularization:
  cardiac
  coronary
  heart muscle   } with catheter stent, prosthesis, or vein graft
  myocardial
Heart revascularization NOS

36.11 Aortocoronary bypass of one coronary artery

36.12 Aortocoronary bypass of two coronary arteries

36.13 Aortocoronary bypass of three coronary arteries

36.14 Aortocoronary bypass of four or more coronary arteries

36.15 Single internal mammary-coronary artery bypass
Anastomosis (single):
  mammary artery to coronary artery
  thoracic artery to coronary artery

36.16 Double internal mammary-coronary artery bypass
Anastomosis, double:
  mammary artery to coronary artery
  thoracic artery to coronary artery

36.19 Other bypass anastomosis for heart revascularization

36.2 Heart revascularization by arterial implant
Implantation of:
  aortic branches [ascending aortic branches] into heart muscle
  blood vessels into myocardium
  internal mammary artery [internal thoracic artery] into:
    heart muscle
    myocardium
    ventricle
    ventricular wall
Indirect heart revascularization NOS

36.3 Other heart revascularization
Abrasion of epicardium
Cardio-omentopexy
Intrapericardial poudrage
Myocardial graft:
  mediastinal fat
  omentum
  pectoral muscles

36.9 Other operations on vessels of heart

Code also cardiopulmonary bypass [extracorporeal circulation] [heart-lung machine] (39.61)

36.91 Repair of aneurysm of coronary vessel

36.99 Other operations on vessels of heart
Exploration
Incision   } of coronary artery
Ligation
Repair of arteriovenous fistula

37 Other operations on heart and pericardium

37.0 Pericardiocentesis

37.1 Cardiotomy and pericardiotomy

Code also cardiopulmonary bypass [extracorporeal circulation] [heart-lung machine] (39.61)

37.10 Incision of heart, not otherwise specified
Cardiolysis NOS

37.11 Cardiotomy
Incision of:
  atrium
  endocardium
  myocardium
  ventricle

37.12 Pericardiotomy
Pericardial window operation
Pericardiolysis
Pericardiotomy

37.2 Diagnostic procedures on heart and pericardium

37.21 Right heart cardiac catheterization NOR
Cardiac catheterization NOS

> Excludes: that with catheterization of left heart (37.23)

37.22 Left heart cardiac catheterization NOR

> Excludes: that with catheterization of right heart (37.23)

37.23 Combined right and left heart cardiac catheterization NOR

37.24 Biopsy of pericardium

37.25 Biopsy of heart

37.26 Cardiac electrophysiologic stimulation and recording studies NOR
Electrophysiologic studies [EPS]
Programmed electrical stimulation

Code also any concomitant procedure

> Excludes: His bundle recording (37.29)

37.27 Cardiac mapping NOR

Code also any concomitant procedure

> Excludes: electrocardiogram (89.52)
> His bundle recording (37.29)

37.29 Other diagnostic procedures on heart and pericardium

> Excludes: angiocardiography (88.50–88.58)
> cardiac function tests (89.41–89.69)
> cardiovascular radioisotopic scan and function study (92.05)
> coronary arteriography (88.55–88.57)
> diagnostic pericardiocentesis (37.0)
> diagnostic ultrasound of heart (88.72)
> x-ray of heart (87.49)

37.3 Pericardiectomy and excision of lesion of heart

Code also cardiopulmonary bypass [extracorporeal circulation] [heart-lung machine] (39.61)

37.31 Pericardiectomy
Excision of:
  adhesions of pericardium
  constricting scar of:
    epicardium
    pericardium

37.32 Excision of aneurysm of heart

OPERATIONS ON THE CARDIOVASCULAR SYSTEM (35-39)

37.33 Excision or destruction of other lesion or tissue of heart

> Excludes: catheter ablation of lesion or tissues of heart (37.34)

37.34 Catheter ablation of lesion or tissues of heart
Cryoablation
Electrocurrent } of lesion or tissues of heart
Resection

37.4 Repair of heart and pericardium

37.5 Heart transplantation

> Excludes: combined heart-lung transplantation (33.6)

37.6 Implantation of heart assist system

37.61 Implant of pulsation balloon

37.62 Implant of other heart assist system
Insertion of heart pump

37.63 Replacement and repair of heart assist system

37.64 Removal of heart assist system

> Excludes: that with replacement of implant (37.63)

37.7 Insertion, revision, replacement, and removal of pacemaker leads, insertion of temporary pacemaker system, or revision of pocket

Code also any insertion and replacement of pacemaker device (37.80–37.87)

* 37.70 Initial insertion of lead [electrode], not otherwise specified

> Excludes: insertion of temporary transvenous pacemaker system (37.78)
> replacement of atrial and/or ventricular lead(s) (37.76)

* 37.71 Initial insertion of transvenous lead [electrode] into ventricle

> Excludes: insertion of temporary transvenous pacemaker system (37.78)
> replacement of atrial and/or ventricular lead(s) (37.76)

* 37.72 Initial insertion of transvenous leads [electrodes] into atrium and ventricle

> Excludes: insertion of temporary transvenous pacemaker system (37.78)
> replacement of atrial and/or ventricular lead(s) (37.76)

* 37.73 Initial insertion of transvenous lead [electrode] into atrium

> Excludes: insertion of temporary transvenous pacemaker system (37.78)
> replacement of atrial and/or ventricular lead(s) (37.76)

37.74 Insertion or replacement of epicardial lead [electrode] into epicardium
Insertion or replacement of epicardial lead by:
sternotomy
thoracotomy

> Excludes: replacement of atrial and/or ventricular lead(s) (37.76)

37.75 Revision of lead [electrode]
Repair of electrode [removal with re-insertion]
Repositioning of lead [electrode]
Revision of lead NOS

> Excludes: repositioning of temporary transvenous pacemaker system—omit code

37.76 Replacement of transvenous atrial and/or ventricular lead(s) [electrode]
Removal or abandonment of existing transvenous or epicardial lead(s) with transvenous lead(s) replacement

> Excludes: replacement of epicardial lead [electrode] (37.74)

37.77 Removal of lead(s) [electrode] without replacement
Removal:
epicardial lead (transthoracic approach)
transvenous lead(s)

> Excludes: removal of temporary transvenous pacemaker system — omit code
> that with replacement of:
> atrial and/or ventricular lead(s) [electrode] (37.76)
> epicardial lead [electrode] (37.74)

37.78 Insertion of temporary transvenous pacemaker system

> Excludes: intraoperative cardiac pacemaker (39.64)

37.79 Revision or relocation of pacemaker pocket
Debridement and reforming pocket (skin and subcutaneous tissue)
Relocation of pocket [creation of new pocket]

37.8 Insertion, replacement, removal, and revision of pacemaker device

Code also any lead insertion, lead replacement, lead removal and/or lead revision (37.70–37.77)

37.80 Insertion of permanent pacemaker, initial or replacement, type of device not specified

* 37.81 Initial insertion of single-chamber device, not specified as rate responsive

> Excludes: replacement of existing pacemaker device (37.85–37.87)

* 37.82 Initial insertion of a single-chamber device, rate responsive
Rate responsive to physiologic stimuli other than atrial rate

> Excludes: replacement of existing pacemaker device (37.85–37.87)

* 37.83 Initial insertion of dual-chamber device
Atrial ventricular sequential device

> Excludes: replacement of existing pacemaker device (37.85–37.87)

37.85 Replacement of any type pacemaker device with single-chamber device, not specified as rate responsive

37.86 Replacement of any type pacemaker device with single-chamber device, rate responsive
Rate responsive to physiologic stimuli other than atrial rate

37.87 Replacement of any type pacemaker device with dual-chamber device
Atrial ventricular sequential device

37.89 Revision or removal of pacemaker device
Repair of pacemaker device

> Excludes: removal of temporary transvenous pacemaker system — omit code
> replacement of existing pacemaker device (37.85–37.87)

---

* Must be used in combination with related codes to be considered an operating room procedure.

37.9 Other operations on heart and pericardium

37.91 Open chest cardiac massage

> Excludes: closed chest cardiac massage (99.63)

37.92 Injection of therapeutic substance into heart

37.93 Injection of therapeutic substance into pericardium

37.94 Implantation or replacement of automatic cardioverter/defibrillator, total system [AICD]

Implantation of defibrillator with leads (epicardial patches), formation of pocket (abdominal fascia) (subcutaneous), any transvenous leads, intraoperative procedures for evaluation of lead signals, and obtaining defibrillator threshold measurements

Techniques: lateral thoracotomy
   medial sternotomy
   subxiphoid procedure

Code also extracorporeal circulation, if performed (39.61)
Code also any concomitant procedure [e.g., coronary bypass] (36.00–36.19)

37.95 Implantation of automatic cardioverter/defibrillator lead(s) only

37.96 Implantation of automatic cardioverter/defibrillator pulse generator only

37.97 Replacement of automatic cardioverter/defibrillator lead(s) only

37.98 Replacement of automatic cardioverter/defibrillator pulse generator only

37.99 Other

Removal of cardioverter/defibrillator pulse generator only without replacement
Repositioning of lead(s) (sensing) (pacing) [electrode]
Repositioning of pulse generator

> Excludes: cardiac retraining (93.36)
> conversion of cardiac rhythm (99.60–99.69)

38 Incision, excision, and occlusion of vessels

Code also cardiopulmonary bypass [extracorporeal circulation] [heart-lung machine] (39.61)

> Excludes: that of coronary vessels (36.01–36.99)

The following fourth-digit subclassification is for use with appropriate categories in section 38, marked with a symbol (§), to identify the site:

0 unspecified site

1 intracranial vessels
   Cerebral (anterior) (middle)
   Circle of Willis
   Posterior communicating artery

2 other vessels of head and neck
   Carotid artery (common) (external) (internal)
   Jugular vein (external) (internal)

3 upper limb vessels
   Axillary   Radial
   Brachial   Ulnar

4 aorta

5 other thoracic vessels
   Innominate   Subclavian
   Pulmonary (artery) Vena cava, superior
     (vein)

6 abdominal arteries
   Celiac   Mesenteric
   Gastric   Renal
   Hepatic   Splenic
   Iliac   Umbilical

> Excludes: abdominal aorta (4)

7 abdominal veins
   Iliac   Splenic
   Portal   Vena cava (inferior)
   Renal

8 lower limb arteries
   Femoral (common) (superficial)
   Popliteal
   Tibial

9 lower limb veins
   Femoral   Saphenous
   Popliteal   Tibial

§ 38.0 Incision of vessel
[0-9] Embolectomy   Thrombectomy

> Excludes: puncture or catheterization of any:
>   artery (38.91, 38.98)
>   vein (38.92–38.95, 38.99)

§ 38.1 Endarterectomy
[0-6,8] Endarterectomy with:
   embolectomy
   patch graft
   temporary bypass during procedure
   thrombectomy

38.2 Diagnostic procedures on blood vessels

38.21 Biopsy of blood vessel

38.22 Percutaneous angioscopy

> Excludes: angioscopy of eye (95.12)

38.29 Other diagnostic procedures on blood vessels

> Excludes: blood vessel thermography (88.86)
>   circulatory monitoring (89.61–89.69)
>   contrast:
>   angiocardiography (88.50–88.58)
>   arteriography (88.40–88.49)
>   phlebography (88.60–88.67)
>   impedance phlebography (88.68)
>   peripheral vascular ultrasonography (88.77)
>   plethysmogram (89.58)

§ 38.3 Resection of vessel with anastomosis
[0-9] Angiectomy
   Excision of:
     aneurysm (arteriovenous) } with anastomosis
     blood vessel (lesion)

---

§ Requires fourth-digit; valid digits are in [brackets] under each code. See above for definitions.

OPERATIONS ON THE CARDIOVASCULAR SYSTEM (35-39)

38.4 Resection of vessel with replacement
    Angiectomy
    Excision of:
        aneurysm (arteriovenous)   } with replacement
        or blood vessel (lesion)
    with vessel replacement

Requires the use of one of the following fourth-digit subclassifications to identify site:

0 unspecified site

1 intracranial vessels
    Cerebral (anterior) (middle)
    Circle of Willis
    Posterior communicating artery

2 other vessels of head and neck
    Carotid artery (common) (external) (internal)
    Jugular vein (external) (internal)

3 upper limb vessels
    Axillary   Radial
    Brachial   Ulnar

4 aorta, abdominal

    Code also any thoracic vessel involvement (thoracoabdominal procedure) (38.45)

5 thoracic vessel
    Aorta (thoracic)   Subclavian
    Innominate   Vena cava, superior
    Pulmonary (artery) (vein)

    Code also any abdominal aorta involvement (thoracoabdominal procedure) (38.44)

6 abdominal arteries
    Celiac   Mesenteric
    Gastric   Renal
    Hepatic   Splenic
    Iliac   Umbilical

    Excludes: abdominal aorta (4)

7 abdominal veins
    Iliac   Splenic
    Portal   Vena cava (inferior)
    Renal

8 lower limb arteries
    Femoral (common) (superficial)
    Popliteal
    Tibial

9 lower limb veins
    Femoral   Saphenous
    Popliteal   Tibial

§ **38.5 Ligation and stripping of varicose veins**
[0-3,5,7,9]
    Excludes: ligation of varices:
            esophageal (42.91)
            gastric (44.91)

§ **38.6 Other excision of vessels**
[0-9] Excision of blood vessel (lesion) NOS

    Excludes: excision of vessel for aortocoronary bypass (36.10-36.14)
            excision with:
                anastomosis (38.30-38.39)
                graft replacement (38.40-38.49)
                implant (38.40-38.49)

38.7 Interruption of the vena cava
    Insertion of implant or sieve in vena cava
    Ligation of vena cava (inferior) (superior)
    Plication of vena cava

§ **38.8 Other surgical occlusion of vessels**
[0-9]   Clamping
       Division   } of blood vessel
       Ligation
       Occlusion

    Excludes: adrenal vessels (07.43)
            esophageal varices (42.91)
            gastric or duodenal vessel for ulcer (44.40-44.49)
            gastric varices (44.91)
            meningeal vessel (02.13)
            spermatic vein for varicocele (63.1)
            surgical occlusion of vena cava (38.7)
            that for control of (postoperative) hemorrhage:
                anus (49.95)
                bladder (57.93)
                following vascular procedure (39.41)
                nose (21.00-21.09)
                prostate (60.94)
                tonsil (28.7)
            thyroid vessel (06.92)

38.9 Puncture of vessel

    Excludes: that for circulatory monitoring (89.61-89.69)

38.91 Arterial catheterization

38.92 Umbilical vein catheterization

38.93 Venous catheterization, not elsewhere classified

    Excludes: that for cardiac catheterization (37.21-37.23)
            that for renal dialysis (38.95)

38.94 Venous cutdown

▲**38.95 Venous catheterization for renal dialysis**

    Excludes: insertion of totally implantable vascular access device [VAD] 86.07

38.98 Other puncture of artery

    Excludes: that for:
            coronary arteriography (88.55-88.57)
            arteriography (88.40-88.49)

▲**38.99 Other puncture of vein**
    Phlebotomy

    Excludes: that for:
            angiography (88.60-88.69)
            extracorporeal circulation (39.61, 50.92)
            injection or infusion of:
                sclerosing solution (39.92)
                therapeutic or prophylactic substance (99.11-99.29)
            perfusion (39.96-39.97)
            phlebography (88.60-88.69)
            transfusion (99.01-99.09)

39 Other operations on vessels

    Excludes: those on coronary vessels 06.0-36.99)

39.0 Systemic to pulmonary artery shunt
    Descending aorta-pulmonary artery }
    Left to right   } anastomosis (graft)
    Subclavian-pulmonary   }

    Code also cardiopulmonary bypass [extracorporeal circulation] [heart-lung machine] (39.61)

---

§ Requires fourth-digit; valid digits are in [brackets] under each code. See above for definitions.

▲ **39.1 Intra-abdominal venous shunt**
Anastomosis:
  mesocaval
  portacaval
  portal vein to inferior vena cava
  splenic and renal veins
  transjugular intrahepatic portosystemic shunt (TIPS)

Excludes: *peritoneovenous shunt (54.94)*

39.2 Other shunt or vascular bypass

39.21 Caval-pulmonary artery anastomosis

Code also cardiopulmonary bypass (39.61)

39.22 Aorta-subclavian-carotid bypass
Bypass (arterial):
  aorta to carotid and brachial
  aorta to subclavian and carotid
  carotid to subclavian

39.23 Other intrathoracic vascular shunt or bypass
Intrathoracic (arterial) bypass graft NOS

Excludes: *coronary artery bypass (36.10–36.19)*

39.24 Aorta-renal bypass

39.25 Aorta-iliac-femoral bypass
Bypass:
  aortofemoral
  aortoiliac, Aortoiliac to popliteal
  aortopopliteal
  iliofemoral [iliac-femoral]

39.26 Other intra-abdominal vascular shunt or bypass
Bypass:
  aortoceliac
  aortic-superior mesenteric
  common hepatic-common iliac-renal
  intra-abdominal arterial bypass graft NOS

Excludes: *peritoneovenous shunt (54.94)*

39.27 Arteriovenostomy for renal dialysis
Anastomosis for renal dialysis
Formation of (peripheral) arteriovenous fistula for renal [kidney] dialysis

Code also any renal dialysis (39.95)

Extracranial-intracranial (EC-IC) vascular bypass

39.29 Other (peripheral) vascular shunt or bypass
Bypass (graft):
  axillary-brachial
  axillary-femoral [axillofemoral] (superficial)
  brachial
  femoral-femoral
  femoroperoneal
  femoropopliteal (arteries)
  femorotibial (anterior) (posterior)
  popliteal
  vascular NOS

Excludes: *peritoneovenous shunt (54.94)*

39.3 Suture of vessel
Repair of laceration of blood vessel

Excludes: *suture of aneurysm (39.52)*
that for control of hemorrhage (postoperative):
  anus (49.95)
  bladder (57.93)
  following vascular procedure (39.41)
  nose (21.00–21.09)
  prostate (60.94)
  tonsil (28.7)

39.30 Suture of unspecified blood vessel

39.31 Suture of artery

39.32 Suture of vein

39.4 Revision of vascular procedure

39.41 Control of hemorrhage following vascular surgery

Excludes: *that for control of hemorrhage (post operative):*
  anus (49.95)
  bladder (57.93)
  nose (21.00–21.09)
  prostate (60.94)
  tonsil (28.7)

39.42 Revision of arteriovenous shunt for renal dialysis
Conversion of renal dialysis:
  end-to-end anastomosis to end-to-side
  end-to-side anastomosis to end-to-end
  vessel-to-vessel cannula to arteriovenous shunt
Removal of old arteriovenous shunt and creation of new shunt

Excludes: *replacement of vessel-to-vessel cannula (39.94)*

39.43 Removal of arteriovenous shunt for renal dialysis

Excludes: *that with replacement [revision] of shunt (39.42)*

39.49 Other revision of vascular procedure
Declotting (graft)
Revision of:
  anastomosis of blood vessel
  vascular procedure (previous)

39.5 Other repair of vessels

39.51 Clipping of aneurysm

Excludes: *clipping of arteriovenous fistula (39.53)*

39.52 Other repair of aneurysm
Repair of aneurysm by:
  coagulation
  electrocoagulation
  filipuncture
  methyl methacrylate
  suture
  wiring
  wrapping

Excludes: *re-entry operation (aorta) (39.54)*
that with:
  graft replacement (38.40–38.49)
  resection (38.30–38.49, 38.60–38.69)

▲ **39.53 Repair of arteriovenous fistula**
Embolization of carotid cavernous fistula
Repair of arteriovenous fistula by:
  clipping
  coagulation
  ligation and division

Excludes: *repair of arteriovenous shunt for renal dialysis (39.42)*
that with:
  graft replacement (38.40–38.49)
  resection (38.30–38.49, 38.60–38.69)

39.54 Re-entry operation (aorta)
Fenestration of dissecting aneurysm of thoracic aorta

Code also cardiopulmonary bypass [extracorporeal circulation] [heart-lung machine] (39.61)

39.55 Reimplantation of aberrant renal vessel

39.56 Repair of blood vessel with tissue patch graft

Excludes: *that with resection (38.40–38.49)*

39.57 Repair of blood vessel with synthetic patch graft

> *Excludes:* that with resection (38.40–38.49)

39.58 Repair of blood vessel with unspecified type of patch graft

> *Excludes:* that with resection (38.40–38.49)

39.59 Other repair of vessel
Aorticopulmonary window operation
Arterioplasty NOS
Construction of venous valves (peripheral)
Plication of vein (peripheral)
Reimplantation of artery

Code also cardiopulmonary bypass [extracorporeal circulation] [heart-lung machine] (39.61)

> *Excludes:* interruption of the vena cava (38.7)
> reimplantation of renal artery (39.55)
> that with:
>   graft (39.56–39.58)
>   resection (38.30–38.49, 38.60–38.69)

39.6 Extracorporeal circulation and procedures auxiliary to open heart surgery

39.61 Extracorporeal circulation auxiliary to open heart surgery
Artificial heart and lung
Cardiopulmonary bypass
Pump oxygenator

> *Excludes:* extracorporeal hepatic assistance (50.92)
> extracorporeal membrane oxygenation [ECMO] (39.65)
> hemodialysis (39.95)
> percutaneous cardiopulmonary bypass (39.66)

39.62 Hypothermia (systemic) incidental to open heart surgery

39.63 Cardioplegia
Arrest:
  anoxic
  circulatory

39.64 Intraoperative cardiac pacemaker
Temporary pacemaker used during and immediately following cardiac surgery

39.65 Extracorporeal membrane oxygenation [ECMO]

> *Excludes:* extracorporeal circulation auxiliary to open heart surgery (39.61)
> percutaneous cardiopulmonary bypass (39.66)

39.66 Percutaneous cardiopulmonary bypass
Closed chest

> *Excludes:* extracorporeal circulation auxiliary to open heart surgery (39.61)
> extracorporeal hepatic assistance (50.92)
> extracorporeal membrane oxygenation [ECMO] (39.65)
> hemodialysis (39.95)

39.7 Periarterial sympathectomy

39.8 Operations on carotid body and other vascular bodies
Chemodectomy
Denervation of:
  aortic body
  carotid body
Glomectomy, carotid
Implantation into carotid body:
  electronic stimulator
  pacemaker

> *Excludes:* excision of glomus jugulare (20.51)

39.9 Other operations on vessels

39.91 Freeing of vessel
Dissection and freeing of adherent tissue:
  artery-vein-nerve bundle
  vascular bundle

39.92 Injection of sclerosing agent into vein

> *Excludes:* injection:
>   esophageal varices (42.33)
>   hemorrhoids (49.42)

39.93 Insertion of vessel-to-vessel cannula
Formation of:
  arteriovenous:
    fistula } by external cannula
    shunt

Code also any renal dialysis (39.95)

39.94 Replacement of vessel-to-vessel cannula
Revision of vessel-to-vessel cannula

39.95 Hemodialysis
Artificial kidney   Hemofiltration
Hemodiafiltration   Renal dialysis

> *Excludes:* peritoneal dialysis (54.98)

39.96 Total body perfusion

Code also substance perfused (99.21–99.29)

39.97 Other perfusion
Perfusion NOS
Perfusion
local [regional] of:
  carotid artery
  coronary artery
  head
  lower limb
  neck
  upper limb

Code also substance perfused (99.21–99.29)

> *Excludes:* perfusion of:
>   kidney (55.95)
>   large intestine (46.96)
>   liver (50.93)
>   small intestine (46.95)

39.98 Control of hemorrhage, not otherwise specified
Angiotripsy
Control of postoperative hemorrhage NOS
Venotripsy

> *Excludes:* control of hemorrhage (postoperative):
>   anus (49.95)
>   bladder (57.93)
>   following vascular procedure (39.41)
>   nose (21.00–21.09)
>   prostate (60.94)
>   tonsil (28.7)
>   that by:
>   ligation (38.80–38.89)
>   suture (39.30–39.32)

39.99 Other operations on vessels

> *Excludes:* injection or infusion of therapeutic or prophylactic substance (99.11–99.29)
> transfusion of blood and blood components (99.01–99.09)

OPERATIONS ON THE HEMIC AND LYMPHATIC SYSTEM (40-41)

8. OPERATIONS ON THE HEMIC AND LYMPHATIC SYSTEM (40–41)

40 Operations on lymphatic system

40.0 Incision of lymphatic structures

40.1 Diagnostic procedures on lymphatic structures

40.11 Biopsy of lymphatic structure

40.19 Other diagnostic procedures on lymphatic structures

> *Excludes:* lymphangiogram:
> abdominal (88.04)
> cervical (87.08)
> intrathoracic (87.34)
> lower limb (88.36)
> upper limb (88.34)
> microscopic examination of specimen (90.71–90.79)
> radioisotope scan (92.16)
> thermography (88.89)

40.2 Simple excision of lymphatic structure

> *Excludes:* biopsy of lymphatic structure (40.11)

40.21 Excision of deep cervical lymph node

40.22 Excision of internal mammary lymph node

40.23 Excision of axillary lymph node

40.24 Excision of inguinal lymph node

40.29 Simple excision of other lymphatic structure
Excision of:
  cystic hygroma
  lymphangioma
Simple lymphadenectomy

40.3 Regional lymph node excision
Extended regional lymph node excision
Regional lymph node excision with excision of lymphatic drainage area including skin, subcutaneous tissue, and fat

40.4 Radical excision of cervical lymph nodes
Resection of cervical lymph nodes down to muscle and deep fascia

> *Excludes:* that associated with radical laryngectomy (30.4)

40.40 Radical neck dissection, not otherwise specified

40.41 Radical neck dissection, unilateral

40.42 Radical neck dissection, bilateral

40.5 Radical excision of other lymph nodes

> *Excludes:* that associated with radical mastectomy (85.45–85.48)

40.50 Radical excision of lymph nodes, not otherwise specified
Radical (lymph) node dissection NOS

40.51 Radical excision of axillary lymph nodes

40.52 Radical excision of periaortic lymph nodes

40.53 Radical excision of iliac lymph nodes

40.54 Radical groin dissection

40.59 Radical excision of other lymph nodes

> *Excludes:* radical neck dissection (40.40–40.42)

40.6 Operations on thoracic duct

40.61 Cannulation of thoracic duct

40.62 Fistulization of thoracic duct

40.63 Closure of fistula of thoracic duct

40.64 Ligation of thoracic duct

40.69 Other operations on thoracic duct

40.9 Other operations on lymphatic structures
Anastomosis
Dilation
Ligation
Obliteration   } of peripheral lymphatics
Reconstruction
Repair
Transplantation
Correction of lymphedema of limb, NOS

> *Excludes:* reduction of elephantiasis of scrotum (61.3)

41 Operations on bone marrow and spleen

▲ 41.0 Bone marrow or hematopoietic stem cell transplant

> *Excludes:* aspiration of bone marrow from donor (41.91)

41.00 Bone marrow transplant, not otherwise specified

41.01 Autologous bone marrow transplant
With extracorporeal purging of malignant cells from marrow
Autograft of bone marrow NOS

41.02 Allogeneic bone marrow transplant with purging
Allograft of bone marrow with in vitro removal (purging) of T-cells

41.03 Allogeneic bone marrow transplant without purging
Allograft of bone marrow NOS

● **41.04** Autologous hematopoietic stem cell transplant [NOR]

41.1 Puncture of spleen

> *Excludes:* aspiration biopsy of spleen (41.32)

41.2 Splenotomy

41.3 Diagnostic procedures on bone marrow and spleen

41.31 Biopsy of bone marrow

41.32 Closed [aspiration] [percutaneous] biopsy of spleen
Needle biopsy of spleen

41.33 Open biopsy of spleen

41.38 Other diagnostic procedures on bone marrow

> *Excludes:* microscopic examination of specimen from bone marrow (90.61–90.69)
> radioisotope scan (92.05)

41.39 Other diagnostic procedures on spleen

> *Excludes:* microscopic examination of specimen from spleen (90.61–90.69)
> radioisotope scan (92.05)

41.4 Excision or destruction of lesion or tissue of spleen

> *Excludes:* excision of accessory spleen (41.93)

41.41 Marsupialization of splenic cyst

41.42 Excision of lesion or tissue of spleen

> *Excludes:* biopsy of spleen (41.32–41.33)

41.43 Partial splenectomy

41.5 Total splenectomy
Splenectomy NOS

41.9 Other operations on spleen and bone marrow

41.91 Aspiration of bone marrow from donor for transplant

> *Excludes:* biopsy of bone marrow (41.31)

41.92 Injection into bone marrow

> Excludes: bone marrow transplant (41.00–41.03)

41.93 Excision of accessory spleen

41.94 Transplantation of spleen

41.95 Repair and plastic operations on spleen

41.98 Other operations on bone marrow

41.99 Other operations on spleen

OPERATIONS ON THE DIGESTIVE SYSTEM (42-54)

9. OPERATIONS ON THE DIGESTIVE SYSTEM (42–54)

42 Operations on esophagus

42.0 Esophagotomy

42.01 Incision of esophageal web

42.09 Other incision of esophagus
Esophagotomy NOS

Excludes: esophagomyotomy (42.7)
esophagostomy (42.10–42.19)

42.1 Esophagostomy

42.10 Esophagostomy, not otherwise specified

42.11 Cervical esophagostomy

42.12 Exteriorization of esophageal pouch

42.19 Other external fistulization of esophagus
Thoracic esophagostomy

Code also any resection (42.40–42.42)

42.2 Diagnostic procedures on esophagus

42.21 Operative esophagoscopy by incision

42.22 Esophagoscopy through artificial stoma NOR

Excludes: that with biopsy (42.24)

42.23 Other esophagoscopy NOR

Excludes: that with biopsy (42.24)

42.24 Closed [endoscopic] biopsy of esophagus NOR
Brushing or washing for specimen collection
Esophagoscopy with biopsy
Suction biopsy of the esophagus

Excludes: esophagogastroduodenoscopy [EGD] with closed biopsy (45.16)

42.25 Open biopsy of esophagus

42.29 Other diagnostic procedures on esophagus

Excludes: barium swallow (87.61)
esophageal manometry (89.32)
microscopic examination of specimen from esophagus (90.81–90.89)

42.3 Local excision or destruction of lesion or tissue of esophagus

42.31 Local excision of esophageal diverticulum

42.32 Local excision of other lesion or tissue of esophagus

Excludes: biopsy of esophagus (42.24–42.25)
esophageal fistulectomy (42.84)

▲ **42.33** Endoscopic excision or destruction of lesion or tissue of esophagus NOR
Ablation of esophageal neoplasm ⎫
Control of esophageal bleeding ⎬ by endoscopic
Esophageal polypectomy ⎪ approach
Esophageal varices by endoscopic approach ⎪
Injection of esophageal varices ⎭

Excludes: biopsy of esophagus (42.24–42.25)
fistulectomy (42.84)
open ligation (open) of esophageal varices (42.91)

42.39 Other destruction of lesion or tissue of esophagus

Excludes: that by endoscopic approach (42.33)

42.4 Excision of esophagus

Excludes: esophagogastrectomy NOS (43.99)

42.40 Esophagectomy, not otherwise specified

42.41 Partial esophagectomy

Code also any synchronous:
anastomosis other than end-to-end (42.51–42.69)
esophagostomy (42.10–42.19)
gastrostomy (43.11–43.19)

42.42 Total esophagectomy

Code also any synchronous:
gastrostomy (43.11–43.19)
interposition or anastomosis other than end-to-end (42.51–42.69)

Excludes: esophagogastrectomy (43.99)

42.5 Intrathoracic anastomosis of esophagus

Code also any synchronous:
esophagectomy (42.40–42.42)
gastrostomy (41.1–43.2)

42.51 Intrathoracic esophagoesophagostomy

42.52 Intrathoracic esophagogastrostomy

42.53 Intrathoracic esophageal anastomosis with interposition of small bowel

42.54 Other intrathoracic esophagoenterostomy
Anastomosis of esophagus to intestinal segment NOS

42.55 Intrathoracic esophageal anastomosis with interposition of colon

42.56 Other intrathoracic esophagocolostomy
Esophagocolostomy NOS

42.58 Intrathoracic esophageal anastomosis with other interposition
Construction of artificial esophagus
Retrosternal formation of reversed gastric tube

42.59 Other intrathoracic anastomosis of esophagus

42.6 Antesternal anastomosis of esophagus

Code also any synchronous:
esophagectomy (42.40–42.42)
gastrostomy (43.1–43.2)

42.61 Antesternal esophagoesophagostomy

42.62 Antesternal esophagogastrostomy

42.63 Antesternal esophageal anastomosis with interposition of small bowel

42.64 Other antesternal esophagoenterostomy
Antethoracic:
esophagoenterostomy
esophagoileostomy
esophagojejunostomy

42.65 Antesternal esophageal anastomosis with interposition of colon

42.66 Other antesternal esophagocolostomy
Antethoracic esophagocolostomy

42.68 Other antesternal esophageal anastomosis with interposition

42.69 Other antesternal anastomosis of esophagus

42.7 Esophagomyotomy

42.8 Other repair of esophagus

42.81 Insertion of permanent tube into esophagus

42.82 Suture of laceration of esophagus

42.83 Closure of esophagostomy

42.84 Repair of esophageal fistula, not elsewhere classified

Excludes: repair of fistula:
bronchoesophageal (33.42)
esophagopleurocutaneous (34.73)
pharyngoesophageal (29.53)
tracheoesophageal (31.73)

42.85 Repair of esophageal stricture

42.86 Production of subcutaneous tunnel without esophageal anastomosis

42.87 Other graft of esophagus

Excludes: antesternal esophageal anastomosis with interposition of:
colon (42.65)
small bowel (42.63)
antesternal esophageal anastomosis with other interposition (42.68)
intrathoracic esophageal anastomosis with interposition of:
colon (42.55)
small bowel (42.53)
intrathoracic esophageal anastomosis with other interposition (42.58)

42.89 Other repair of esophagus

42.9 Other operations on esophagus

▲**42.91 Ligation of esophageal varices**

Excludes: that by endoscopic approach (42.33)

42.92 Dilation of esophagus
Dilation of cardiac sphincter

Excludes: intubation of esophagus (96.03, 96.06–96.08)

42.99 Other

Excludes: insertion of Sengstaken tube (96.06)
intubation of esophagus (96.03, 96.06–96.08)
removal of intraluminal foreign body from esophagus without incision (98.02)
tamponade of esophagus (96.06)

43. Incision and excision of stomach

43.0 Gastrotomy

Excludes: gastrostomy (43.11–43.19)
that for control of hemorrhage (44.49)

43.1 Gastrostomy

43.11 Percutaneous [endoscopic] gastrostomy [PEG]
Percutaneous transabdominal gastrostomy

43.19 Other gastrostomy

Excludes: percutaneous [endoscopic] gastrostomy [PEG] (43.11)

43.3 Pyloromyotomy

43.4 Local excision or destruction of lesion or tissue of stomach

▲**43.41 Endoscopic excision or destruction of lesion or tissue of stomach** NOR
Gastric polypectomy by endoscopic approach
Gastric varices by endoscopic approach

Excludes: biopsy of stomach (44.14–44.15)
control of hemorrhage (44.43)
open ligation of gastric varices (44.91)

43.42 Local excision of other lesion or tissue of stomach

Excludes: biopsy of stomach (44.14–44.15)
gastric fistulectomy (44.62–44.63)
partial gastrectomy (43.5–43.89)

43.49 Other destruction of lesion or tissue of stomach

Excludes: that by endoscopic approach (43.41)

43.5 Partial gastrectomy with anastomosis to esophagus
Proximal gastrectomy

43.6 Partial gastrectomy with anastomosis to duodenum
Billroth I operation
Distal gastrectomy
Gastropylorectomy

43.7 Partial gastrectomy with anastomosis to jejunum
Billroth II operation

43.8 Other partial gastrectomy

43.81 Partial gastrectomy with jejunal transposition
Henley jejunal transposition operation

Code also any synchronous intestinal resection (45.51)

43.89 Other
Partial gastrectomy with bypass gastrogastrostomy
Sleeve resection of stomach

43.9 Total gastrectomy

43.91 Total gastrectomy with intestinal interposition

43.99 Other total gastrectomy
Complete gastroduodenectomy
Esophagoduodenostomy with complete gastrectomy
Esophagogastrectomy NOS
Esophagojejunostomy with complete gastrectomy
Radical gastrectomy

44. Other operations on stomach

44.0 Vagotomy

44.00 Vagotomy, not otherwise specified
Division of vagus nerve NOS

44.01 Truncal vagotomy

44.02 Highly selective vagotomy
Parietal cell vagotomy
Selective proximal vagotomy

44.03 Other selective vagotomy

44.1 Diagnostic procedures on stomach

44.11 Transabdominal gastroscopy
Intraoperative gastroscopy

Excludes: that with biopsy (44.14)

44.12 Gastroscopy through artificial stoma NOR

Excludes: that with biopsy (44.14)

44.13 Other gastroscopy NOR

Excludes: that with biopsy (44.14)

44.14 Closed [endoscopic] biopsy of stomach NOR
Brushing or washing for specimen collection

Excludes: esophagogastroduodenoscopy [EGD] with closed biopsy (45.16)

44.15 Open biopsy of stomach

44.19 Other diagnostic procedures on stomach

Excludes: gastric lavage (96.33)
microscopic examination of specimen from stomach (90.81–90.89)
upper GI series (87.62)

OPERATIONS ON THE DIGESTIVE SYSTEM (42-54)

44.2 Pyloroplasty

44.21 Dilation of pylorus by incision

44.22 Endoscopic dilation of pylorus
Dilation with balloon endoscope
Endoscopic dilation of gastrojejunostomy site

44.29 Other pyloroplasty
Pyloroplasty NOS
Revision of pylorus

44.3 Gastroenterostomy without gastrectomy

44.31 High gastric bypass
Printen and Mason gastric bypass

44.39 Other gastroenterostomy
Bypass:
  gastroduodenostomy
  gastroenterostomy
  gastrogastrostomy
Gastrojejunostomy without gastrectomy NOS

44.4 Control of hemorrhage and suture of ulcer of stomach or duodenum

44.40 Suture of peptic ulcer, not otherwise specified

44.41 Suture of gastric ulcer site

> *Excludes:* ligation of gastric varices (44.91)

44.42 Suture of duodenal ulcer site

44.43 Endoscopic control of gastric or duodenal bleeding

44.44 Transcatheter embolization for gastric or duodenal bleeding

> *Excludes:* surgical occlusion of abdominal vessels (38.86–38.87)

44.49 Other control of hemorrhage of stomach or duodenum
That with gastrotomy

44.5 Revision of gastric anastomosis
Closure of:
  gastric anastomosis
  gastroduodenostomy
  gastrojejunostomy
Pantaloon operation

44.6 Other repair of stomach

44.61 Suture of laceration of stomach

> *Excludes:* that of ulcer site (44.41)

44.62 Closure of gastrostomy

44.63 Closure of other gastric fistula
Closure of:
  gastrocolic fistula
  gastrojejunocolic fistula

44.64 Gastropexy

44.65 Esophagogastroplasty
Belsey operation
Esophagus and stomach cardioplasty

44.66 Other procedures for creation of esophagogastric sphincteric competence
Fundoplication
Gastric cardioplasty
Nissen's fundoplication
Restoration of cardio-esophageal angle

44.69 Other
Inversion of gastric diverticulum
Repair of stomach NOS

44.9 Other operations on stomach

▲**44.91 Ligation of gastric varices**

> *Excludes:* that by endoscopic approach (43.41)

44.92 Intraoperative manipulation of stomach
Reduction of gastric volvulus

Insertion of gastric bubble (balloon)

44.94 Removal of gastric bubble (balloon)

44.99 Other

> *Excludes:* change of gastrostomy tube (97.02)
> dilation of cardiac sphincter (42.92)
> gastric:
>   cooling (96.31)
>   freezing (96.32)
>   gavage (96.35)
>   hypothermia (96.31)
>   lavage (96.33)
> insertion of nasogastric tube (96.07)
> irrigation of gastrostomy (96.36)
> irrigation of nasogastric tube (96.34)
> removal of:
>   gastrostomy tube (97.51)
>   intraluminal foreign body from stomach without incision (98.03)
> replacement of:
>   gastrostomy tube (97.02)
>   (naso-)gastric tube (97.01)

45. Incision, excision, and anastomosis of intestine

45.0 Enterotomy

> *Excludes:* duodenocholedochotomy (51.41–51.42, 51.51)
> that for destruction of lesion (45.30–45.34)
> that of exteriorized intestine (46.14, 46.24, 46.31)

45.00 Incision of intestine, not otherwise specified

45.01 Incision of duodenum

45.02 Other incision of small intestine

45.03 Incision of large intestine

> *Excludes:* proctotomy (48.0)

45.1 Diagnostic procedures on small intestine

Code also any laparotomy (54.11–54.19)

45.11 Transabdominal endoscopy of small intestine
Intraoperative endoscopy of small intestine

> *Excludes:* that with biopsy (45.14)

45.12 Endoscopy of small intestine through artificial stoma NOR

> *Excludes:* that with biopsy (45.14)

45.13 Other endoscopy of small intestine NOR
Esophagogastroduodenoscopy [EGD]

> *Excludes:* that with biopsy (45.14, 45.16)

45.14 Closed [endoscopic] biopsy of small intestine NOR
Brushing or washing for specimen collection

> *Excludes:* esophagogastroduodenoscopy [EGD] with closed biopsy (45.16)

45.15 Open biopsy of small intestine

45.16 Esophagogastroduodenoscopy [EGD] with closed biopsy NOR
Biopsy of one or more sites involving esophagus, stomach, and duodenum

45.19 Other diagnostic procedures on small intestine

> Excludes: microscopic examination of specimen from small intestine (90.91–90.99)
> radioisotope scan (92.04)
> ultrasonography (88.74)
> x-ray (87.61–87.69)

45.2 Diagnostic procedures on large intestine

Code also any laparotomy (54.11–54.19)

45.21 Transabdominal endoscopy of large intestine
Intraoperative endoscopy of large intestine

> Excludes: that with biopsy (45.25)

45.22 Endoscopy of large intestine through artificial stoma NOR

> Excludes: that with biopsy (45.25)

45.23 Colonoscopy NOR
Flexible fiberoptic colonoscopy

> Excludes: endoscopy of large intestine through artificial stoma (45.22)
> flexible sigmoidoscopy (45.24)
> rigid proctosigmoidoscopy (48.23)
> transabdominal endoscopy of large intestine (45.21)

45.24 Flexible sigmoidoscopy NOR
Endoscopy of descending colon

> Excludes: rigid proctosigmoidoscopy (48.23)

45.25 Closed [endoscopic] biopsy of large intestine NOR
Biopsy, closed, of unspecified intestinal site
Brushing or washing for specimen collection
Colonoscopy with biopsy

> Excludes: proctosigmoidoscopy with biopsy (48.24)

45.26 Open biopsy of large intestine

45.27 Intestinal biopsy, site unspecified

45.28 Other diagnostic procedures on large intestine

45.29 Other diagnostic procedures on intestine, site unspecified

> Excludes: microscopic examination of specimen (90.91–90.99)
> scan and radioisotope function study (92.04)
> ultrasonography (88.74)
> x-ray (87.61–87.69)

45.3 Local excision or destruction of lesion or tissue of small intestine

45.30 Endoscopic excision or destruction of lesion of duodenum NOR

> Excludes: biopsy of duodenum (45.14–45.15)
> control of hemorrhage (44.43)
> fistulectomy (46.72)

45.31 Other local excision of lesion of duodenum

> Excludes: biopsy of duodenum (45.14–45.15)
> fistulectomy (46.72)
> multiple segmental resection (45.61)
> that by endoscopic approach (45.30)

45.32 Other destruction of lesion of duodenum

> Excludes: that by endoscopic approach (45.30)

45.33 Local excision of lesion or tissue of small intestine, except duodenum
Excision of redundant mucosa of ileostomy

> Excludes: biopsy of small intestine (45.14–45.15)
> fistulectomy (46.74)
> multiple segmental resection (45.61)

45.34 Other destruction of lesion of small intestine, except duodenum

45.4 Local excision or destruction of lesion or tissue of large intestine

45.41 Excision of lesion or tissue of large intestine
Excision of redundant mucosa of colostomy

> Excludes: biopsy of large intestine (45.25–45.27)
> endoscopic polypectomy of large intestine (45.42)
> fistulectomy (46.76)
> multiple segmental resection (45.71)
> that by endoscopic approach (45.42–45.43)

45.42 Endoscopic polypectomy of large intestine NOR

> Excludes: that by open approach (45.41)

45.43 Endoscopic destruction of other lesion or tissue of large intestine NOR
Endoscopic ablation of tumor of large intestine
Endoscopic control of colonic bleeding

> Excludes: endoscopic polypectomy of large intestine (45.42)

45.49 Other destruction of lesion of large intestine

> Excludes: that by endoscopic approach (45.43)

45.5 Isolation of intestinal segment

Code also any synchronous:
anastomosis other than end-to-end (45.90–45.94)
enterostomy (46.10–46.39)

45.50 Isolation of intestinal segment, not otherwise specified
Isolation of intestinal pedicle flap
Reversal of intestinal segment

45.51 Isolation of segment of small intestine
Isolation of ileal loop
Resection of small intestine for interposition

45.52 Isolation of segment of large intestine
Resection of colon for interposition

45.6 Other excision of small intestine

Code also any synchronous:
anastomosis other than end-to-end (45.90–45.93, 45.95)
colostomy (46.10–46.13)
enterostomy (46.10–46.39)

> Excludes: cecectomy (45.72)
> enterocolectomy (45.79)
> gastroduodenectomy (43.6–43.99)
> ileocolectomy (45.73)
> pancreatoduodenectomy (52.51–52.7)

45.61 Multiple segmental resection of small intestine
Segmental resection for multiple traumatic lesions of small intestine

45.62 Other partial resection of small intestine
Duodenectomy
Ileectomy
Jejunectomy

> Excludes: duodenectomy with synchronous pancreatectomy (52.51–52.7)
> resection of cecum and terminal ileum (45.72)

45.63 Total removal of small intestine

OPERATIONS ON THE DIGESTIVE SYSTEM (42-54)

45.7 Partial excision of large intestine

> Code also any synchronous:
> anastomosis other than end-to-end (45.92–45.94)
> enterostomy (46.10–46.39)

45.71 Multiple segmental resection of large intestine
Segmental resection for multiple traumatic lesions of large intestine

45.72 Cecectomy
Resection of cecum and terminal ileum

45.73 Right hemicolectomy
Ileocolectomy   Right radical colectomy

45.74 Resection of transverse colon

45.75 Left hemicolectomy

> Excludes: proctosigmoidectomy (48.41–48.69)
> second stage Mikulicz operation (46.04)

45.76 Sigmoidectomy

45.79 Other partial excision of large intestine
Enterocolectomy NEC

45.8 Total intra-abdominal colectomy
Excision of cecum, colon, and sigmoid

> Excludes: coloproctectomy (48.41–48.69)

45.9 Intestinal anastomosis

> Code also any synchronous resection (45.31–45.8, 48.41–48.69)

> Excludes: end-to-end anastomosis — omit code

45.90 Intestinal anastomosis, not otherwise specified

45.91 Small-to-small intestinal anastomosis

45.92 Anastomosis of small intestine to rectal stump
Hampton procedure

45.93 Other small-to-large intestinal anastomosis

45.94 Large-to-large intestinal anastomosis

> Excludes: rectorectostomy (48.74)

45.95 Anastomosis to anus
Formation of endorectal ileal pouch (J-pouch) (H-pouch) (S-pouch) with anastomosis of small intestine to anus

46 Other operations on intestine

46.0 Exteriorization of intestine
Includes: loop enterostomy
multiple stage resection of intestine

46.01 Exteriorization of small intestine
Loop ileostomy

46.02 Resection of exteriorized segment of small intestine

46.03 Exteriorization of large intestine
Exteriorization of intestine NOS
First stage Mikulicz exteriorization of intestine
Loop colostomy

46.04 Resection of exteriorized segment of large intestine
Resection of exteriorized segment of intestine NOS
Second stage Mikulicz operation

46.1 Colostomy

> Code also any synchronous resection (45.49, 45.71–45.79, 45.8)

> Excludes: loop colostomy (46.03)
> that with synchronous anterior rectal resection (48.62)

46.10 Colostomy, not otherwise specified

46.11 Temporary colostomy

46.13 Permanent colostomy

46.14 Delayed opening of colostomy

46.2 Ileostomy

> Code also any synchronous resection (45.34, 45.61–45.63)

> Excludes: loop ileostomy (46.01)

46.20 Ileostomy, not otherwise specified

46.21 Temporary ileostomy

46.22 Continent ileostomy

46.23 Other permanent ileostomy

46.24 Delayed opening of ileostomy

46.3 Other enterostomy

> Code also any synchronous resection (45.61–45.8)

46.31 Delayed opening of other enterostomy

46.32 Percutaneous [endoscopic] jejunostomy [PEJ]
Endoscopic conversion of gastrostomy to jejunostomy

46.39 Other
Duodenostomy
Feeding enterostomy

46.4 Revision of intestinal stoma

46.40 Revision of intestinal stoma, not otherwise specified
Plastic enlargement of intestinal stoma
Reconstruction of stoma of intestine
Release of scar tissue of intestinal stoma

> Excludes: excision of redundant mucosa (45.41)

46.41 Revision of stoma of small intestine

> Excludes: excision of redundant mucosa (45.33)

46.42 Repair of pericolostomy hernia

46.43 Other revision of stoma of large intestine

> Excludes: excision of redundant mucosa (45.41)

46.5 Closure of intestinal stoma

> Code also any synchronous resection (45.34, 45.49, 45.61–45.8)

46.50 Closure of intestinal stoma, not otherwise specified

46.51 Closure of stoma of small intestine

46.52 Closure of stoma of large intestine
Closure or take-down of:
cecostomy
colostomy
sigmoidostomy

46.6 Fixation of intestine

46.60 Fixation of intestine, not otherwise specified
Fixation of intestine to abdominal wall

46.61 Fixation of small intestine to abdominal wall
  Ileopexy

46.62 Other fixation of small intestine
  Noble plication of small intestine
  Plication of jejunum

46.63 Fixation of large intestine to abdominal wall
  Cecocoloplicopexy   Sigmoidopexy (Moschowitz)

46.64 Other fixation of large intestine
  Cecofixation   Colofixation

46.7 Other repair of intestine

> *Excludes:* closure of:
>   ulcer of duodenum (44.42)
>   vesicoenteric fistula (57.83)

46.71 Suture of laceration of duodenum

46.72 Closure of fistula of duodenum

46.73 Suture of laceration of small intestine, except duodenum

46.74 Closure of fistula of small intestine, except duodenum

> *Excludes:* closure of:
>   artificial stoma (46.51)
>   vaginal fistula (70.74)
>   repair of gastrojejunocolic fistula (44.63)

46.75 Suture of laceration of large intestine

46.76 Closure of fistula of large intestine

> *Excludes:* closure of:
>   gastrocolic fistula (44.63)
>   rectal fistula (48.73)
>   sigmoidovesical fistula (57.83)
>   stoma (46.52)
>   vaginal fistula (70.72–70.73)
>   vesicocolic fistula (57.83)
>   vesicosigmoidovaginal fistula (57.83)

46.79 Other repair of intestine

46.8 Dilation and manipulation of intestine

46.80 Intra-abdominal manipulation of intestine, not otherwise specified
  Correction of intestinal malrotation
  Reduction of:
    intestinal torsion
    intestinal volvulus
    intussusception

46.81 Intra-abdominal manipulation of small intestine

46.82 Intra-abdominal manipulation of large intestine

46.85 Dilation of colon
  Dilation (balloon) of duodenum
  Dilation (balloon) of jejunum
  Endoscopic dilation (balloon) of large intestine
  That through rectum or colostomy

46.9 Other operations on intestines

46.91 Myotomy of sigmoid colon

46.92 Myotomy of other parts of colon

46.93 Revision of anastomosis of small intestine

46.94 Revision of anastomosis of large intestine

46.95 Local perfusion of small intestine

  Code also substance perfused (99.21–99.29)

46.96 Local perfusion of large intestine

  Code also substance perfused (99.21–99.29)

46.99 Other
  Ileoentectropy

> *Excludes:* diagnostic procedures on intestine (45.11–45.29)
>   dilation of enterostomy stoma (96.24)
>   intestinal intubation (96.08)
>   removal of:
>   intraluminal foreign body from large intestine without incision (98.04)
>   intraluminal foreign body from small intestine without incision (98.03)
>   tube from large intestine (97.53)
>   tube from small intestine (97.52)
>   replacement of:
>   large intestine tube or enterostomy device (97.04)
>   small intestine tube or enterostomy device (97.03)

47 Operations on appendix

Includes: appendiceal stump

47.0 Appendectomy

> *Excludes:* incidental appendectomy, so described (47.1)

47.1 Incidental appendectomy

47.2 Drainage of appendiceal abscess

> *Excludes:* that with appendectomy (47.0)

47.9 Other operations on appendix

47.91 Appendicostomy

47.92 Closure of appendiceal fistula

47.99 Other
  Anastomosis of appendix

> *Excludes:* diagnostic procedures on appendix (45.21–45.29)

48 Operations on rectum, rectosigmoid, and perirectal tissue

48.0 Proctotomy
  Decompression of imperforate anus
  Panas' operation [linear proctotomy]

> *Excludes:* incision of perirectal tissue (48.81)

48.1 Proctostomy

48.2 Diagnostic procedures on rectum, rectosigmoid, and perirectal tissue

48.21 Transabdominal proctosigmoidoscopy
  Intraoperative proctosigmoidoscopy

> *Excludes:* that with biopsy (48.24)

48.22 Proctosigmoidoscopy through artificial stoma `NOR`

> *Excludes:* that with biopsy (48.24)

48.23 Rigid proctosigmoidoscopy `NOR`

> *Excludes:* flexible sigmoidoscopy (45.24)

48.24 Closed [endoscopic] biopsy of rectum `NOR`
  Brushing or washing for specimen collection
  Proctosigmoidoscopy with biopsy

48.25 Open biopsy of rectum

48.26 Biopsy of perirectal tissue

48.29 Other diagnostic procedures on rectum, rectosigmoid, and perirectal tissue

> *Excludes:* digital examination of rectum (89.34)
>   lower GI series (87.64)
>   microscopic examination of specimen from rectum (90.91–90.99)

OPERATIONS ON THE DIGESTIVE SYSTEM (42-54)

48.3 Local excision or destruction of lesion or tissue of rectum

    48.31 Radical electrocoagulation of rectal lesion or tissue

    48.32 Other electrocoagulation of rectal lesion or tissue

    48.33 Destruction of rectal lesion or tissue by laser

    48.34 Destruction of rectal lesion or tissue by cryosurgery

    48.35 Local excision of rectal lesion or tissue

> Excludes: biopsy of rectum (48.24–48.25)
> excision of perirectal tissue (48.82)
> hemorrhoidectomy (49.46)
> rectal fistulectomy (48.73)

48.4 Pull-through resection of rectum

Code also any synchronous anastomosis other than end-to-end (45.90, 45.92–45.95)

    48.41 Soave submucosal resection of rectum
Endorectal pull-through operation

    48.49 Other pull-through resection of rectum
Abdominoperineal pull-through
Altemeier operation
Swenson proctectomy

> Excludes: Duhamel abdominoperineal pull-through (48.65)

48.5 Abdominoperineal resection of rectum
Combined abdominoendorectal resection
Complete proctectomy
Code also any synchronous anastomosis other than end-to-end (45.90, 45.92–45.95)

> Excludes: duhamel abdominoperineal pull-through (48.65)
> that as part of pelvic exenteration (68.8)

48.6 Other resection of rectum

Code also any synchronous anastomosis other than end-to-end (45.90, 45.92–45.95)

    48.61 Transsacral rectosigmoidectomy

    48.62 Anterior resection of rectum with synchronous colostomy

    48.63 Other anterior resection of rectum

> Excludes: that with synchronous colostomy (48.62)

    48.64 Posterior resection of rectum

    48.65 Duhamel resection of rectum
Duhamel abdominoperineal pull-through

    48.69 Other
Partial proctectomy
Rectal resection NOS

48.7 Repair of rectum

> Excludes: repair of:
> current obstetric laceration (75.62)
> vaginal rectocele (70.50, 70.52)

    48.71 Suture of laceration of rectum

    48.72 Closure of proctostomy

    48.73 Closure of other rectal fistula

> Excludes: fistulectomy:
> perirectal (48.93)
> rectourethral (58.43)
> rectovaginal (70.73)
> rectovesical (57.83)
> rectovesicovaginal (57.83)

    48.74 Rectorectostomy
Rectal anastomosis NOS

    48.75 Abdominal proctopexy
Frickman procedure
Ripstein repair of rectal prolapse

    48.76 Other proctopexy
Delorme repair of prolapsed rectum
Proctosigmoidopexy
Puborectalis sling operation

> Excludes: manual reduction of rectal prolapse (96.26)

    48.79 Other repair of rectum
Repair of old obstetric laceration of rectum

> Excludes: anastomosis to:
> large intestine (45.94)
> small intestine (45.92–45.93)
> repair of:
> current obstetrical laceration (75.62)
> vaginal rectocele (70.50, 70.52)

48.8 Incision or excision of perirectal tissue or lesion
Includes: pelvirectal tissue
rectovaginal septum

    48.81 Incision of perirectal tissue
Incision of rectovaginal septum

    48.82 Excision of perirectal tissue

> Excludes: perirectal biopsy (48.26)
> perirectofistulectomy (48.93)
> rectal fistulectomy (48.73)

48.9 Other operations on rectum and perirectal tissue

    48.91 Incision of rectal stricture

    48.92 Anorectal myectomy

    48.93 Repair of perirectal fistula

> Excludes: that opening into rectum (48.73)

    48.99 Other

> Excludes: digital examination of rectum (89.34)
> dilation of rectum (96.22)
> insertion of rectal tube (96.09)
> irrigation of rectum (96.38–96.39)
> manual reduction of rectal prolapse (96.26)
> proctoclysis (96.37)
> rectal massage (99.93)
> rectal packing (96.19)
> removal of:
> impacted feces (96.38)
> intraluminal foreign body from rectum without incision (98.05)
> rectal packing (97.59)
> transanal enema (96.39)

49 Operations on anus

49.0 Incision or excision of perianal tissue

    49.01 Incision of perianal abscess

    49.02 Other incision of perianal tissue
Undercutting of perianal tissue

> Excludes: anal fistulotomy (49.11)

    49.03 Excision of perianal skin tags

    49.04 Other excision of perianal tissue

> Excludes: anal fistulectomy (49.12)
> biopsy of perianal tissue (49.22)

49.1 Incision or excision of anal fistula

> Excludes: closure of anal fistula (49.73)

    49.11 Anal fistulotomy

    49.12 Anal fistulectomy

49.2 Diagnostic procedures on anus and perianal tissue

- **49.21 Anoscopy** NOR
- **49.22 Biopsy of perianal tissue**
- **49.23 Biopsy of anus**
- **49.29 Other diagnostic procedures on anus and perianal tissue**

    Excludes: microscopic examination of specimen from anus (90.91–90.99)

49.3 Local excision or destruction of other lesion or tissue of anus
Anal cryptotomy
Cauterization of lesion of anus

Excludes: biopsy of anus (49.23)
control of (postoperative) hemorrhage of anus (49.95)
hemorrhoidectomy (49.46)

- **49.31 Endoscopic excision or destruction of lesion or tissue of anus** NOR
- **49.39 Other local excision or destruction of lesion or tissue of anus**

    Excludes: that by endoscopic approach (49.31)

49.4 Procedures on hemorrhoids

- **49.41 Reduction of hemorrhoids**
- **49.42 Injection of hemorrhoids**
- **49.43 Cauterization of hemorrhoids**
  Clamp and cautery of hemorrhoids
- **49.44 Destruction of hemorrhoids by cryotherapy**
- **49.45 Ligation of hemorrhoids**
- **49.46 Excision of hemorrhoids**
  Hemorrhoidectomy NOS
- **49.47 Evacuation of thrombosed hemorrhoids**
- **49.49 Other procedures on hemorrhoids**
  Lord procedure

49.5 Division of anal sphincter

- **49.51 Left lateral anal sphincterotomy**
- **49.52 Posterior anal sphincterotomy**
- **49.59 Other anal sphincterotomy**
  Division of sphincter NOS

49.6 Excision of anus

49.7 Repair of anus

Excludes: repair of current obstetric laceration (75.62)

- **49.71 Suture of laceration of anus**
- **49.72 Anal cerclage**
- **49.73 Closure of anal fistula**

    Excludes: excision of anal fistula (49.12)

- **49.74 Gracilis muscle transplant for anal incontinence**
- **49.79 Other repair of anal sphincter**
  Repair of old obstetric laceration of anus

    Excludes: anoplasty with synchronous hemorrhoidectomy (49.46)
    repair of current obstetric laceration (75.62)

49.9 Other operations on anus

Excludes: dilation of anus (sphincter) (96.23)

- **49.91 Incision of anal septum**
- **49.92 Insertion of subcutaneous electrical anal stimulator**
- **49.93 Other incision of anus**
  Removal of:
    foreign body from anus with incision
    seton from anus

    Excludes: anal fistulotomy (49.11)
    removal of intraluminal foreign body without incision (98.05)

- **49.94 Reduction of anal prolapse**

    Excludes: manual reduction of rectal prolapse (96.26)

- **49.95 Control of (postoperative) hemorrhage of anus**
- **49.99 Other**

50 Operations on liver

50.0 Hepatotomy
Incision of abscess of liver
Removal of gallstones from liver
Stromeyer-Little operation

50.1 Diagnostic procedures on liver

- **50.11 Closed (percutaneous) [needle] biopsy of liver**
  Diagnostic aspiration of liver
- **50.12 Open biopsy of liver**
  Wedge biopsy
- **50.19 Other diagnostic procedures on liver**

    Excludes: liver scan and radioisotope function study (92.02)
    microscopic examination of specimen from liver (91.01–91.09)

50.2 Local excision or destruction of liver tissue or lesion

- **50.21 Marsupialization of lesion of liver**
- **50.22 Partial hepatectomy**
  Wedge resection of liver

    Excludes: biopsy of liver (50.11–50.12)
    hepatic lobectomy (50.3)

- **50.29 Other destruction of lesion of liver**
  Cauterization ⎫
  Enucleation ⎬ of hepatic lesion
  Evacuation   ⎭

    Excludes: percutaneous aspiration of lesion (50.91)

50.3 Lobectomy of liver
Total hepatic lobectomy with partial excision of other lobe

50.4 Total hepatectomy

50.5 Liver transplant

Auxiliary liver transplant
Auxiliary hepatic transplantation leaving patient's own liver in situ

Other transplant of liver

50.6 Repair of liver

- **50.61 Closure of laceration of liver**
- **50.69 Other repair of liver**
  Hepatopexy

50.9 Other operations on liver

Excludes: lysis of adhesions (54.5)

- **50.91 Percutaneous aspiration of liver**

    Excludes: percutaneous biopsy (50.11)

50.92 Extracorporeal hepatic assistance

50.93 Localized perfusion of liver

50.94 Other injection of therapeutic substance into liver

50.99 Other

51 Operations on gallbladder and biliary tract

Includes: operations on:
- ampulla of Vater
- common bile duct
- cystic duct
- hepatic duct
- intrahepatic bile duct
- sphincter of Oddi

51.0 Cholecystotomy and cholecystostomy

51.01 Percutaneous aspiration of gallbladder

> Excludes: needle biopsy (51.12)

51.02 Trocar cholecystostomy

51.03 Other cholecystostomy

51.04 Other cholecystotomy
Cholelithotomy NOS

51.1 Diagnostic procedures on biliary tract

> Excludes: that for endoscopic procedures classifiable to 51.64, 51.84–51.88, 52.14, 52.21, 52.93–52.94, 52.97–52.98

51.10 Endoscopic retrograde cholangiopancreatography [ERCP] NOR

> Excludes: endoscopic retrograde:
> cholangiography [ERC] (51.11)
> pancreatography [ERP] (52.13)

51.11 Endoscopic retrograde cholangiography [ERC] NOR

> Excludes: endoscopic retrograde:
> cholangiopancreatography [ERCP] (51.10)
> pancreatography [ERP] (52.13)

51.12 Percutaneous biopsy of gallbladder or bile ducts NOR
Needle biopsy of gallbladder

51.13 Open biopsy of gallbladder or bile ducts

51.14 Other closed [endoscopic] biopsy of biliary duct or sphincter of Oddi NOR
Brushing or washing for specimen collection
Closed biopsy of biliary duct or sphincter of Oddi by procedures classifiable to 51.10–51.11, 52.13

51.15 Pressure measurement of sphincter of Oddi
Pressure measurement of sphincter by procedures classifiable to 51.10–51.11, 52.13

51.19 Other diagnostic procedures on biliary tract

> Excludes: biliary tract x-ray (87.51–87.59)
> microscopic examination of specimen from biliary tract (91.01–91.09)

51.2 Cholecystectomy

51.22 Total cholecystectomy

> Excludes: laparoscopic cholecystectomy (51.23)

51.23 Laparoscopic cholecystectomy
That by laser

51.3 Anastomosis of gallbladder or bile duct

> Excludes: resection with end-to-end anastomosis (51.61–51.69)

51.31 Anastomosis of gallbladder to hepatic ducts

51.32 Anastomosis of gallbladder to intestine

51.33 Anastomosis of gallbladder to pancreas

51.34 Anastomosis of gallbladder to stomach

51.35 Other gallbladder anastomosis
Gallbladder anastomosis NOS

51.36 Choledochoenterostomy

51.37 Anastomosis of hepatic duct to gastrointestinal tract

51.39 Other bile duct anastomosis
Anastomosis of bile duct NOS
Anastomosis of unspecified bile duct to:
- intestine
- liver
- pancreas
- stomach

51.4 Incision of bile duct for relief of obstruction

51.41 Common duct exploration for removal of calculus

> Excludes: percutaneous extraction (51.96)

51.42 Common duct exploration for relief of other obstruction

51.43 Insertion of choledochohepatic tube for decompression
Hepatocholedochostomy

51.49 Incision of other bile ducts for relief of obstruction

51.5 Other incision of bile duct

> Excludes: that for relief of obstruction (51.41–51.49)

51.51 Exploration of common duct
Incision of common bile duct

51.59 Incision of other bile duct

51.6 Local excision or destruction of lesion or tissue of biliary ducts and sphincter of Oddi

Code also anastomosis other than end-to-end (51.31, 51.36–51.39)

> Excludes: biopsy of bile duct (51.12–51.13)

51.61 Excision of cystic duct remnant

51.62 Excision of ampulla of Vater (with reimplantation of common duct)

51.63 Other excision of common duct
Choledochectomy

> Excludes: fistulectomy (51.72)

51.64 Endoscopic excision or destruction of lesion of biliary ducts or sphincter of Oddi NOR
Excision or destruction of lesion of biliary duct by procedures classifiable to 51.10–51.11, 52.13

51.69 Excision of other bile duct
Excision of lesion of bile duct NOS

> Excludes: fistulectomy (51.79)

51.7 Repair of bile ducts

51.71 Simple suture of common bile duct

51.72 Choledochoplasty
Repair of fistula of common bile duct

51.79 Repair of other bile ducts
Closure of artificial opening of bile duct NOS
Suture of bile duct NOS

> Excludes: operative removal of prosthetic device (51.95)

51.8 Other operations on biliary ducts and sphincter of Oddi

51.81 Dilation of sphincter of Oddi
Dilation of ampulla of Vater

> Excludes: that by endoscopic approach (51.84)

51.82 Pancreatic sphincterotomy
Incision of pancreatic sphincter
Transduodenal ampullary sphincterotomy

> Excludes: that by endoscopic approach (51.85)

51.83 Pancreatic sphincteroplasty

51.84 Endoscopic dilation of ampulla and biliary duct NOR
Dilation of ampulla and biliary duct by procedures classifiable to 51.10–51.11, 52.13

51.85 Endoscopic sphincterotomy and papillotomy NOR
Sphincterotomy and papillotomy by procedures classifiable to 51.10–51.11, 52.13

51.86 Endoscopic insertion of nasobiliary drainage tube NOR
Insertion of nasobiliary tube by procedures classifiable to 51.10–51.11, 52.13

51.87 Endoscopic insertion of stent (tube) into bile duct NOR
Endoprosthesis of bile duct
Insertion of stent into bile duct by procedures classifiable to 51.10–51.11, 52.13

> Excludes: nasobiliary drainage tube (51.86)
> replacement of stent (tube) (97.05)

51.88 Endoscopic removal of stone(s) from biliary tract
Removal of biliary tract stone(s) by procedures classifiable to 51.10–51.11, 52.13

> Excludes: percutaneous extraction of common duct stones (51.96)

51.89 Other operations on sphincter of Oddi

51.9 Other operations on biliary tract

51.91 Repair of laceration of gallbladder

51.92 Closure of cholecystostomy

51.93 Closure of other biliary fistula
Cholecystogastroenteric fistulectomy

51.94 Revision of anastomosis of biliary tract

51.95 Removal of prosthetic device from bile duct

> Excludes: nonoperative removal (97.55)

51.96 Percutaneous extraction of common duct stones

51.98 Other percutaneous procedures on biliary tract
Percutaneous biliary endoscopy via existing T-tube or other tract for:
  dilation of biliary duct stricture
  removal of stone(s) except common duct stone
  exploration (postoperative)
percutaneous transhepatic biliary drainage

> Excludes: percutaneous aspiration of gallbladder (51.01)
> percutaneous biopsy and/or collection of specimen by brushing or washing (51.12)
> removal of common duct stone(s) (51.96)

51.99 Other
Insertion or replacement of biliary tract prosthesis

> Excludes: biopsy of gallbladder (51.12–51.13)
> irrigation of cholecystostomy and other biliary tube (96.41)
> lysis of peritoneal adhesions (54.5)
> nonoperative removal of:
>   cholecystostomy tube (97.54)
>   tube from biliary tract or liver (97.55)

52 Operations on pancreas
Includes: operations on pancreatic duct

52.0 Pancreatotomy

52.01 Drainage of pancreatic cyst by catheter

52.09 Other pancreatotomy
Pancreatolithotomy

> Excludes: drainage by anastomosis (52.4, 52.96)
> incision of pancreatic sphincter (51.82)
> marsupialization of cyst (52.3)

52.1 Diagnostic procedures on pancreas

52.11 Closed [aspiration] [needle] [percutaneous] biopsy of pancreas

52.12 Open biopsy of pancreas

52.13 Endoscopic retrograde pancreatography [ERP] NOR

> Excludes: endoscopic retrograde:
>   cholangiography [ERC] (51.11)
>   cholangiopancreatography [ERP] (51.10)
> that for procedures classifiable to 51.14–51.15, 51.64, 51.84–51.88, 52.14, 52.21, 52.92–52.94, 52.97–52.98

52.14 Closed [endoscopic] biopsy of pancreatic duct NOR
Closed biopsy of pancreatic duct by procedures classifiable to 51.10–51.11, 52.13

52.19 Other diagnostic procedures on pancreas

> Excludes: contrast pancreatogram (87.66)
> endoscopic retrograde pancreatography [ERP] (52.13)
> microscopic examination of specimen from pancreas (91.01–91.09)

52.2 Local excision or destruction of pancreas and pancreatic duct

> Excludes: biopsy of pancreas (52.11–52.12, 52.14)
> pancreatic fistulectomy (52.95)

52.21 Endoscopic excision or destruction of lesion or tissue of pancreatic duct NOR
Excision or destruction of lesion or tissue of pancreatic duct by procedures classifiable to 51.10–51.11, 52.13

52.22 Other excision or destruction of lesion or tissue of pancreas or pancreatic duct

52.3 Marsupialization of pancreatic cyst

> Excludes: drainage of cyst by catheter (52.01)

52.4 Internal drainage of pancreatic cyst
Pancreaticocystoduodenostomy
Pancreaticocystogastrostomy
Pancreaticocystojejunostomy

52.5 Partial pancreatectomy

> Excludes: pancreatic fistulectomy (52.95)

52.51 Proximal pancreatectomy
Excision of head of pancreas (with part of body)
Proximal pancreatectomy with synchronous duodenectomy

52.52 Distal pancreatectomy
Excision of tail of pancreas (with part of body)

52.53 Radical subtotal pancreatectomy

52.59 Other partial pancreatectomy

52.6 Total pancreatectomy
Pancreatectomy with synchronous duodenectomy

OPERATIONS ON THE DIGESTIVE SYSTEM (42-54)

52.7 Radical pancreaticoduodenectomy
One-stage pancreaticoduodenal resection with choledochojejunal anastomosis, pancreaticojejunal anastontosis, and gastrojejunostomy
Two-stage pancreaticoduodenal resection (first stage) (second stage)
Radical resection of the pancreas
Whipple procedure

Excludes: radical subtotal pancreatectomy (52.53)

52.8 Transplant of pancreas

52. Pancreatic transplant, not otherwise specified

52.81 Reimplantation of pancreatic tissue

52.82 Homotransplant of pancreas
Heterotransplant of pancreas

52.9 Other operations on pancreas

52.92 Cannulation of pancreatic duct

Excludes: that by endoscopic approach (52.93)

52.93 **Endoscopic insertion of stent (tube) into pancreatic duct** NOR
Insertion of cannula or stent into pancreatic duct by procedures classifiable to 51.10–51,11, 52.13

Excludes: endoscopic insertion of nasopancreatic drainage tube (52.97)
replacement of stent (tube) (97.05)

52.94 **Endoscopic removal of stone(s) from pancreatic duct**
Removal of stone(s) from pancreatic duct by procedures classifiable to 51.10–51.11, 52.13

52.95 Other repair of pancreas
Fistulectomy } of pancreas
Simple suture

52.96 Anastomosis of pancreas
Anastomosis of pancreas (duct) to:
  intestine
  jejunum
  stomach

Excludes: anastomosis to:
  bile duct (51.39)
  gallbladder (51.33)

52.97 **Endoscopic insertion of nasopancreatic drainage tube** NOR
Insertion of nasopancreatic drainage tube by procedures classifiable to 51.10–51.11, 52.13

Excludes: drainage of pancreatic cyst by catheter (52.01)
replacement of stent (tube) (97.05)

52.98 **Endoscopic dilation of pancreatic duct** NOR
Dilation of Wirsung's duct by procedures classifiable to 51.10–51.11, 52.13

52.99 Other
Dilation of pancreatic [Wirsung's] duct } by open
Repair of pancreatic [Wirsung's] duct   approach

Excludes: irrigation of pancreatic tube (96.42)
removal of pancreatic tube (97.56)

53 Repair of hernia

Includes: hernioplasty
herniorrhaphy
herniotomy

Excludes: manual reduction of hernia (96.27)

53.0 Unilateral repair of inguinal hernia

53.00 Unilateral repair of inguinal hernia, not otherwise specified
Inguinal herniorrhaphy NOS

53.01 Repair of direct inguinal hernia

53.02 Repair of indirect inguinal hernia

53.03 Repair of direct inguinal hernia with graft or prosthesis

53.04 Repair of indirect inguinal hernia with graft or prosthesis

53.05 Repair of inguinal hernia with graft or prosthesis, not otherwise specified

53.1 Bilateral repair of inguinal hernia

53.10 Bilateral repair of inguinal hernia, not otherwise specified

53.11 Bilateral repair of direct inguinal hernia

53.12 Bilateral repair of indirect inguinal hernia

53.13 Bilateral repair of inguinal hernia, one direct and one indirect

53.14 Bilateral repair of direct inguinal hernia with graft or prosthesis

53.15 Bilateral repair of indirect inguinal hernia with graft or prosthesis

53.16 Bilateral repair of inguinal hernia, one direct and one indirect, with graft or prosthesis

53.17 Bilateral inguinal hernia repair with graft or prosthesis, not otherwise specified

53.2 Unilateral repair of femoral hernia

53.21 Unilateral repair of femoral hernia with graft or prosthesis

53.29 Other unilateral femoral herniorrhaphy

53.3 Bilateral repair of femoral hernia

53.31 Bilateral repair of femoral hernia with graft or prosthesis

53.39 Other bilateral femoral herniorrhaphy

53.4 Repair of umbilical hernia

Excludes: repair of gastroschisis (54.71)

53.41 Repair of umbilical hernia with prosthesis

53.49 Other umbilical herniorrhaphy

53.5 Repair of other hernia of anterior abdominal wall (without graft or prosthesis)

53.51 Incisional hernia repair

53.59 Repair of other hernia of anterior abdominal wall
Repair of hernia:
  epigastric
  hypogastric
  spigelian
  ventral

53.6 Repair of other hernia of anterior abdominal wall with graft or prosthesis

53.61 Incisional hernia repair with prosthesis

53.69 Repair of other hernia of anterior abdominal wall with prosthesis

53.7 Repair of diaphragmatic hernia, abdominal approach

53.8 Repair of diaphragmatic hernia, thoracic approach

53.80 Repair of diaphragmatic hernia with thoracic approach, not otherwise specified
Thoracoabdominal repair of diaphragmatic hernia

53.81 Plication of the diaphragm

53.82 Repair of parasternal hernia

53.9 Other hernia repair
Repair of hernia:
ischiatic
ischiorectal
lumbar
obturator
omental
retroperitoneal
sciatic

> Excludes: relief of strangulated hernia with exteriorization of intestine (46.01, 46.03)
> repair of pericolostomy hernia (46.42)
> repair of vaginal enterocele (70.8)

54 Other operations on abdominal region
Includes: operations on:
epigastric region
flank
groin region
hypochondrium
inguinal region
loin region
male pelvic cavity
mesentery
omentum
peritoneum
retroperitoneal tissue space

> Excludes: female pelvic cavity (69.01–70.92)
> hernia repair (53.00–53.9)
> obliteration of cul-de-sac (70.8)
> retroperitoneal tissue dissection (59.00–59.09)
> skin and subcutaneous tissue of abdominal wall (86.01–86.99)

54.0 Incision of abdominal wall
Drainage of:
abdominal wall
extraperitoneal abscess
retroperitoneal abscess

> Excludes: incision of peritoneum (54.95)
> laparotomy (54.11–54.19)

54.1 Laparotomy

54.11 Exploratory laparotomy

> Excludes: exploration incidental to intra-abdominal surgery — omit code

54.12 Reopening of recent laparotomy site
Reopening of recent laparotomy site for:
control of hemorrhage
exploration
incision of hematoma

54.19 Other laparotomy
Drainage of intraperitoneal abscess or hematoma

> Excludes: culdocentesis (70.0)
> drainage of appendiceal abscess (47.2)
> exploration incidental to intra-abdominal surgery — omit code
> Ladd operation (54.95)
> removal of foreign body (54.92)

54.2 Diagnostic procedures of abdominal region

54.21 Laparoscopy
Peritoneoscopy

> Excludes: laparoscopic cholecystectomy (51.23)
> that incidental to destruction of fallopian tubes (66.21–66.29)

54.22 Biopsy of abdominal wall or umbilicus

54.23 Biopsy of peritoneum
Biopsy of:
mesentery
omentum
peritoneal implant

54.24 Closed [percutaneous] [needle] biopsy of intra-abdominal mass

> Excludes: that of:
> fallopian tube (66.11)
> ovary (65.11) Peritoneum (54.23)
> uterine ligaments (68.15)
> uterus (68.16)

54.25 Peritoneal lavage
Diagnostic peritoneal lavage

> Excludes: peritoneal dialysis (54.98)

54.29 Other diagnostic procedures on abdominal region

> Excludes: abdominal lymphangiogram (88.04)
> abdominal x-ray NEC (88.19)
> angiocardiography of venae cavae (88.51)
> C.A.T. scan of abdomen (88.01)
> contrast x-ray of abdominal cavity (88.11–88.15)
> intra-abdominal arteriography NEC (88.47)
> microscopic examination of peritoneal and retroperitoneal specimen (91.11–91.19)
> phlebography of:
> intra-abdominal vessels NEC (88.65)
> portal venous system (88.64)
> sinogram of abdominal wall (88.03)
> soft tissue x-ray of abdominal wall NEC (88.09)
> tomography of abdomen NEC (88.02)
> ultrasonography of abdomen and retroperitoneum (88.76)

54.3 Excision or destruction of lesion or tissue of abdominal wall or umbilicus
Debridement of abdominal wall
Omphalectomy

> Excludes: biopsy of abdominal wall or umbilicus (54.22)
> size reduction operation (86.83)
> that of skin of abdominal wall (86.22, 86.26, 86.3)

54.4 Excision or destruction of peritoneal tissue
Excision of:
appendices epiploicae
falciform ligament
gastrocolic ligament
lesion of:
mesentery
omentum
peritoneum
presacral lesion NOS
retroperitoneal lesion NOS

> Excludes: biopsy of peritoneum (54.23)
> endometrectomy of cul-de-sac (70.32)

54.5 Lysis of peritoneal adhesions
Freeing of adhesions of:
biliary tract
intestines
liver
pelvic peritoneum
peritoneum
spleen
uterus

> Excludes: lysis of adhesions of:
> bladder (59.11)
> fallopian tube and ovary (65.8)
> kidney (59.02)
> ureter (59.01–59.02)

54.6 Suture of abdominal wall and peritoneum

54.61 Reclosure of postoperative disruption of abdominal wall

54.62 Delayed closure of granulating abdominal wound
Tertiary subcutaneous wound closure

54.63 Other suture of abdominal wall
Suture of laceration of abdominal wall

> Excludes: closure of operative wound — omit code

54.64 Suture of peritoneum
Secondary suture of peritoneum

> Excludes: closure of operative wound — omit code

54.7 Other repair of abdominal wall and peritoneum

54.71 Repair of gastroschisis

54.72 Other repair of abdominal wall

54.73 Other repair of peritoneum
Suture of gastrocolic ligament

54.74 Other repair of omentum
Epiplorrhaphy
Graft of omentum
Omentopexy
Reduction of torsion of omentum

> Excludes: cardio-omentopexy (36.3)

54.75 Other repair of mesentery
Mesenteric plication
Mesenteropexy

54.9 Other operations of abdominal region

> Excludes: removal of ectopic pregnancy (74.3)

54.91 Percutaneous abdominal drainage
Paracentesis

> Excludes: creation of cutaneoperitoneal fistula (54.93)

54.92 Removal of foreign body from peritoneal cavity

54.93 Creation of cutaneoperitoneal fistula

54.94 Creation of peritoneovascular shunt
Peritoneovenous shunt

54.95 Incision of peritoneum
Ladd operation

> Excludes: that incidental to laparotomy (54.11–54.19)

54.96 Injection of air into peritoneal cavity
Pneumoperitoneum

> Excludes: that for:
> collapse of lung (33.33)
> radiography (88.12–88.13, 88.15)

54.97 Injection of locally-acting therapeutic substance into peritoneal cavity

> Excludes: peritoneal dialysis (54.98)

54.98 Peritoneal dialysis

> Excludes: peritoneal lavage (diagnostic) (54.25)

54.99 Other

> Excludes: removal of:
> abdominal wall sutures (97.83)
> peritoneal drainage device (97.82)
> retroperitoneal drainage device (97.81)

10. OPERATIONS ON THE URINARY SYSTEM (55–59)

55 Operations on kidney

Includes: operations on renal pelvis

Excludes: perirenal tissue (59.00–59.09, 59.21–59.29, 59.91–59.92)

55.0 Nephrotomy and nephrostomy

Excludes: drainage by:
anastomosis (55.86)
aspiration (55.92)
incision of kidney pelvis (55.11–55.12)

55.01 Nephrotomy
Evacuation of renal cyst
Exploration of kidney
Nephrolithotomy

55.02 Nephrostomy

55.03 Percutaneous nephrotomy without fragmentation
Nephrostolithotomy, percutaneous (nephroscopic)
Percutaneous removal of kidney stone(s) by:
  forceps extraction (nephroscopic)
  basket extraction
Pyelostolithotomy, percutaneous (nephroscopic)
With placement of catheter down ureter

Excludes: percutaneous removal by fragmentation (55.04)
repeat nephroscopic removal during current episode (55.92)

55.04 Percutaneous nephrostomy with fragmentation
Percutaneous nephrostomy with disruption of kidney stone by ultrasonic energy and extraction (suction) through endoscope
With placement of catheter down ureter
With fluoroscopic guidance

Excludes: repeat fragmentation during current episode (59.95)

55.1 Pyelotomy and pyelostomy

Excludes: drainage by anastomosis (55.86)
percutaneous pyelostolithotomy (55.03)
removal of calculus without incision (56.0)

55.11 Pyelotomy
Exploration of renal pelvis
Pyelolithotomy

55.12 Pyelostomy
Insertion of drainage tube into renal pelvis

55.2 Diagnostic procedures on kidney

55.21 Nephroscopy NOR
55.22 Pyeloscopy NOR
55.23 Closed [percutaneous] [needle] biopsy of kidney
Endoscopic biopsy via existing nephrostomy, nephrotomy, pyelostomy, or pyelotomy

55.24 Open biopsy of kidney

55.29 Other diagnostic procedures on kidney

Excludes: microscopic examination of specimen from kidney (91.21–91.29)
pyelogram:
  intravenous (87.73)
  percutaneous (87.75)
  retrograde (87.74)
radioisotope scan (92.03)
renal arteriography (88.45)
tomography:
  C.A.T. scan (87.71)
  other (87.72)

55.3 Local excision or destruction of lesion or tissue of kidney

55.31 Marsupialization of kidney lesion

55.39 Other local destruction or excision of renal lesion or tissue
Obliteration of calyceal diverticulum

Excludes: biopsy of kidney (55.23–55.24)
partial nephrectomy (55.4)
percutaneous aspiration of kidney (55.92)
wedge resection of kidney (55.4)

55.4 Partial nephrectomy
Calycectomy
Wedge resection of kidney

Code also any synchronous resection of ureter (56.40–56.42)

55.5 Complete nephrectomy

Code also any synchronous excision of:
bladder segment (57.6)
lymph nodes (40.3, 40.52–40.59)

55.51 Nephroureterectomy
Nephroureterectomy with bladder cuff
Total nephrectomy (unilateral)

Excludes: removal of transplanted kidney (55.53)

55.52 Nephrectomy of remaining kidney
Removal of solitary kidney

Excludes: removal of transplanted kidney (55.53)

55.53 Removal of transplanted or rejected kidney

55.54 Bilateral nephrectomy

Excludes: complete nephrectomy NOS (55.51)

55.6 Transplant of kidney

55.61 Renal autotransplantation

55.69 Other kidney transplantation

55.7 Nephropexy
Fixation or suspension of movable [floating] kidney

55.8 Other repair of kidney

55.81 Suture of laceration of kidney

55.82 Closure of nephrostomy and pyelostomy

55.83 Closure of other fistula of kidney

55.84 Reduction of torsion of renal pedicle

55.85 Symphysiotomy for horseshoe kidney

55.86 Anastomosis of kidney
Nephropyeloureterostomy
Pyeloureterovesical anastomosis
Ureterocalyceal anastomosis

Excludes: nephrocystanastomosis NOS (56.73)

55.87 Correction of ureteropelvic junction

55.89 Other

55.9 Other operations on kidney

Excludes: lysis of perirenal adhesions (59.02)

55.91 Decapsulation of kidney
Capsulectomy } of kidney
Decortication

55.92 Percutaneous aspiration of kidney (pelvis)
Aspiration of renal cyst
Renipuncture

> Excludes: percutaneous biopsy of kidney (55.23)

55.93 Replacement of nephrostomy tube

55.94 Replacement of pyelostomy tube

55.95 Local perfusion of kidney

55.96 Other injection of therapeutic substance into kidney
Injection into renal cyst

55.97 Implantation or replacement of mechanical kidney

55.98 Removal of mechanical kidney

55.99 Other

> Excludes: removal of pyelostomy or nephrostomy tube (97.61)

56 Operations on ureter

56.0 Transurethral removal of obstruction from ureter and renal pelvis
Removal of:
  blood clot
  calculus   } from ureter or renal pelvis without incision
  foreign body

> Excludes: that by incision (55.11, 56.2)
> transurethral insertion of ureteral stent for passage of calculus (59.8)

56.1 Ureteral meatotomy

56.2 Ureterotomy
Incision of ureter for:
  drainage
  exploration
  removal of calculus

> Excludes: cutting of ureterovesical orifice (56.1)
> removal of calculus without incision (56.0)
> transurethral insertion of ureteral stent for passage of calculus (59.8)
> urinary diversion (56.51–56.79)

56.3 Diagnostic procedures on ureter

56.31 Ureteroscopy NOR

56.32 Closed percutaneous biopsy of ureter

> Excludes: endoscopic biopsy of ureter (56.33)

56.33 Closed endoscopic biopsy of ureter
Cystourethroscopy with ureteral biopsy
Transurethral biopsy of ureter
Ureteral endoscopy with biopsy through ureterotomy
Ureteroscopy with biopsy

> Excludes: percutaneous biopsy of ureter (56.32)

56.34 Open biopsy of ureter

56.35 Endoscopy (cystoscopy) (looposcopy) of ileal conduit

56.39 Other diagnostic procedures on ureter

> Excludes: microscopic examination of specimen from ureter (91.21–91.29)

56.4 Ureterectomy

Code also anastomosis other than end-to-end (56.51–56.79)

> Excludes: fistulectomy (56.84)
> nephroureterectomy (55.31–55.54)

56.40 Ureterectomy, not otherwise specified

56.41 Partial ureterectomy
Excision of lesion of ureter
Shortening of ureter with reimplantation

> Excludes: biopsy of ureter (56.32–56.34)

56.42 Total ureterectomy

56.5 Cutaneous uretero-ileostomy

56.51 Formation of cutaneous uretero-ileostomy
Construction of ileal conduit
External ureteral ileostomy
Formation of open ileal bladder
Ileal loop operation
Ileoureterostomy (Bricker's) (ileal bladder)
Transplantation of ureter into ileum with external diversion

> Excludes: closed ileal bladder (57.87)
> replacement of ureteral defect by ileal segment (56.89)

56.52 Revision of cutaneous uretero-ileostomy

56.6 Other external urinary diversion

56.61 Formation of other cutaneous ureterostomy
Anastomosis of ureter to skin
Ureterostomy NOS

56.62 Revision of other cutaneous ureterostomy
Revision of ureterostomy stoma

> Excludes: nonoperative removal of ureterostomy tube (97.62)

56.7 Other anastomosis or bypass of ureter

> Excludes: ureteropyelostomy (55.86)

56.71 Urinary diversion to intestine
Anastomosis of ureter to intestine
Internal urinary diversion NOS

Code also any synchronous colostomy (46.10–46.13)

> Excludes: external ureteral ileostomy (56.51)

56.72 Revision of ureterointestinal anastomosis

> Excludes: revision of external ureteral ileostomy (56.52)

56.73 Nephrocystanastomosis, not otherwise specified

56.74 Ureteroneocystostomy
Replacement of ureter with bladder flap
Ureterovesical anastomosis

56.75 Transureteroureterostomy

> Excludes: ureteroureterostomy associated with partial resection (56.41)

56.79 Other

56.8 Repair of ureter

56.81 Lysis of intraluminal adhesions of ureter

> Excludes: lysis of periureteral adhesions (59.01–59.02)
> ureterolysis (59.01–59.02)

56.82 Suture of laceration of ureter

56.83 Closure of ureterostomy

56.84 Closure of other fistula of ureter

56.85 Ureteropexy

56.86 Removal of ligature from ureter

OPERATIONS ON THE URINARY SYSTEM (55-59)

56.89 Other repair of ureter
Graft of ureter
Replacement of ureter with ileal segment implanted into bladder
Ureteroplication

56.9 Other operations on ureter

56.91 Dilation of ureteral meatus

56.92 Implantation of electronic ureteral stimulator

56.93 Replacement of electronic ureteral stimulator

56.94 Removal of electronic ureteral stimulator

> Excludes: that with synchronous replacement (56.93)

56.95 Ligation of ureter

56.99 Other

> Excludes: removal of ureterostomy tube and ureteral catheter (97.62)
> ureteral catheterization (59.8)

57 Operations on urinary bladder

> Excludes: perivesical tissue (59.11–59.29, 59.91–59.92)
> ureterovesical orifice (56.0–56.99)

57.0 Transurethral clearance of bladder
Drainage of bladder without incision
Removal of:
  blood clots
  calculus   } from bladder without incision
  foreign body

> Excludes: that by incision (57.19)

57.1 Cystotomy and cystostomy

> Excludes: cystotomy and cystostomy as operative approach — omit code

57.11 Percutaneous aspiration of bladder

57.12 Lysis of intraluminal adhesions with incision into bladder

> Excludes: transurethral lysis of intraluminal adhesions (57.41)

57.17 Percutaneous cystostomy
Closed cystostomy
Percutaneous suprapubic cystostomy

> Excludes: removal of cystostomy tube (97.61)
> replacement of cystostomy tube (59.94)

57.18 Other suprapubic cystostomy

> Excludes: percutaneous cystostomy (57.17)
> removal of cystostomy tube (97.63)
> replacement of cystostomy tube (59.94)

57.19 Other cystotomy
Cystolithotomy

> Excludes: percutaneous cystostomy (57.17)
> suprapubic cystostomy (57.18)

57.2 Vesicostomy

> Excludes: percutaneous cystostomy (57.17)
> suprapubic cystostomy (57.18)

57.21 Vesicostomy
Creation of permanent opening from bladder to skin using a bladder flap

57.22 Revision or closure of vesicostomy

> Excludes: closure of cystostomy (57.82)

57.3 Diagnostic procedures on bladder

57.31 Cystoscopy through artificial stoma NOR

57.32 Other cystoscopy NOR
Transurethral cystoscopy

> Excludes: cystourethroscopy with ureteral biopsy (56.33)
> retrograde pyelogram (87.74)
> that for control of hemorrhage (postoperative):
>   bladder (57.93)
>   prostate (60.94)

57.33 Closed [transurethral] biopsy of bladder

57.34 Open biopsy of bladder

57.39 Other diagnostic procedures on bladder

> Excludes: cystogram NEC (87.77)
> microscopic examination of specimen from bladder (91.31–91.39)
> retrograde cystourethrogram (87.76)

57.4 Transurethral excision or destruction of bladder tissue

57.41 Transurethral lysis of intraluminal adhesions

57.49 Other transurethral excision or destruction of lesion or tissue of bladder
Endoscopic resection of bladder lesion

> Excludes: transurethral biopsy of bladder (57.33)
> transurethral fistulectomy (57.83–57.84)

57.5 Other excision or destruction of bladder tissue

> Excludes: that with transurethral approach (57.41–57.49)

57.51 Excision of urachus
Excision of urachal sinus of bladder

> Excludes: excision of urachal cyst of abdominal wall (54.3)

57.59 Open excision or destruction of other lesion or tissue of bladder
Endometrectomy of bladder
Suprapubic excision of bladder lesion

> Excludes: biopsy of bladder (57.33–57.34)
> fistulectomy of bladder (57.83–57.84)

57.6 Partial cystectomy
Excision of bladder dome
Trigonectomy
Wedge resection of bladder

57.7 Total cystectomy
Includes: total cystectomy with urethrectomy

57.71 Radical cystectomy
Pelvic exenteration in male
Removal of bladder, prostate, seminal vesicles and fat
Removal of bladder, urethra, and fat in a female

Code also any:
  lymph node dissection (40.3, 40.5)
  urinary diversion (56.51–56.79)

> Excludes: that as part of pelvic exenteration in female (68.8)

57.79 Other total cystectomy

57.8 Other repair of urinary bladder

> Excludes: repair of:
>   current obstetric laceration (75.61)
>   cystocele (70.50–70.51)
>   that for stress incontinence (59.3–59.79)

57.81 Suture of laceration of bladder

57.82 Closure of cystostomy

57.83 Repair of fistula involving bladder and intestine
Rectovesicovaginal ⎫
Vesicosigmoidovaginal ⎬ fistulectomy

57.84 Repair of other fistula of bladder
Cervicovesical ⎫
Urethroperineovesical ⎬ fistulectomy
Vaginovesical ⎭

Excludes: *vesicoureterovaginal fistulectomy (56.84)*

57.85 Cystourethroplasty and plastic repair of bladder neck
Plication of sphincter of urinary bladder
V-Y plasty of bladder neck

57.86 Repair of bladder exstrophy

57.87 Reconstruction of urinary bladder
Anastomosis of bladder with isolated segment of ileum
Augmentation of bladder
Replacement of bladder with ileum or sigmoid [closed ileal bladder]

Code also resection of intestine (45.50–45.52)

57.88 Other anastomosis of bladder
Anastomosis of bladder to intestine NOS
Cystocolic anastomosis

Excludes: *formation of closed ileal bladder (57.87)*

57.89 Other repair of bladder
Bladder suspension, not elsewhere classified
Cystopexy NOS
Repair of old obstetric laceration of bladder

Excludes: *repair of current obstetric laceration (75.61)*

57.9 Other operations on bladder

57.91 Sphincterotomy of bladder
Division of bladder neck

57.92 Dilation of bladder neck

57.93 Control of (postoperative) hemorrhage of bladder

57.94 Insertion of indwelling urinary catheter

57.95 Replacement of indwelling urinary catheter

Implantation of electronic bladder stimulator

Replacement of electronic bladder stimulator

57.98 Removal of electronic bladder stimulator

Excludes: *that with synchronous replacement (57.97)*

57.99 Other

Excludes: *irrigation of:*
cystostomy (96.47)
other indwelling urinary catheter (96.48)
lysis of external adhesions (59.11)
removal of:
cystostomy tube (97.63)
other urinary drainage device (97.64)
therapeutic distention of bladder (96.25)

58 Operations on urethra
Includes: operations on:
bulbourethral gland [Cowper's gland]
periurethral tissue

58.0 Urethrotomy
Excision of urethral septum
Formation of urethrovaginal fistula
Perineal urethrostomy
Removal of calculus from urethra by incision

Excludes: *drainage of bulbourethral gland or periurethral tissue (58.91)*
internal urethral meatotomy (58.5)
removal of urethral calculus without incision (58.6)

58.1 Urethral meatotomy

Excludes: *internal urethral meatotomy (58.5)*

58.2 Diagnostic procedures on urethra

58.21 Perineal urethroscopy

58.22 Other urethroscopy NOR

58.23 Biopsy of urethra

58.24 Biopsy of periurethral tissue

58.29 Other diagnostic procedures on urethra and periurethral tissue

Excludes: *microscopic examination of specimen from urethra (91.31–91.39)*
retrograde cystourethrogram (87.76)
urethral pressure profile (89.25)
urethral sphincter electromyogram (89.23)

58.3 Excision or destruction of lesion or tissue of urethra

Excludes: *biopsy of urethra (58.23)*
excision of bulbourethral gland (58.92)
fistulectomy (58.43)
urethrectomy as part of:
complete cystectomy (57.79)
pelvic exenteration (68.8)
radical cystectomy (57.71)

58.31 Endoscopic excision or destruction of lesion or tissue of urethra
Fulguration of urethral lesion

58.39 Other local excision or destruction of lesion or tissue of urethra
Excision of:
congenital valve ⎫
lesion ⎬ of urethra
stricture ⎭
Urethrectomy

Excludes: *that by endoscopic approach (58.31)*

58.4 Repair of urethra

Excludes: *repair of current obstetric laceration (75.61)*

58.41 Suture of laceration of urethra

58.42 Closure of urethrostomy

58.43 Closure of other fistula of urethra

Excludes: *repair of urethroperineovesical fistula (57.84)*

58.44 Reanastomosis of urethra
Anastomosis of urethra

58.45 Repair of hypospadias or epispadias

58.46 Other reconstruction of urethra
Urethral construction

58.47 Urethral meatoplasty

OPERATIONS ON THE URINARY SYSTEM (55-59)

58.49 Other repair of urethra
Benenenti rotation of bulbous urethra
Repair of old obstetric laceration of urethra
Urethral plication

> Excludes: repair of:
> current obstetric laceration (75.61)
> urethrocele (70.50–70.51)

58.5 Release of urethral stricture
Cutting of urethral sphincter
Internal urethral meatotomy
Urethrolysis

58.6 Dilation of urethra
Dilation of urethrovesical junction
Passage of sounds through urethra
Removal of calculus from urethra without incision

> Excludes: urethral calibration (89.29)

58.9 Other operations on urethra and periurethral tissue

58.91 Incision of periurethral tissue
Drainage of bulbourethral gland

58.92 Excision of periurethral tissue

> Excludes: biopsy of periurethral tissue (58.24)

58.93 Implantation of artificial urinary sphincter [AUS]
Placement of inflatable:
urethral sphincter
bladder sphincter
With pump and/or reservoir
Removal with replacement of sphincter device [AUS]

58.99 Other
Repair of inflatable sphincter pump and/or reservoir
Surgical correction of hydraulic pressure of inflatable sphincter device
Removal of inflatable urinary sphincter without replacement

> Excludes: removal of:
> intraluminal foreign body from urethra without incision (98.19)
> urethral stent (97.65)

59 Other operations on urinary tract

59.0 Dissection of retroperitoneal tissue

59.00 Retroperitoneal dissection, not otherwise specified

59.01 Ureterolysis with freeing or repositioning of ureter for retroperitoneal fibrosis

59.02 Other lysis of perirenal or periureteral adhesions

59.09 Other incision of perirenal or periureteral tissue
Exploration of perinephric area
Incision of perirenal abscess

59.1 Incision of perivesical tissue

59.11 Lysis of perivesical adhesions

59.19 Other incision of perivesical tissue
Exploration of perivesical tissue
Incision of hematoma of space of Retzius
Retropubic exploration

59.2 Diagnostic procedures on perirenal and perivesical tissue

59.21 Biopsy of perirenal or perivesical tissue

59.29 Other diagnostic procedures on perirenal tissue, perivesical tissue, and retroperitoneum

> Excludes: microscopic examination of specimen from:
> perirenal tissue (91.21–91.29)
> perivesical tissue (91.31–91.39)
> retroperitoneum NEC (91.11–91.19)
> retroperitoneal x-ray (88.14–88.16)

59.3 Plication of urethrovesical junction
Kelly-Kennedy operation on urethra
Kelly-Stoeckel urethral plication

59.4 Suprapubic sling operation
Goebel-Frangenheim-Stoeckel urethrovesical suspension
Millin-Read urethrovesical suspension
Oxford operation for urinary incontinence
Urethrocystopexy by suprapubic suspension

59.5 Retropubic urethral suspension
Marshall-Marthetti-Krantz operation
Suture of periurethral tissue to symphysis pubis
Urethral suspension NOS

59.6 Paraurethral suspension
Pereyra paraurethral suspension
Periurethral suspension

59.7 Other repair of urinary stress incontinence

59.71 Levator muscle operation for urethrovesical suspension
Cystourethropexy with levator muscle sling
Gracilis muscle transplant for urethrovesical suspension
Pubococcygeal sling

59.79 Other
Anterior urethropexy
Polytef augmentation urethroplasty
Repair of stress incontinence NOS
Tudor "rabbit ear" urethropexy

59.8 Ureteral catheterization
Drainage of kidney by catheter
Insertion of ureteral stent
Ureterovesical orifice dilation

Code also any ureterotomy (56.2)

> Excludes: that for:
> transurethral removal of calculus or clot from ureter and renal pelvis (56.0)
> retrograde pyelogram (87.74)

59.9 Other operations on urinary system

> Excludes: nonoperative removal of therapeutic device (97.61–97.69)

59.91 Excision of perirenal or perivesical tissue

> Excludes: biopsy of perirenal or perivesical tissue (59.21)

59.92 Other operations on perirenal or perivesical tissue

59.93 Replacement of ureterostomy tube
Change of ureterostomy tube
Reinsertion of ureterostomy tube

> Excludes: nonoperative removal of ureterostomy tube (97.62)

59.94 Replacement of cystostomy tube

> Excludes: nonoperative removal of cystostomy tube (97.63)

59.95 Ultrasonic fragmentation of urinary stones
Shattered urinary stones

> Excludes: percutaneous nephrostomy with fragmentation (55.04)
> shockwave disintegration (98.51)

59.99 Other

> Excludes: installation of medication into urinary tract (96.49)
> irrigation of urinary tract (96.45–96.48)

11. OPERATIONS ON THE MALE GENITAL ORGANS (60–64)

60 Operations on prostate and seminal vesicles

Includes: operations on periprostatic tissue

> Excludes: that associated with radical cystectomy (57.71)

60.0 Incision of prostate ♂
Drainage of prostatic abscess
Prostatolithotomy

> Excludes: drainage of periprostatic tissue only (60.81)

60.1 Diagnostic procedures on prostate and seminal vesicles

60.11 Closed [percutaneous] [needle] biopsy of prostate ♂
Approach:
 transrectal
 transurethral
Punch biopsy

60.12 Open biopsy of prostate ♂

60.13 Closed [percutaneous] biopsy of seminal vesicles ♂
Needle biopsy of seminal vesicles

60.14 Open biopsy of seminal vesicles ♂

60.15 Biopsy of periprostatic tissue ♂

60.18 Other diagnostic procedures on prostate and periprostatic tissue ♂

> Excludes: microscopic examination of specimen from prostate (91.31–91.39)
> x-ray of prostate (87.92)

60.19 Other diagnostic procedures on seminal vesicles ♂

> Excludes: microscopic examination of specimen from seminal vesicles (91.31–91.39)
> x-ray:
> contrast seminal vesiculogram (87.91)
> other (87.92)

60.2 Transurethral prostatectomy ♂
Excision of median bar by transurethral approach
Transurethral enucleative procedure

> Excludes: local excision of lesion of prostate (60.61)

60.3 Suprapubic prostatectomy ♂
Transvesical prostatectomy

> Excludes: local excision of lesion of prostate (60.61)
> radical prostatectomy (60.5)

60.4 Retropubic prostatectomy ♂

> Excludes: local excision of lesion of prostate (60.61)
> radical prostatectomy (60.5)

60.5 Radical prostatectomy ♂
Prostatovesiculectomy
Radical prostatectomy by any approach

> Excludes: cystoprostatectomy (57.71)

60.6 Other prostatectomy

60.61 Local excision of lesion of prostate ♂
Excision of prostatic lesion by any approach

> Excludes: biopsy of prostate (60.11–60.12)

60.62 Perineal prostatectomy ♂

60.69 Other ♂

60.7 Operations on seminal vesicles

60.71 Percutaneous aspiration of seminal vesicle ♂

> Excludes: needle biopsy of seminal vesicle (60.13)

60.72 Incision of seminal vesicle ♂

60.73 Excision of seminal vesicle ♂
Excision of Mullerian duct cyst
Spermatocystectomy

> Excludes: biopsy of seminal vesicle (60.13–60.14)
> prostatovesiculectomy (60.5)

60.79 Other operations on seminal vesicles ♂

60.8 Incision or excision of periprostatic tissue

60.81 Incision of periprostatic tissue ♂
Drainage of periprostatic abscess

60.82 Excision of periprostatic tissue ♂
Excision of lesion of periprostatic tissue

> Excludes: biopsy of periprostatic tissue (60.15)

60.9 Other operations on prostate

60.91 Percutaneous aspiration of prostate ♂

> Excludes: needle biopsy of prostate (60.11)

60.92 Injection into prostate ♂

60.93 Repair of prostate ♂

60.94 Control of (postoperative) hemorrhage of prostate ♂
Coagulation of prostatic bed
Cystoscopy for control of prostate hemorrhage

60.95 Transurethral balloon dilation of the prostatic urethra ♂

60.99 Other ♂

> Excludes: prostatic massage (99.94)

61 Operations on scrotum and tunica vaginalis

61.0 Incision and drainage of scrotum and tunica vaginalis ♂

> Excludes: percutaneous aspiration of hydrocele (61.91)

61.1 Diagnostic procedures on scrotum and tunica vaginalis

61.11 Biopsy of scrotum or tunica vaginalis ♂

61.19 Other diagnostic procedures on scrotum and tunica vaginalis ♂

61.2 Excision of hydrocele (of tunica vaginalis) ♂
Bottle repair of hydrocele of tunica vaginalis

> Excludes: percutaneous aspiration of hydrocele (61.91)

61.3 Excision or destruction of lesion or tissue of scrotum ♂
Fulguration of lesion } of scrotum
Reduction of elephantiasis
Partial scrotectomy

> Excludes: biopsy of scrotum (61.11)
> scrotal fistulectomy (61.42)

61.4 Repair of scrotum and tunica vaginalis

61.41 Suture of laceration of scrotum and tunica vaginalis ♂

61.42 Repair of scrotal fistula ♂

61.49 Other repair of scrotum and tunica vaginalis ♂
Reconstruction with rotational or pedicle flaps

61.9 Other operations on scrotum and tunica vaginalis

61.91 Percutaneous aspiration of tunica vaginalis ♂
Aspiration of hydrocele of tunica vaginalis

61.92 Excision of lesion of tunica vaginalis other than hydrocele ♂
Excision of hematocele of tunica vaginalis

61.99 Other ♂

> Excludes: removal of foreign body from scrotum without incision (98.24)

62. Operations on testes

62.0 Incision of testis ♂

62.1 Diagnostic procedures on testes

62.11 Closed [percutaneous] [needle] biopsy of testis ♂

62.12 Open biopsy of testis ♂

62.19 Other diagnostic procedures on testes ♂

62.2 Excision or destruction of testicular lesion ♂
Excision of appendix testis
Excision of cyst of Morgagni in the male

> Excludes: biopsy of testis (62.11–62.12)

62.3 Unilateral orchiectomy ♂
Orchidectomy (with epididymectomy) NOS

62.4 Bilateral orchiectomy
Male castration
Radical bilateral orchiectomy (with epididymectomy)

Code also any synchronous lymph node dissection (40.3, 40.5)

62.41 Removal of both testes at same operative episode ♂
Bilateral orchidectomy NOS

62.42 Removal of remaining testis ♂
Removal of solitary testis

▲ **62.5 Orchiopexy** ♂
Mobilization and replacement of testis in scrotum
Orchiopexy with detorsion of testis
Torek (Bevan) operation (first stage) (second stage)
Transplantation to and fixation of testis in scrotum

62.6 Repair of testes

> Excludes: reduction of torsion (63.52)

62.61 Suture of laceration of testis ♂

62.69 Other repair of testis ♂
Testicular graft

62.7 Insertion of testicular prosthesis ♂

62.9 Other operations on testes

62.91 Aspiration of testis ♂

> Excludes: percutaneous biopsy of testis (62.11)

62.92 Injection of therapeutic substance into testis ♂

62.99 Other ♂

63. Operations on spermatic cord, epididymis, and vas deferens

63.0 Diagnostic procedures on spermatic cord, epididymis, and vas deferens

63.01 Biopsy of spermatic cord, epididymis, or vas deferens ♂

63.09 Other diagnostic procedures on spermatic cord, epididymis, and vas deferens ♂

> Excludes: contrast epididymogram (87.93)
> contrast vasogram (87.94)
> other x-ray of epididymis and vas deferens (87.95)

63.1 Excision of varicocele and hydrocele of spermatic cord ♂
High ligation of spermatic vein
Hydrocelectomy of canal of Nuck

63.2 Excision of cyst of epididymis ♂
Spermatocelectomy

63.3 Excision of other lesion or tissue of spermatic cord and epididymis ♂
Excision of appendix epididymis

> Excludes: biopsy of spermatic cord or epididymis (63.01)

63.4 Epididymectomy ♂

> Excludes: that synchronous with orchiectomy (62.3–62.42)

63.5 Repair of spermatic cord and epididymis

63.51 Suture of laceration of spermatic cord and epididymis ♂

63.52 Reduction of torsion of testis or spermatic cord ♂

> Excludes: that associated with orchiopexy (62.5)

63.53 Transplantation of spermatic cord ♂

63.59 Other repair of spermatic cord and epididymis ♂

63.6 Vasotomy ♂
Vasostomy

63.7 Vasectomy and ligation of vas deferens

63. Male sterilization procedure, not otherwise specified ♂

Ligation of vas deferens ♂
Crushing of vas deferens
Division of vas deferens

Ligation of spermatic cord ♂

Vasectomy ♂

63.8 Repair of vas deferens and epididymis

63.81 Suture of laceration of vas deferens and epididymis ♂

63.82 Reconstruction of surgically divided vas deferens ♂

63.83 Epididymovasostomy ♂

63.84 Removal of ligature from vas deferens ♂

63.85 Removal of valve from vas deferens ♂

63.89 Other repair of vas deferens and epididymis ♂

63.9 Other operations on spermatic cord, epididymis, and vas deferens

63.91 Aspiration of spermatocele ♂

63.92 Epididymotomy ♂

63.93 Incision of spermatic cord ♂

63.94 Lysis of adhesions of spermatic cord ♂

63.95 Insertion of valve in vas deferens ♂

63.99 Other ♂

OPERATIONS ON THE MALE GENITAL ORGANS (60-64)

64 Operations on penis

Includes: operations on:
corpora cavernosa
glans penis
prepuce

64.0 Circumcision ♂

64.1 Diagnostic procedures on the penis

64.11 Biopsy of penis ♂

64.19 Other diagnostic procedures on penis ♂

64.2 Local excision or destruction of lesion of penis ♂

Excludes: biopsy of penis (64.11)

64.3 Amputation of penis ♂

64.4 Repair and plastic operation on penis

64.41 Suture of laceration of penis ♂

64.42 Release of chordee ♂

64.43 Construction of penis ♂

64.44 Reconstruction of penis ♂

64.45 Replantation of penis
Reattachment of amputated penis ♂

64.49 Other repair of penis ♂

Excludes: repair of epispadias and hypospadias (58.45)

64 Operations for sex transformation, not elsewhere classified ♂

64.9 Other operations on male genital organs

64.91 Dorsal or lateral slit of prepuce ♂

64.92 Incision of penis ♂

64.93 Division of penile adhesions ♂

64.94 Fitting of external prosthesis of penis ♂
Penile prosthesis NOS

64.95 Insertion or replacement of non-inflatable penile prosthesis ♂
insertion of semi-rigid rod prosthesis into shaft of penis

Excludes: external penile prosthesis (64.94)
inflatable penile prosthesis (64.97)
plastic repair
penis (64.43–64.49)
that associated with:
construction (64.43)
reconstruction (64.44)

64.96 Removal of internal prosthesis of penis ♂
Removal without replacement of non-inflatable or inflatable penile prosthesis

64.97 Insertion or replacement of inflatable penile prosthesis ♂
Insertion of cylinders into shaft of penis and placement of pump and reservoir

Excludes: external penile prosthesis (64.94)
non-inflatable penile prosthesis (64.95)
plastic repair, penis (64.43–64.49)

64.98 Other operations on penis ♂
Corpora cavernosa-corpus spongiosum shunt
Corpora-saphenous shunt
Irrigation of corpus cavernosum

Excludes: removal of foreign body:
intraluminal (98.19)
without incision (98.24)
stretching of foreskin (99.95)

64.99 Other ♂

Excludes: collection of sperm for artificial insemination (99.96)

OPERATIONS ON THE FEMALE GENITAL ORGANS (65-71)

12. OPERATIONS ON THE FEMALE GENITAL ORGANS (65–71)

65 Operations on ovary

65.0 Oophorotomy ♀
  Salpingo-oophorotomy

65.1 Diagnostic procedures on ovaries

  65.11 Aspiration biopsy of ovary ♀

  65.12 Other biopsy of ovary ♀

  65.19 Other diagnostic procedures on ovaries ♀

  > Excludes: microscopic examination of specimen from ovary (91.41–91.49)

65.2 Local excision or destruction of ovarian lesion or tissue

  65.21 Marsupialization of ovarian cyst ♀

  65.22 Wedge resection of ovary ♀

  65.29 Other local excision or destruction of ovary ♀
   Bisection
   Cauterization } of ovary
   Partial excision

  > Excludes: biopsy of ovary (65.11–65.12)

65.3 Unilateral oophorectomy ♀

65.4 Unilateral salpingo-oophorectomy ♀

65.5 Bilateral oophorectomy

  65.51 Removal of both ovaries at same operative episode ♀
   Female castration

  65.52 Removal of remaining ovary ♀
   Removal of solitary ovary

65.6 Bilateral salpingo-oophorectomy

  65.61 Removal of both ovaries and tubes at same operative episode ♀

  65.62 Removal of remaining ovary and tube ♀
   Removal of solitary ovary and tube

65.7 Repair of ovary

  > Excludes: salpingo-oophorostomy (66.72)

  65.71 Simple suture of ovary ♀

  65.72 Reimplantation of ovary ♀

  65.73 Salpingo-oophoroplasty ♀

  65.79 Other repair of ovary ♀
   Oophoropexy

65.8 Lysis of adhesions of ovary and fallopian tube ♀

65.9 Other operations on ovary

  65.91 Aspiration of ovary ♀

  > Excludes: aspiration biopsy of ovary (65.11)

  65.92 Transplantation of ovary ♀

  > Excludes: reimplantation of ovary (65.72)

  65.93 Manual rupture of ovarian cyst ♀

  65.94 Ovarian denervation ♀

  65.95 Release of torsion of ovary ♀

  65.99 Other ♀

66 Operations on fallopian tubes

66.0 Salpingotomy and salpingostomy

  66.01 Salpingotomy ♀

  66.02 Salpingostomy ♀

66.1 Diagnostic procedures on fallopian tubes

  66.11 Biopsy of fallopian tube ♀

  66.19 Other diagnostic procedures on fallopian tubes ♀

  > Excludes: microscopic examination of specimen from fallopian tubes (91.41–91.49)
  > radiography of fallopian tubes (87.82–87.83, 87.85)
  > Rubin's test (66.8)

66.2 Bilateral endoscopic destruction or occlusion of fallopian tubes
  Includes: bilateral endoscopic destruction or occlusion of fallopian tubes by:
   culdoscopy
   endoscopy
   hysteroscopy
   laparoscopy
   peritoneoscopy
  endoscopic destruction of solitary fallopian tube

  66.21 Bilateral endoscopic ligation and crushing of fallopian tubes ♀

  66.22 Bilateral endoscopic ligation and division of fallopian tubes ♀

  66.29 Other bilateral endoscopic destruction or occlusion of fallopian tubes ♀

66.3 Other bilateral destruction or occlusion of fallopian tubes
  Includes: destruction of solitary fallopian tube

  > Excludes: endoscopic destruction or occlusion of fallopian tubes (66.21–66.29)

  66.31 Other bilateral ligation and crushing of fallopian tubes ♀

  66.32 Other bilateral ligation and division of fallopian tubes ♀
   Pomeroy operation

  66.39 Other bilateral destruction or occlusion of fallopian tubes ♀
   Female sterilization operation NOS

66.4 Total unilateral salpingectomy ♀

66.5 Total bilateral salpingectomy

  > Excludes: bilateral partial salpingectomy for sterilization (66.39)
  > that with oophorectomy (65.61–65.62)

  66.51 Removal of both fallopian tubes at same operative episode ♀

  66.52 Removal of remaining fallopian tube ♀
   Removal of solitary fallopian tube

66.6 Other salpingectomy
  Includes: salpingectomy by:
   cauterization
   coagulation
   electrocoagulation
   excision

  > Excludes: fistulectomy (66.73)

  66.61 Excision or destruction of lesion of fallopian tube ♀

  > Excludes: biopsy of fallopian tube (66.11)

66.62 Salpingectomy with removal of tubal pregnancy ♀

Code also any synchronous oophorectomy (65.3)

66.63 Bilateral partial salpingectomy, not otherwise specified ♀

66.69 Other partial salpingectomy ♀

66.7 Repair of fallopian tube

66.71 Simple suture of fallopian tube ♀

66.72 Salpingo-oophorostomy ♀

66.73 Salpingo-salpingostomy ♀

66.74 Salpingo-uterostomy ♀

66.79 Other repair of fallopian tube ♀
Graft of fallopian tube
Reopening of divided fallopian tube
Salpingoplasty

66.8 Insufflation of fallopian tube ♀

Insufflation of fallopian tube with:
   air
   dye
   gas
   saline
Rubin's test

| Excludes: | insufflation of therapeutic agent (66.95)
that for hysterosalpingography (87.82–87.83) |

66.9 Other operations on fallopian tubes

66.91 Aspiration of fallopian tube ♀

66.92 Unilateral destruction or occlusion of fallopian tube ♀

| Excludes: | that of solitary tube (66.21–66.39) |

66.93 Implantation or replacement of prosthesis of fallopian tube ♀

66.94 Removal of prosthesis of fallopian tube ♀

66.95 Insufflation of therapeutic agent into fallopian tubes ♀

66.96 Dilation of fallopian tube ♀

66.97 Burying of fimbriae in uterine wall ♀

66.99 Other ♀

| Excludes: | lysis of adhesions of ovary and tube (65.8) |

67. Operations on cervix

67.0 Dilation of cervical canal ♀

| Excludes: | dilation and curettage (69.01–69.09)
that for induction of labor (73.1) |

67.1 Diagnostic procedures on cervix

67.11 Endocervical biopsy ♀

| Excludes: | conization of cervix (67.2) |

67.12 Other cervical biopsy ♀
Punch biopsy of cervix NOS

| Excludes: | conization of cervix (67.2) |

67.19 Other diagnostic procedures on cervix ♀

| Excludes: | microscopic examination of specimen from cervix (91.41–91.49) |

67.2 Conization of cervix ♀

| Excludes: | that by:
cryosurgery (67.33)
electrosurgery (67.32) |

67.3 Other excision or destruction of lesion or tissue of cervix

67.31 Marsupialization of cervical cyst ♀

67.32 Destruction of lesion of cervix by cauterization ♀
Electroconization of cervix

67.33 Destruction of lesion of cervix by cryosurgery ♀
Cryoconization of cervix

67.39 Other excision or destruction of lesion or tissue of cervix ♀

| Excludes: | biopsy of cervix (67.11, 67.12)
cervical fistulectomy (67.62)
conization of cervix (67.2) |

67.4 Amputation of cervix ♀
Cervicectomy with synchronous colporrhaphy

67.5 Repair of internal cervical os ♀
Cerclage of isthmus uteri
Shirodkar operation

67.6 Other repair of cervix

| Excludes: | repair of current obstetric laceration (75.51) |

67.61 Suture of laceration of cervix ♀

67.62 Repair of fistula of cervix ♀
Cervicosigmoidal fistulectomy

| Excludes: | fistulectomy:
cervicovesical (57.84)
ureterocervical (56.84)
vesicocervicovaginal (57.84) |

67.69 Other repair of cervix ♀
Repair of old obstetric laceration of cervix

68. Other incision and excision of uterus

68.0 Hysterotomy ♀
Hysterotomy with removal of hydatidiform mole

| Excludes: | hysterotomy for termination of pregnancy (74.91) |

68.1 Diagnostic procedures on uterus and supporting structures

68.11 Distal examination of uterus ♀

| Excludes: | pelvic examination, so described (89.26)
postpartal manual exploration of uterine cavity (75.7) |

68.12 Hysteroscopy ♀ NOR

| Excludes: | that with biopsy (68.16) |

68.13 Open biopsy of uterus ♀

| Excludes: | closed biopsy of uterus (68.16) |

68.14 Open biopsy of uterine ligaments ♀

| Excludes: | closed biopsy of uterine ligaments (68.15) |

68.15 Closed biopsy of uterine ligaments ♀
Endoscopic (laparoscopy) biopsy of uterine adnexa, except ovary and fallopian tube

68.16 Closed biopsy of uterus ♀
Endoscopic (laparoscopy) (hysteroscopy) biopsy of uterus

| Excludes: | open biopsy of uterus (68.13) |

OPERATIONS ON THE FEMALE GENITAL ORGANS (65-71)

68.19 Other diagnostic procedures on uterus and supporting structures ♀

   Excludes: diagnostic:
   aspiration curettage (69.59)
   dilation and curettage (69.09)
   microscopic examination of specimen from uterus (91.41–91.49)
   pelvic examination (89.26)
   radioisotope scan of:
   placenta (92.17)
   uterus (92.19)
   ultrasonography of uterus (88.78–88.79)
   x-ray of uterus (87.81–87.89)

68.2 Excision or destruction of lesion or tissue of uterus

   68.21 Division of endometrial synechiae ♀
   Lysis of intraluminal uterine adhesions

   68.22 Incision or excision of congenital septum of uterus ♀

   68.29 Other excision or destruction of lesion of uterus ♀
   Uterine myomectomy

   Excludes: biopsy of uterus (68.13)
   uterine fistulectomy (69.42)

68.3 Subtotal abdominal hysterectomy ♀
   Supracervical hysterectomy

68.4 Total abdominal hysterectomy ♀
   Hysterectomy:
   extended

   Code also any synchronous removal of tubes and ovaries (65.3–65.6)

68.5 Vaginal hysterectomy ♀

   Code also any synchronous:
   Removal of tubes and ovaries (65.3–65.6)
   Repair of cystocele or rectocele (70.50–70.52)
   Repair of pelvic floor (70.79)

68.6 Radical abdominal hysterectomy ♀
   Modified radical hysterectomy
   Wertheim's operation

   Code also any synchronous:
   lymph gland dissection (40.3, 40.5)
   removal of tubes and ovaries (65.61–65.62)

   Excludes: pelvic evisceration (68.8)

68.7 Radical vaginal hysterectomy ♀
   Schauta operation

   Code also any synchronous:
   lymph gland dissection (40.3, 40.5)
   removal of tubes and ovaries (65.61–65.62)

68.8 Pelvic evisceration ♀
   Removal of ovaries, tubes, uterus, vagina, bladder, and urethra (with removal of sigmoid colon and rectum)

   Code also any synchronous:
   colostomy (46.12–46.13)
   lymph gland dissection (40.3, 40.5)
   urinary diversion (56.51–56.79)

68.9 Other and unspecified hysterectomy ♀
   Hysterectomy NOS

   Excludes: abdominal hysterectomy, any approach (68.3, 68.4, 68.6)
   vaginal hysterectomy, any approach (68.5, 68.7)

69 Other operations on uterus and supporting structures

   69.0 Dilation and curettage of uterus

   Excludes: aspiration curettage of uterus (69.51–69.59)

   69.01 Dilation and curettage for termination of pregnancy ♀

   69.02 Dilation and curettage following delivery or abortion ♀

   69.09 Other dilation and curettage ♀
   Diagnostic D and C

   69.1 Excision or destruction of lesion or tissue of uterus and supporting structures

   69.19 Other excision or destruction of uterus and supporting structures ♀

   Excludes: biopsy of uterine ligament (68.14)

   69.2 Repair of uterine supporting structures

   69.21 Interposition operation ♀
   Watkins procedure

   69.22 Other uterine suspension ♀
   Hysteropexy
   Manchester operation
   Plication of uterine ligament

   69.23 Vaginal repair of chronic inversion of uterus ♀

   69.29 Other repair of uterus and supporting structures ♀

   69.3 Paracervical uterine denervation ♀

   69.4 Uterine repair

   Excludes: repair of current obstetric laceration (75.50–75.52)

   69.41 Suture of laceration of uterus ♀

   69.42 Closure of fistula of uterus ♀

   Excludes: uterovesical fistulectomy (57.84)

   69.49 Other repair of uterus ♀
   Repair of old obstetric laceration of uterus

   69.5 Aspiration curettage of uterus

   Excludes: menstrual extraction (69.6)

   69.51 Aspiration curettage of uterus for termination of pregnancy ♀
   Therapeutic abortion NOS

   69.52 Aspiration curettage following delivery or abortion ♀

   69.59 Other aspiration curettage of uterus ♀

   69.6 Menstrual extraction or regulation ♀

   69.7 Insertion of intrauterine contraceptive device ♀

   69.9 Other operations on uterus, cervix, and supporting structures

   Excludes: obstetric dilation or incision of cervix (73.1, 73.93)

   69.91 Insertion of therapeutic device into uterus ♀

   Excludes: insertion of:
   intrauterine contraceptive device (69.7)
   laminaria (69.93)
   obstetric insertion of bag, bougie, or pack (73.1)

   69.92 Artificial insemination ♀

   69.93 Insertion of laminaria ♀

69.94 Manual replacement of inverted uterus ♀

>   Excludes: *that immediate postpartal period (75.94)*

69.95 Incision of cervix ♀

>   Excludes: *that to assist delivery (73.93)*

69.96 Removal of cerclage material from cervix ♀

69.97 Removal of other penetrating foreign body from cervix ♀

>   Excludes: *removal of intraluminal foreign body from cervix (98.16)*

69.98 Other operations on supporting structures of uterus ♀

>   Excludes: *biopsy of uterine ligament (68.14)*

69.99 Other operations on cervix and uterus ♀

>   Excludes: *removal of:*
>   *foreign body (98.16)*
>   *intrauterine contraceptive device (97.71)*
>   *obstetric bag, bougie, or pack (97.72)*
>   *packing (97.72)*

70 Operations on vagina and cul-de-sac

70.0 Culdocentesis ♀

70.1 Incision of vagina and cul-de-sac

    70.11 Hymenotomy ♀

    70.12 Culdotomy ♀

    70.13 Lysis of intraluminal adhesions of vagina ♀

    70.14 Other vaginotomy ♀
Division of vaginal septum
Drainage of hematoma of vaginal cuff

70.2 Diagnostic procedures on vagina and cul-de-sac

    70.21 Vaginoscopy ♀ NOR
    70.22 Culdoscopy ♀ NOR
    70.23 Biopsy of cul-de-sac ♀
    70.24 Vaginal biopsy ♀
    70.29 Other diagnostic procedures on vagina and cul-de-sac ♀

70.3 Local excision or destruction of vagina and cul-de-sac

    70.31 Hymenectomy ♀

    70.32 Excision or destruction of lesion of cul-de-sac ♀
Endometrectomy of cul-de-sac

>   Excludes: *biopsy of cul-de-sac (70.23)*

    70.33 Excision or destruction of lesion of vagina ♀

>   Excludes: *biopsy of vagina (70.24)*
>   *vaginal fistulectomy (70.72–70.75)*

▲ **70.4** Obliteration and total excision of vagina ♀
Vaginectomy

>   Excludes: *obliteration of vaginal vault (70.8)*

70.5 Repair of cystocele and rectocele

    70.50 Repair of cystocele and rectocele ♀

    70.51 Repair of cystocele ♀
Anterior colporrhaphy (with urethrocele repair)

    70.52 Repair of rectocele ♀
Posterior colporrhaphy

70.6 Vaginal construction and reconstruction

    70.61 Vaginal construction ♀
    70.62 Vaginal reconstruction ♀

70.7 Other repair of vagina

>   Excludes: *lysis of intraluminal adhesions (70.13)*
>   *repair of current obstetric laceration (75.69)*
>   *that associated with cervical amputation (67.4)*

    70.71 Suture of laceration of vagina ♀
    70.72 Repair of colovaginal fistula ♀
    70.73 Repair of rectovaginal fistula ♀
    70.74 Repair of other vaginoenteric fistula ♀
    70.75 Repair of other fistula of vagina ♀

>   Excludes: *repair of fistula:*
>   *rectovesicovaginal (57.83)*
>   *ureterovaginal (56.84)*
>   *urethrovaginal (58.43)*
>   *uterovaginal (69.42)*
>   *vesicocervicovaginal (57.84)*
>   *vesicosigmoidovaginal (57.83)*
>   *vesicoureterovaginal (56.84)*
>   *vesicovaginal (57.84)*

    70.76 Hymenorrhaphy ♀
    70.77 Vaginal suspension and fixation ♀
    70.79 Other repair of vagina ♀
Colpoperineoplasty
Repair of old obstetric laceration of vagina

▲ **70.8** Obliteration of vaginal vault ♀
LeFort operation

70.9 Other operations on vagina and cul-de-sac

    70.91 Other operations on vagina ♀

>   Excludes: *insertion of:*
>   *diaphragm (96.17)*
>   *mold (96.15)*
>   *pack (96.14)*
>   *pessary (96.18)*
>   *suppository (96.49)*
>   *removal of:*
>   *diaphragm (97.73)*
>   *foreign body (98.17)*
>   *pack (97.75)*
>   *pessary (97.74)*
>   *replacement of:*
>   *diaphragm (97.24)*
>   *pack (97.26)*
>   *pessary (97.25)*
>   *vaginal dilation (96.16)*
>   *vaginal douche (96.44)*

▲**70.92** Other operations on cul-de-sac ♀
Obliteration of cul-de-sac
Repair of vaginal enterocele

71 Operations on vulva and perineum

71.0 Incision of vulva and perineum

    71.01 Lysis of vulvar adhesions ♀

    71.09 Other incision of vulva and perineum ♀
Enlargement of introitus NOS

>   Excludes: *removal of foreign body without incision (98.23)*

71.1 Diagnostic procedures on vulva

    71.11 Biopsy of vulva ♀
    71.19 Other diagnostic procedures on vulva ♀

71.2 Operations on Bartholin's gland

71.21 Percutaneous aspiration of Bartholin's gland (cyst) ♀

71.22 Incision of Bartholin's gland (cyst) ♀

71.23 Marsupialization of Bartholin's gland (cyst) ♀

71.24 Excision or other destruction of Bartholin's gland (cyst) ♀

71.29 Other operations on Bartholin's gland ♀

71.3 Other local excision or destruction of vulva and perineum ♀
Division of Skene's gland

> Excludes: biopsy of vulva (71.11)
> vulvar fistulectomy (71.72)

71.4 Operations on clitoris ♀
Amputation of clitoris
Clitoridotomy
Female circumcision

71.5 Radical vulvectomy ♀
Code also any synchronous lymph gland dissection (40.3, 40.5)

71.6 Other vulvectomy

71.61 Unilateral vulvectomy ♀

71.62 Bilateral vulvectomy ♀
Vulvectomy NOS

71.7 Repair of vulva and perineum

> Excludes: repair of current obstetric laceration (75.69)

71.71 Suture of laceration of vulva or perineum ♀

71.72 Repair of fistula of vulva or perineum ♀

> Excludes: repair of fistula:
> urethroperineal (58.43)
> urethroperineovesical (57.84)
> vaginoperineal (70.75)

71.79 Other repair of vulva and perineum ♀
Repair of old obstetric laceration of vulva or perineum

71.8 Other operations on vulva ♀

> Excludes: removal of:
> foreign body without incision (98.23)
> packing (97.75)
> replacement of packing (97.26)

71.9 Other operations on female genital organs ♀

13. OBSTETRICAL PROCEDURES (72–75)

72 Forceps, vacuum, and breech delivery

- **72.0 Low forceps operation** ♀
  - Outlet forceps operation

- **72.1 Low forceps operation with episiotomy** ♀
  - Outlet forceps operation with episiotomy

- **72.2 Mid forceps operation**
  - **72.21 Mid forceps operation with episiotomy** ♀
  - **72.29 Other mid forceps operation** ♀

- **72.3 High forceps operation**
  - **72.31 High forceps operation with episiotomy** ♀
  - **72.39 Other high forceps operation** ♀

- **72.4 Forceps rotation of fetal head** ♀
  - DeLee maneuver
  - Key-in-lock rotation
  - Kielland rotation
  - Scanzoni's maneuver

  Code also any associated forceps extraction (72.0–72.39)

- **72.5 Breech extraction**
  - **72.51 Partial breech extraction with forceps to aftercoming head** ♀
  - **72.52 Other partial breech extraction** ♀
  - **72.53 Total breech extraction with forceps to aftercoming head** ♀
  - **72.54 Other total breech extraction** ♀

- **72.6 Forceps application to aftercoming head** ♀
  - Piper forceps operation

  Excludes: partial breech extraction with forceps to aftercoming head (72.51)
  total breech extraction with forceps to aftercoming head (72.53)

- **72.7 Vacuum extraction**
  - Includes: Malström's extraction
  - **72.71 Vacuum extraction with episiotomy** ♀
  - **72.79 Other vacuum extraction** ♀

- **72.8 Other specified instrumental delivery** ♀

- **72.9 Unspecified instrumental delivery** ♀

73 Other procedures inducing or assisting delivery

- **73.0 Artificial rupture of membranes**
  - **73.01 Induction of labor by artificial rupture of membranes** ♀
    - Surgical induction NOS

    Excludes: artificial rupture of membranes after onset of labor (73.09)

  - **73.09 Other artificial rupture of membranes** ♀
    - Artificial rupture of membranes at time of delivery

- **73.1 Other surgical induction of labor** ♀
  - Induction by cervical dilation

  Excludes: injection for abortion (75.0)
  insertion of suppository for abortion (96.49)

- **73.2 Internal and combined version and extraction**
  - **73.21 Internal and combined version without extraction** ♀
    - Version NOS
  - **73.22 Internal and combined version with extraction** ♀

- **73.3 Failed forceps** ♀
  - Application of forceps without delivery
  - Trial forceps

- **73.4 Medical induction of labor** ♀

  Excludes: medication to augment active labor — omit code

- **73.5 Manually assisted delivery**
  - **73.51 Manual rotation of fetal head** ♀
  - **73.59 Other manually assisted delivery** ♀
    - Assisted spontaneous delivery
    - Credé maneuver

- **73.6 Episiotomy** ♀
  - Episioproctotomy
  - Episiotomy with subsequent episiorrhaphy

  Excludes: that with:
  high forceps (72.31)
  low forceps (72.1)
  mid forceps (72.21)
  outlet forceps (72.1)
  vacuum extraction (72.71)

- **73.8 Operations on fetus to facilitate delivery** ♀
  - Clavicotomy on fetus
  - Destruction of fetus
  - Needling of hydrocephalic head

- **73.9 Other operations assisting delivery**
  - **73.91 External version** ♀
  - **73.92 Replacement of prolapsed umbilical cord** ♀
  - **73.93 Excision of cervix to assist delivery** ♀
    - Dührssen's incisions
  - **73.94 Pubiotomy to assist delivery** ♀
    - Obstetrical symphysiotomy
  - **73.99 Other** ♀

    Excludes: dilation of cervix obstetrical, to induce labor (73.1)
    insertion of bag or bougie to induce labor (73.1)
    removal of cerclage material (69.96)

74 Cesarean section and removal of fetus

Code also any synchronous:
hysterectomy (68.3–68.4, 68.6, 68.8)
myomectomy (68.29)
sterilization (66.31–66.39, 66.63)

- **74.0 Classical cesarean section** ♀
  - Transperitoneal classical cesarean section

- **74.1 Low cervical cesarean section** ♀
  - Lower uterine segment cesarean section

- **74.2 Extraperitoneal cesarean section** ♀
  - Supravesical cesarean section

74.3 Removal of extratubal ectopic pregnancy ♀
    Removal of:
      ectopic abdominal pregnancy
      fetus from peritoneal or extraperitoneal cavity following uterine or tubal rupture

> *Excludes:* that by salpingostomy (66.02)
> that by salpingotomy (66.01)
> that with synchronous salpingectomy (66.62)

74.4 Cesarean section of other specified type ♀
    Peritoneal exclusion cesarean section
    Transperitoneal cesarean section NOS
    Vaginal cesarean section

74.9 Cesarean section of unspecified type

  74.91 Hysterotomy to terminate pregnancy ♀
    Therapeutic abortion by hysterotomy

  74.99 Other cesarean section of unspecified type ♀
    Cesarean section NOS
    Obstetrical abdominouterotomy
    Obstetrical hysterotomy

75 Other obstetric operations

75.0 Intra-amniotic injection for abortion ♀
    Injection of:
      prostaglandin } for induction of abortion
      saline
    Termination of pregnancy by intrauterine injection

> *Excludes:* insertion of prostaglandin suppository for abortion (96.49)

75.1 Diagnostic amniocentesis ♀

75.2 Intrauterine transfusion ♀
    Exchange transfusion in utero
    Insertion of catheter into abdomen of fetus for transfusion

    Code also any hysterotomy approach (68.0)

75.3 Other intrauterine operations on fetus and amnion

    Code also any hysterotomy approach (68.0)

  75.31 Amnioscopy ♀
    Fetoscopy
    Laparoamnioscopy

  75.32 Fetal EKG (scalp) ♀

  75.33 Fetal blood sampling and biopsy ♀

  75.34 Fetal monitoring, not otherwise specified ♀

  75.35 Other diagnostic procedures on fetus and amnion ♀
    Intrauterine pressure determination

> *Excludes:* amniocentesis (75.1)
> diagnostic procedures on gravid uterus and placenta (87.81, 88.46, 88.78, 92.17)

  75.36 Correction of fetal defect ♀

75.4 Manual removal of retained placenta ♀

> *Excludes:* aspiration curettage (69.52)
> dilation and curettage (69.02)

75.5 Repair of current obstetric laceration of uterus

  75.50 Repair of current obstetric laceration of uterus, not otherwise specified ♀

  75.51 Repair of current obstetric laceration of cervix ♀

  75.52 Repair of current obstetric laceration of corpus uteri ♀

75.6 Repair of other current obstetric laceration

  75.61 Repair of current obstetric laceration of bladder and urethra ♀

  75.62 Repair of current obstetric laceration of rectum and sphincter ani ♀

  75.69 Repair of other current obstetric laceration ♀
    Episioperineorrhaphy
    Repair of:
      pelvic floor
      perineum
      vagina
      vulva
    Secondary repair of episiotomy

> *Excludes:* repair of routine episiotomy (73.6)

75.7 Manual exploration of uterine cavity, postpartum ♀

> *Excludes:* antepartum tamponade (73.1)

75.8 Obstetric tamponade of uterus or vagina ♀

> *Excludes:* antepartum tamponade (73.1)

75.9 Other obstetric operations

  75.91 Evacuation of obstetrical incisional hematoma of perineum ♀
    Evacuation of hematoma of:
      episiotomy
      perineorrhaphy

  75.92 Evacuation of other hematoma of vulva or vagina ♀

  75.93 Surgical correction of inverted uterus ♀
    Spintelli operation

> *Excludes:* vaginal repair of chronic inversion of uterus (69.23)

  75.94 Manual replacement of inverted uterus ♀

  75.99 Other ♀

14. OPERATIONS ON THE MUSCULOSKELETAL SYSTEM (76–84)

76 Operations on facial bones and joints

Excludes: accessory sinuses (22.00–22.9)
nasal bones (21.00–21.99)
skull (01.01–02.99)

76.0 Incision of facial bone without division

76.01 Sequestrectomy of facial bone
Removal of necrotic bone chip from facial bone

76.09 Other incision of facial bone
Reopening of osteotomy site of facial bone

Excludes: osteotomy associated with orthognathic surgery (76.61–76.69)
removal of internal fixation device (76.97)

76.1 Diagnostic procedures on facial bones and joints

76.11 Biopsy of facial bone

76.19 Other diagnostic procedures on facial bones and joints

Excludes: contrast arthrogram of temporomandibular joint (87.11)
other x-ray (87.11–87.12, 87.14–87.16)

76.2 Local excision or destruction of lesion of facial bone

Excludes: biopsy of facial bone (76.11)
excision of odontogenic lesion (24.4)

76.3 Partial ostectomy of facial bone

76.31 Partial mandibulectomy
Hemimandibulectomy

Excludes: that associated with temporomandibular arthroplasty (76.5)

76.39 Partial ostectomy of other facial bone
Hemimaxillectomy (with bone graft or prosthesis)

76.4 Excision and reconstruction of facial bones

76.41 Total mandibulectomy with synchronous reconstruction

76.42 Other total mandibulectomy

76.43 Other reconstruction of mandible

Excludes: genioplasty (76.67–76.68)
that with synchronous total mandibulectomy (76.41)

76.44 Total ostectomy of other facial bone with synchronous reconstruction

76.45 Other total ostectomy of other facial bone

76.46 Other reconstruction of other facial bone

Excludes: that with synchronous total ostectomy (76.44)

76.5 Temporomandibular arthroplasty

76.6 Other facial bone repair and orthognathic surgery

Code also any synchronous:
bone graft (76.91)
synthetic implant (76.92)

Excludes: reconstruction of facial bones (76.41–76.46)

76.61 Closed osteoplasty [osteotomy] of mandibular ramus
Gigli saw osteotomy

76.62 Open osteoplasty [osteotomy] of mandibular ramus

76.63 Osteoplasty [osteotomy] of body of mandible

76.64 Other orthognathic surgery on mandible
Mandibular osteoplasty NOS
Segmental or subapical osteotomy

76.65 Segmental osteoplasty [osteotomy] of maxilla
Maxillary osteoplasty NOS

76.66 Total osteoplasty [osteotomy] of maxilla

76.67 Reduction genioplasty
Reduction mentoplasty

76.68 Augmentation genioplasty
Mentoplasty:
NOS
with graft or implant

76.69 Other facial bone repair
Osteoplasty of facial bone NOS

76.7 Reduction of facial fracture

Includes: internal fixation

Code also any synchronous:
bone graft (76.91)
synthetic implant (76.92)

Excludes: that of nasal bones (21.71–21.72)

76.70 Reduction of facial fracture, not otherwise specified

76.71 Closed reduction of malar and zygomatic fracture

76.72 Open reduction of malar and zygomatic fracture

76.73 Closed reduction of maxillary fracture

76.74 Open reduction of maxillary fracture

76.75 Closed reduction of mandibular fracture

76.76 Open reduction of mandibular fracture

76.77 Open reduction of alveolar fracture
Reduction of alveolar fracture with stabilization of teeth

76.78 Other closed reduction of facial fracture
Closed reduction of orbital fracture

Excludes: nasal bone (21.71)

76.79 Other open reduction of facial fracture
Open reduction of orbit rim or wall

Excludes: nasal bone (21.72)

76.9 Other operations on facial bones and joints

76.91 Bone graft to facial bone
Autogenous
Bone bank } graft to facial bone
Heterogenous

76.92 Insertion of synthetic implant in facial bone
Alloplastic implant to facial bone

76.93 Closed reduction of temporomandibular dislocation

76.94 Open reduction of temporomandibular dislocation

76.95 Other manipulation of temporomandibular joint

76.96 Injection of therapeutic substance into temporomandibular joint

76.97 Removal of internal fixation device from facial bone

Excludes: removal of:
dental wiring (97.33)
external mandibular fixation device NEC (97.36)

76.99 Other

77 Incision, excision, and division of other bones

Excludes: laminectomy for decompression (03.09)
operations on:
accessory sinuses (22.00–22.9)
ear ossicles (19.0–19.55)
facial bones (76.01–76.99)
joint structures (80.00–81.99)
mastoid (19.9–20.99)
nasal bones (21.00–21.99)
skull (01.01–02.99)

The following fourth-digit subclassification is for use with appropriate categories in section 77, marked with a symbol (§), to identify the site:

- 0 unspecified site
- 1 scapula, clavicle, and thorax [ribs and sternum]
- 2 humerus
- 3 radius and ulna
- 4 carpals and metacarpals
- 5 femur
- 6 patella
- 7 tibia and fibula
- 8 tarsals and metatarsals
- 9 other
    Pelvic bones
    Phalanges (of foot) (of hand)
    Vertebrae

§ 77.0 Sequestrectomy
[0-9]

§ 77.1 Other incision of bone without division
[0-9] Reopening of osteotomy site

Excludes: aspiration of bone marrow (41.31, 41.91)
removal of internal fixation device (78.60–78.69)

§ 77.2 Wedge osteotomy
[0-9]

Excludes: that for hallux valgus (77.51)

§ 77.3 Other division of bone
[0-9] Osteoarthrotomy

Excludes: clavicotomy of fetus (73.8)
laminotomy or incision of vertebra (03.01–03.09)
pubiotomy to assist delivery (73.94)
sternotomy incidental to thoracic operation — omit code

§ 77.4 Biopsy of bone
[0-9]

77.5 Excision and repair of bunion and other toe deformities

77.51 Bunionectomy with soft tissue correction and osteotomy of the first metatarsal

77.52 Bunionectomy with soft tissue correction and arthrodesis

77.53 Other bunionectomy with soft tissue correction

77.54 Excision or correction of bunionette that with osteotomy

77.56 Repair of hammer toe
Fusion
Phalangectomy (partial) } of hammer toe
Filleting

77.57 Repair of claw toe
Fusion
Phalangectomy (partial)
Capsulotomy } of claw toe
Tendon lengthening

77.58 Other excision, fusion, and repair of toes
Cockup toe repair
Overlapping toe repair
That with use of prosthetic materials

77.59 Other bunionectomy
Resection of hallux valgus joint with insertion of prosthesis

§ 77.6 Local excision of lesion or tissue of bone
[0-9]

Excludes: biopsy of bone (77.40–77.49)
debridement of compound fracture (79.60–79,69)

§ 77.7 Excision of bone for graft
[0-9]

§ 77.8 Other partial ostectomy
[0-9] Condylectomy

Excludes: amputation (84.00–84.19, 84.91)
arthrectomy (80.90–80.99)
excision of bone ends associated with:
  arthrodesis (81.00–81.29)
  arthroplasty (81.51–81.59, 81.71–81.81, 81.84)
excision of cartilage (80.5–80.6, 80.80–80.99)
excision of head of femur with synchronous replacement (81.51–81.53)
hemilaminectomy (03.01–03.09)
laminectomy (03.01–03.09)
ostectomy for hallux valgus (77.51–77.59)
partial amputation:
  finger (84.01)
  thumb (84.02)
  toe (84.11)
resection of ribs incidental to thoracic operation — omit code
that incidental to other operation — omit code

§ 77.9 Total ostectomy
[0-9]

Excludes: amputation of limb (84.00–84.19, 84.91)
that incidental to other operation — omit code

OPERATIONS ON THE MUSCULOSKELETAL SYSTEM (76-84)

78 Other operations on bones, except facial bones

> Excludes: operations on:
> accessory sinuses (22.00–22.9)
> facial bones (76.01–76.99)
> joint structures (80.00–81.99)
> nasal bones (21.00–21.99)
> skull (01.01–02.99)

The following fourth-digit subclassification is for use with categories in section 78 to identify the site:

 0 unspecified site
 1 scapula, clavicle, and thorax [ribs and sternum]
 2 humerus
 3 radius and ulna
 4 carpals and metacarpals
 5 femur
 6 patella
 7 tibia and fibula
 8 tarsals and metatarsals
 9 other
    Pelvic bones
    Phalanges (of foot) (of hand)
    Vertebrae

§ 78.0 Bone graft
[0-9] Bone:
   bank graft
   graft (autogenous) (heterogenous)
That with debridement of bone graft site (removal of sclerosed, fibrous, or necrotic bone or tissue)
Transplantation of bone

Code also any excision of bone for graft (77.70–77.79)

> Excludes: that for bone lengthening (78.30–78.39)

§ 78.1 Application of external fixation device
[0-9] Minifixator with insertion of pins/wires/screws into bone

> Excludes: other immobilization, pressure and attention to wound (93.51–93.59)

§ 78.2 Limb shortening procedures
[0,2,3,5,7,9] Epiphyseal stapling
Open epiphysiodesis
Percutaneous epiphysiodesis
Resection/osteotomy

§ 78.3 Limb lengthening procedures
[0-5,7-9] Bone graft with or without internal fixation devices or osteotomy
Distraction technique with or without corticotomy/osteotomy
Code also any application of an external fixation device (78.10–78.19)

§ 78.4 Other repair or plastic operations on bone
[0-9] Other operation on bone NEC
Repair of malunion or nonunion fracture NEC

> Excludes: application of external fixation device (78.10–78.19)
> limb lengthening procedures (78.30–78.39)
> limb shortening procedures (78.20–78.29)
> osteotomy (77.3), Reconstruction of thumb (82.61–82.69)
> repair of pectus deformity (34.74)
> repair with bone graft (78.00–78.09)

§ 78.5 Internal fixation of bone without fracture reduction
[0-9] Internal fixation of bone (prophylactic)
Reinsertion of internal fixation device
Revision of displaced or broken fixation device

> Excludes: arthroplasty and arthrodesis (81.00–81.87)
> bone graft (78.00–78.09)
> limb shortening procedures (78.20–78.29)
> that for fracture reduction (79.10–79.19, 79.30–79.59)

§ 78.6 Removal of implanted devices from bone
[0-9] External fixator device (invasive)
Internal fixation device
Removal of bone growth stimulator (invasive)

> Excludes: removal of cast, splint, and traction device (Kirschner wire) (Steinmann pin) (97.88)
> removal of skull tongs or halo traction device (02.95)

§ 78.7 Osteoclasis
[0-9]

§ 78.8 Diagnostic procedures on bone, not elsewhere classified
[0-9]

> Excludes: biopsy of bone (77.40–77.49)
> magnetic resonance imaging (88.94)
> microscopic examination of specimen from bone (91.51–91.59)
> radioisotope scan (92.14)
> skeletal x-ray (87.21–87.29, 87.43, 88.21–88.33)
> thermography (88.83)

§ 78.9 Insertion of bone growth stimulator
[0-9] Insertion of:
   bone stimulator (electrical) to aid bone healing
   osteogenic electrodes for bone growth stimulation
   totally implanted device (invasive)

> Excludes: non-invasive (transcutaneous) (surface) stimulator (99.86)

---

§ Requires fourth-digit; valid digits are in [brackets] under each code. See above for definitions.

79 Reduction of fracture and dislocation

Includes: application of cast or splint
reduction with insertion of traction device (Kirschner wire) (Steinmann pin)

Code also any application of external fixation device (78.10–78.19)

Excludes: *external fixation alone for immobilization of fracture (93.51–93.56, 93.59)*
internal fixation without reduction of fracture (78.50–78.59)
operations on:
 facial bones (76.70–76.79)
 nasal bones (21.71–21.72)
 orbit (76.78–76.79)
 skull (02.02)
 vertebrae (03.53)
removal of cast or splint (97.88)
replacement of cast or splint (97.11–97.14)
traction alone for reduction of fracture (93.41–93.46)

The following fourth-digit subclassification is for use with appropriate categories in section 79, marked with a symbol (§), to identify the site:

0 unspecified site

1 humerus

2 radius and ulna
 Arm NOS

3 carpals and metacarpals
 Hand NOS

4 phalanges of hand

5 femur

6 tibia and fibula
 Leg NOS

7 tarsals and metatarsals
 Foot NOS

8 phalanges of foot

9 other specified bone

§ **79.0 Closed reduction of fracture without internal fixation**
[0-9]

Excludes: *that for separation of epiphysis (79.40–79.49)*

§ **79.1 Closed reduction of fracture with internal fixation**
[0-9]

Excludes: *that for separation of epiphysis (79.40–79.49)*

§ **79.2 Open reduction of fracture without internal fixation**
[0-9]

Excludes: *that for separation of epiphysis (79.50–79.59)*

§ **79.3 Open reduction of fracture with internal fixation**
[0-9]

Excludes: *that for separation of epiphysis (79.50–79.59)*

§ **79.4 Closed reduction of separated epiphysis reduction with or without internal fixation**
[0-2,5,6,9]

§ **79.5 Open reduction of separated epiphysis reduction with or without internal fixation**
[0-2,5,6,9]

§ **79.6 Debridement of open fracture site**
[0-9] Debridement of compound fracture

79.7 Closed reduction of dislocation
Includes: Closed reduction (with external traction device)

Excludes: *closed reduction of dislocation of temporomandibular joint (76.93)*

79.70 Closed reduction of dislocation of unspecified site
79.71 Closed reduction of dislocation of shoulder
79.72 Closed reduction of dislocation of elbow
79.73 Closed reduction of dislocation of wrist
79.74 Closed reduction of dislocation of hand and finger
79.75 Closed reduction of dislocation of hip
79.76 Closed reduction of dislocation of knee
79.77 Closed reduction of dislocation of ankle
79.78 Closed reduction of dislocation of foot and toe
79.79 Closed reduction of dislocation of other specified sites

79.8 Open reduction of dislocation
Includes: open reduction (with internal and external fixation devices)

Excludes: *open reduction of dislocation of temporomandibular joint (76.94)*

79.80 Open reduction of dislocation of unspecified site
79.81 Open reduction of dislocation of shoulder
79.82 Open reduction of dislocation of elbow
79.83 Open reduction of dislocation of wrist
79.84 Open reduction of dislocation of hand and finger
79.85 Open reduction of dislocation of hip
79.86 Open reduction of dislocation of knee
79.87 Open reduction of dislocation of ankle
79.88 Open reduction of dislocation of foot and toe
79.89 Open reduction of dislocation of other specified sites

§ **79.9 Unspecified operation on bone injury**
[0-9]

---

§ Requires fourth-digit; valid digits are in [brackets] under each code. See above for definitions.

OPERATIONS ON THE MUSCULOSKELETAL SYSTEM (76-84)

80 Incision and excision of joint structures

Includes: operations on:
- capsule of joint
- cartilage
- condyle
- ligament
- meniscus
- synovial membrane

Excludes: cartilage of:
- ear (18.01–18.9)
- nose (21.00–21.99)
- temporomandibular joint (76.01–76.99)

The following fourth-digit subclassification is for use with appropriate categories in section 80, marked with a symbol (§), to identify the site:

0 unspecified site
1 shoulder
2 elbow
3 wrist
4 hand and finger
5 hip
6 knee
7 ankle
8 foot and toe
9 other specified sites
   Spine

§ 80.0 Arthrotomy for removal of prosthesis

§ 80.1 Other arthrotomy
   Arthrostomy

   Excludes: that for:
   - arthrography (88.32)
   - arthroscopy (80.20–80.29)
   - injection of drug (81.92)
   - operative approach — omit code

§ 80.2 Arthroscopy

§ 80.3 Biopsy of joint structure
   Aspiration biopsy

§ 80.4 Division of joint capsule, ligament, or cartilage
   Goldner clubfoot release
   Heyman-Herndon (-Strong) correction of metatarsus varus
   Release of:
   - adherent or constrictive joint capsule
   - joint
   - ligament

   Excludes: symphysiotomy to assist delivery (73.94)
   that for:
   - carpal tunnel syndrome (04.43)
   - tarsal tunnel syndrome (04.44)

80.5 Excision or destruction of intervertebral disc

   80.50 Excision or destruction of intervertebral disc, unspecified
   Unspecified as to excision or destruction

   80.51 Excision of intervertebral disc
   Diskectomy
   Removal of herniated nucleus pulposus
   Level: cervical
         thoracic
         lumbar (lumbosacral)
   That by laminotomy or hemilaminectomy
   That with decompression of spinal nerve root at same level

   Requires additional code for any concomitant decompression of spinal nerve root at different level from excision site

   Excludes: intervertebral chemonucleolysis (80.52)
   laminectomy for exploration of intraspinal canal (03.09)
   laminotomy for decompression of spinal nerve root only (03.09)

   80.52 Intervertebral chemonucleolysis
   With aspiration of disc fragments
   With diskography
   Injection of proteolytic enzyme into intervertebral space (chymopapain)

   Excludes: injection of anesthetic substance (03.91)
   injection of other substances (03.92)

   80.59 Other destruction of intervertebral disc
   Destruction NEC
   That by laser

80.6 Excision of semilunar cartilage of knee
   Excision of meniscus of knee

§ 80.7 Synovectomy
   Complete or partial resection of synovial membrane

   Excludes: excision of Baker's cyst (83.39)

§ 80.8 Other local excision or destruction of lesion of joint

§ 80.9 Other excision of joint

   Excludes: cheilectomy of joint (77.80–77.89)
   excision of bone ends (77.80–77.89)

81 Repair and plastic operations on joint structures

81.0 Spinal fusion
   Includes: arthrodesis of spine with:
   - bone graft
   - internal fixation

   81.00 Spinal fusion, not otherwise specified

   81.01 Atlas-axis spine fusion
   Craniocervical fusion
   C1-C2 fusion   } by anterior transoral or
   Occiput-C2 fusion   } posterior technique

   Excludes: that for pseudarthrosis (81.09)

   81.02 Other cervical fusion, anterior technique
   Arthrodesis of C2 level or below:
   - anterior (interbody) technique
   - anterolateral technique

   Excludes: that for pseudarthrosis (81.09)

   81.03 Other cervical fusion, posterior technique
   Arthrodesis of C2 level or below:
   - posterior (interbody) technique
   - posterolateral technique

   Excludes: that for pseudarthrosis (81.09)

---

§ Requires fourth-digit. See above for definitions.

81.04 Dorsal and dorsolumbar fusion, anterior technique
Arthrodesis of thoracic or thoracolumbar region:
anterior (interbody) technique
anterolateral technique

> Excludes: that for pseudarthrosis (81.09)

81.05 Dorsal and dorsolumbar fusion, posterior technique
Arthrodesis of thoracic or thoracolumbar region:
posterior (interbody) technique
posterolateral technique

> Excludes: that for pseudarthrosis (81.09)

81.06 Lumbar and lumbosacral fusion, anterior technique
Arthrodesis of lumbar or lumbosacral region:
anterior (interbody) technique
anterolateral technique

> Excludes: that for pseudarthrosis (81.09)

81.07 Lumbar and lumbosacral fusion, lateral transverse process technique

> Excludes: that for pseudarthrosis (81.09)

81.08 Lumbar and lumbosacral fusion, posterior technique
Arthrodesis of lumbar or lumbosacral region:
posterior (interbody) technique
posterolateral technique

81.09 Refusion of spine, any level or technique
Correction of pseudarthrosis of spine

81.1 Arthrodesis of foot and ankle
Includes: arthrodesis of foot and ankle with:
bone graft
external fixation device

81.11 Ankle fusion
Tibiotalar fusion

81.12 Triple arthrodesis
Talus to calcaneus and calcaneus to cuboid and navicular

81.13 Subtalar fusion

81.14 Midtarsal fusion

81.15 Tarsometatarsal fusion

81.16 Metatarsophalangeal fusion

81.17 Other fusion of foot

81.2 Arthrodesis of other joint
Includes: arthrodesis with:
bone graft
external fixation device
excision of bone ends and compression

81.20 Arthrodesis of unspecified joint

81.21 Arthrodesis of hip

81.22 Arthrodesis of knee

81.23 Arthrodesis of shoulder

81.24 Arthrodesis of elbow

81.25 Carporadial fusion

81.26 Metacarpocarpal fusion

81.27 Metacarpophalangeal fusion

81.28 Interphalangeal fusion

81.29 Arthrodesis of other specified joints

81.4 Other repair of joint of lower extremity
Includes: arthroplasty of lower extremity with:
external traction or fixation
graft of bone (chips) or cartilage
internal fixation device

81.40 Repair of hip, not elsewhere classified

81.42 Five-in-one repair of knee
Medial meniscectomy, medial collateral ligament repair, vastus medialis advancement, semitendinosus advancement, and pes anserinus transfer

81.43 Triad knee repair
Medial meniscectomy with repair of the anterior cruciate ligament and the medial collateral ligament
O'Donoghue procedure

81.44 Patellar stabilization
Roux-Goldthwait operation for recurrent dislocation of patella

81.45 Other repair of the cruciate ligaments

81.46 Other repair of the collateral ligaments

81.47 Other repair of knee

81.49 Other repair of ankle

81.5 Joint replacement of lower extremity
Includes: arthroplasty of lower extremity with:
external traction or fixation
graft of bone (chips) or cartilage
internal fixation device or prosthesis

81.51 Total hip replacement BIL
Replacement of both femoral head and acetabulum by prosthesis
Total reconstruction of hip

81.52 Partial hip replacement BIL
Bipolar endoprosthesis

81.53 Revision of hip replacement BIL
Partial
Total

81.54 Total knee replacement BIL
Bicompartmental
Tricompartmental
Unicompartmental (hemijoint)

81.55 Revision of knee replacement BIL

> Excludes: arthrodesis of knee (81.22)

81.56 Total ankle replacement

81.57 Replacement of joint of foot and toe

81.59 Revision of joint replacement of lower extremity, not elsewhere classified

81.7 Arthroplasty and repair of hand, fingers, and wrist
Includes: arthroplasty of hand and finger with:
external traction or fixation
graft of bone (chips) or cartilage
internal fixation device or prosthesis

> Excludes: operations on muscle, tendon, and fascia of hand (82.01–82.99)

81.71 Arthroplasty of metacarpophalangeal and interphalangeal joint with implant

81.72 Arthroplasty of metacarpophalangeal and interphalangeal joint without implant

81.73 Total wrist replacement

81.74 Arthroplasty of carpocarpal or carpometacarpal joint with implant

81.75 Arthroplasty of carpocarpal or carpometacarpal joint without implant

81.79 Other repair of hand, fingers, and wrist

81.8 Arthroplasty and repair of shoulder and elbow
Includes: arthroplasty of upper limb NEC with:
  external traction or fixation
  graft of bone (chips) or cartilage
  internal fixation device or prosthesis

81.80 Total shoulder replacement
81.81 Partial shoulder replacement
81.82 Repair of recurrent dislocation of shoulder
81.83 Other repair of shoulder
Revision of arthroplasty of shoulder
81.84 Total elbow replacement
81.85 Other repair of elbow

81.9 Other operations on joint structures

81.91 Arthrocentesis
Joint aspiration

Excludes: that for:
  arthrography (88.32)
  biopsy of joint structure (80.30–80.39)
  injection of drug (81.92)

81.92 Injection of therapeutic substance into joint or ligament

81.93 Suture of capsule or ligament of upper extremity

Excludes: that associated with arthroplasty
  (81.71–81.75, 81.80–81.81, 81.84)

81.94 Suture of capsule or ligament of ankle and foot

Excludes: that associated with arthroplasty
  (81.56–81.59)

81.95 Suture of capsule or ligament of other lower extremity

Excludes: that associated with arthroplasty
  (81.51–81.55, 81.59)

81.96 Other repair of joint

81.97 Revision of joint replacement of upper extremity
Partial
Total

81.98 Other diagnostic procedures on joint structures

Excludes: arthroscopy (80.20–80.29)
  biopsy of joint structure (80.30–80.39)
  microscopic examination of specimen from
    joint (91.51–91.59)
  thermography (88.83)
  x-ray (87.21–87.29, 88.21–88.33)

81.99 Other

82 Operations on muscle, tendon, and fascia of hand
Includes: operations on:
  aponeurosis
  synovial membrane (tendon sheath)
  tendon sheath

82.0 Incision of muscle, tendon, fascia, and bursa of hand

82.01 Exploration of tendon sheath of hand
Incision of tendon sheath } tendon sheath of hand
Removal of rice bodies in

Excludes: division of tendon (82.11)

82.02 Myotomy of hand

Excludes: myotomy for division (82.19)

82.03 Bursotomy of hand
82.04 Incision and drainage of palmar or thenar space
82.09 Other incision of soft tissue of hand

Excludes: incision of skin and subcutaneous tissue
  alone (86.01–86.09)

82.1 Division of muscle, tendon, and fascia of hand

82.11 Tenotomy of hand
Division of tendon of hand

82.12 Fasciotomy of hand
Division of fascia of hand

82.19 Other division of soft tissue of hand
Division of muscle of hand

82.2 Excision of lesion of muscle, tendon, and fascia of hand

82.21 Excision of lesion of tendon sheath of hand
Ganglionectomy of tendon sheath (wrist)

82.22 Excision of lesion of muscle of hand

82.29 Excision of other lesion of soft tissue of hand

Excludes: excision of lesion of skin and
  subcutaneous tissue (86.21–86.3)

82.3 Other excision of soft tissue of hand

Code also any skin graft (86.61–86.62, 86.73)

Excludes: excision of skin and subcutaneous tissue
  (86.21–86.3)

82.31 Bursectomy of hand
82.32 Excision of tendon of hand for graft
82.33 Other tenonectomy of hand
Tenosynovectomy of hand

Excludes: excision of lesion of:
  tendon (82.29)
  sheath (82.21)

82.34 Excision of muscle or fascia of hand for graft
82.35 Other fasciectomy of hand
Release of Dupuytren's contracture

Excludes: excision of lesion of fascia (82.29)

82.36 Other myectomy of hand

Excludes: excision of lesion of muscle (82.22)

82.39 Other excision of soft tissue of hand

Excludes: excision of skin (86.21–86.3)
  excision of soft tissue lesion (82.29)

82.4 Suture of muscle, tendon, and fascia of hand

82.41 Suture of tendon sheath of hand
82.42 Delayed suture of flexor tendon of hand
82.43 Delayed suture of other tendon of hand
82.44 Other suture of flexor tendon of hand

Excludes: delayed suture of flexor tendon of hand
  (82.42)

82.45 Other suture of other tendon of hand

Excludes: delayed suture of other tendon of hand
  (82.43)

82.46 Suture of muscle or fascia of hand

82.5 Transplantation of muscle and tendon of hand

82.51 Advancement of tendon of hand
82.52 Recession of tendon of hand
82.53 Reattachment of tendon of hand
82.54 Reattachment of muscle of hand
82.55 Other change in hand muscle or tendon length

82.56 Other hand tendon transfer or transplantation

> Excludes: pollicization of thumb (82.61)
> transfer of finger, except thumb (82.81)

82.57 Other hand tendon transposition

82.58 Other hand muscle transfer or transplantation

82.59 Other hand muscle transposition

82.6 Reconstruction of thumb
Includes: digital transfer to act as thumb

Code also any amputation for digital transfer (84.01, 84.11)

82.61 Pollicization operation carrying over nerves and blood supply

82.69 Other reconstruction of thumb
"Cocked-hat" procedure [skin flap and bone]
Grafts:
bone
skin (pedicle) } to thumb

82.7 Plastic operation on hand with graft or implant

82.71 Tendon pulley reconstruction
Reconstruction for opponensplasty

82.72 Plastic operation on hand with graft of muscle or fascia

82.79 Plastic operation on hand with other graft or implant
Tendon graft to hand

82.8 Other plastic operations on hand

82.81 Transfer of finger, except thumb

> Excludes: pollicization of thumb (82.61)

82.82 Repair of cleft hand

82.83 Repair of macrodactyly

82.84 Repair of mallet finger

82.85 Other tenodesis of hand
Tendon fixation of hand NOS

82.86 Other tenoplasty of hand
Myotenoplasty of hand

82.89 Other plastic operations on hand
Plication of fascia
Repair of fascial hernia

> Excludes: that with graft or implant (82.71–82.79)

82.9 Other operations on muscle, tendon, and fascia of hand

> Excludes: diagnostic procedures on soft tissue of hand (83.21–83.29)

82.91 Lysis of adhesions of hand
Freeing of adhesions of fascia, muscle, and tendon of hand

> Excludes: decompression of carpal tunnel (04.43)
> that by stretching or manipulation only (93.26)

82.92 Aspiration of bursa of hand

82.93 Aspiration of other soft tissue of hand

> Excludes: skin and subcutaneous tissue (86.01)

82.94 Injection of therapeutic substance into bursa of hand

82.95 Injection of therapeutic substance into tendon of hand

82.96 Other injection of locally acting therapeutic substance into soft tissue of hand

> Excludes: subcutaneous or intramuscular injection (99.11–99.29)

82.99 Other operations on muscle, tendon, and fascia of hand

83 Operations on muscle, tendon, fascia, and bursa, except hand
Includes: operations on:
aponeurosis
synovial membrane of bursa and tendon sheaths
tendon sheaths

> Excludes: diaphragm (34.81–34.89)
> hand (82.01–82.99)
> muscles of eye (15.01–15.9)

83.0 Incision of muscle, tendon, fascia, and bursa

83.01 Exploration of tendon sheath
Incision of tendon sheath
Removal of rice bodies from tendon sheath

83.02 Myotomy

> Excludes: cricopharyngeal myotomy (29.31)

83.03 Bursotomy
Removal of calcareous deposit of bursa

> Excludes: aspiration of bursa (percutaneous) (83.94)

83.09 Other incision of soft tissue
Incision of fascia

> Excludes: incision of skin and subcutaneous tissue alone (86.01–86.09)

83.1 Division of muscle, tendon, and fascia

83.11 Achillotenotomy

83.12 Adductor tenotomy of hip

83.13 Other tenotomy
Aponeurotomy
Division of tendon
Tendon release
Tendon transection
Tenotomy for thoracic outlet decompression

83.14 Fasciotomy
Division of fascia
Division of iliotibial band
Fascia stripping
Release of Volkmann's contracture by fasciotomy

83.19 Other division of soft tissue
Division of muscle
Muscle release
Myotomy for thoracic outlet decompression
Myotomy with division
Scalenotomy
Transection of muscle

83.2 Diagnostic procedures on muscle, tendon, fascia, and bursa, including that of hand

83.21 Biopsy of soft tissue

> Excludes: biopsy of chest wall (34.23)
> biopsy of skin and subcutaneous tissue (86.11)

83.29 Other diagnostic procedures on muscle, tendon, fascia, and bursa, including that of hand

> Excludes: microscopic examination of specimen (91.51–91.59)
> soft tissue x-ray (87.09, 87.38–87.39, 88.09, 88.35, 88.37)
> thermography of muscle (88.84)

83.3 Excision of lesion of muscle, tendon, fascia, and bursa

> Excludes: biopsy of soft tissue (83.21)

83.31 Excision of lesion of tendon sheath
Excision of ganglion of tendon sheath, except of hand

OPERATIONS ON THE MUSCULOSKELETAL SYSTEM (76-84)

83.32 Excision of lesion of muscle
Excision of:
heterotopic bone
muscle scar for release of Volkmann's contracture
myositis ossificans

83.39 Excision of lesion of other soft tissue
Excision of Baker's cyst

Excludes: bursectomy (83.5)
excision of lesion of skin and subcutaneous tissue (86.3)
synovectomy (80.70–80.79)

83.4 Other excision of muscle, tendon, and fascia

83.41 Excision of tendon for graft

83.42 Other tenonectomy
Excision of:
aponeurosis
tendon sheath
Tenosynovectomy

83.43 Excision of muscle or fascia for graft

83.44 Other fasciectomy

83.45 Other myectomy
Debridement of muscle NOS
Scalenectomy

83.49 Other excision of soft tissue

83.5 Bursectomy

83.6 Suture of muscle, tendon, and fascia

83.61 Suture of tendon sheath

83.62 Delayed suture of tendon

83.63 Rotator cuff repair

83.64 Other suture of tendon
Achillorrhaphy
Aponeurorrhaphy

Excludes: delayed suture of tendon (83.62)

83.65 Other suture of muscle or fascia
Repair of diastasis recti

83.7 Reconstruction of muscle and tendon

Excludes: reconstruction of muscle and tendon associated with arthroplasty

83.71 Advancement of tendon

83.72 Recession of tendon

83.73 Reattachment of tendon

83.74 Reattachment of muscle

83.75 Tendon transfer or transplantation

83.76 Other tendon transposition

83.77 Muscle transfer or transplantation
Release of Volkmann's contracture by muscle transplantation

83.79 Other muscle transposition

83.8 Other plastic operations on muscle, tendon, and fascia

Excludes: plastic operations on muscle, tendon, and fascia associated with arthroplasty

83.81 Tendon graft

83.82 Graft of muscle or fascia

83.83 Tendon pulley reconstruction

83.84 Release of clubfoot, not elsewhere classified
Evans operation on clubfoot

83.85 Other change in muscle or tendon length
Hamstring lengthening
Heel cord shortening
Plastic achillotenotomy
Tendon plication

83.86 Quadricepsplasty

83.87 Other plastic operations on muscle
Musculoplasty
Myoplasty

83.88 Other plastic operations on tendon
Myotenoplasty
Tendon fixation
Tenodesis
Tenoplasty

83.89 Other plastic operations on fascia
Fascia lengthening
Fascioplasty
Plication of fascia

83.9 Other operations on muscle, tendon, fascia, and bursa

Excludes: nonoperative:
manipulation (93.24–93.29)
stretching (93.27–93.29)

83.91 Lysis of adhesions of muscle, tendon, fascia, and bursa

Excludes: that for tarsal tunnel syndrome (04.44)

83.92 Insertion or replacement of skeletal muscle stimulator

83.93 Removal of skeletal muscle stimulator

83.94 Aspiration of bursa

83.95 Aspiration of other soft tissue

Excludes: that of skin and subcutaneous tissue (86.01)

83.96 Injection of therapeutic substance into bursa

83.97 Injection of therapeutic substance into tendon

83.98 Injection of locally-acting therapeutic substance into other soft tissue

Excludes: subcutaneous or intramuscular injection (99.11–99.29)

83.99 Other operations on muscle, tendon, fascia, and bursa
Suture of bursa

84 Other procedures on musculoskeletal system

84.0 Amputation of upper limb

Excludes: revision of amputation stump (84.3)

84.00 Upper limb amputation, not otherwise specified
Closed flap amputation
Kineplastic amputation
Open or guillotine amputation } of upper limb NOS
Revision of current traumatic amputation

84.01 Amputation and disarticulation of finger

Excludes: ligation of supernumerary finger (86.26)

84.02 Amputation and disarticulation of thumb

84.03 Amputation through hand
Amputation through carpals

84.04 Disarticulation of wrist

84.05 Amputation through forearm
Forearm amputation

84.06 Disarticulation of elbow

84.07 Amputation through humerus
Upper arm amputation

84.08 Disarticulation of shoulder

84.09 Interthoracoscapular amputation
Forequarter amputation

84.1 Amputation of lower limb

> Excludes: revision of amputation stump (84.3)

84.10 Lower limb amputation, not otherwise specified
Closed flap amputation
Kineplastic amputation
Open or guillotine amputation } of lower limb NOS
Revision of current traumatic amputation

84.11 Amputation of toe
Amputation through metatarsophalangeal joint
Disarticulation of toe

> Excludes: ligation of supernumerary toe (86.26)

84.12 Amputation through forefoot
Amputation of forefoot
Amputation through middle of foot
Chopart's amputation
Midtarsal amputation
Transmetatarsal amputation

84.13 Disarticulation of ankle

84.14 Amputation of ankle through malleoli of tibia and fibula

84.15 Other amputation below knee
Amputation of leg through tibia and fibula NOS

84.16 Disarticulation of knee
Batch, Spitler, and McFaddin amputation
Mazet amputation
S.P. Roger's amputation

84.17 Amputation above knee
Amputation of leg through femur
Amputation of thigh
Conversion of below-knee amputation into above-knee amputation
Supracondylar above-knee amputation

84.18 Disarticulation of hip

84.19 Abdominopelvic amputation
Hemipelvectomy
Hindquarter amputation

84.2 Reattachment of extremity

84.21 Thumb reattachment

84.22 Finger reattachment

84.23 Forearm, wrist, or hand reattachment

84.24 Upper arm reattachment
Reattachment of arm NOS

84.25 Toe reattachment

84.26 Foot reattachment

84.27 Lower leg or ankle reattachment
Reattachment of leg NOS

84.28 Thigh reattachment

84.29 Other reattachment

84.3 Revision of amputation stump
Reamputation
Secondary closure } of stump
Trimming

> Excludes: revision of current traumatic amputation [revision by further amputation of current injury] (84.00–84.19, 84.91)

84.4 Implantation or fitting of prosthetic limb device

84.40 Implantation or fitting of prosthetic limb device, not otherwise specified

84.41 Fitting of prosthesis of upper arm and shoulder

84.42 Fitting of prosthesis of lower arm and hand

84.43 Fitting of prosthesis of arm, not otherwise specified

84.44 Implantation of prosthetic device of arm

84.45 Fitting of prosthesis above knee

84.46 Fitting of prosthesis below knee

84.47 Fitting of prosthesis of leg, not otherwise specified

84.48 Implantation of prosthetic device of leg

84.9 Other operations on musculoskeletal system

> Excludes: nonoperative manipulation (93.25–93.29)

84.91 Amputation, not otherwise specified

84.92 Separation of equal conjoined twins

84.93 Separation of unequal conjoined twins
Separation of conjoined twins NOS

84.99 Other

15. OPERATIONS ON THE INTEGUMENTARY SYSTEM (85–86)

85 Operations on the breast

Includes: operations on the skin and subcutaneous tissue of:
 breast
 previous mastectomy site } female or male
 revision of previous mastectomy site

85.0 Mastotomy
Incision of breast (skin)
Mammotomy

Excludes: aspiration of breast (85.91)
 removal of implant (85.94)

85.1 Diagnostic procedures on breast

85.11 Closed [percutaneous] [needle] biopsy of breast

85.12 Open biopsy of breast

85.19 Other diagnostic procedures on breast

Excludes: mammary ductogram (87.35)
 mammography NEC (87.37)
 manual examination (89.36)
 microscopic examination of specimen (91.61–91.69)
 thermography (88.85)
 ultrasonography (88.73)
 xerography (87.36)

85.2 Excision or destruction of breast tissue

Excludes: mastectomy (85.41–85.48)
 reduction mammoplasty (85.31–85.32)

85.20 Excision or destruction of breast tissue, not otherwise specified

85.21 Local excision of lesion of breast
Lumpectomy
Removal of area of fibrosis from breast

Excludes: biopsy of breast (85.11–85.12)

85.22 Resection of quadrant of breast

85.23 Subtotal mastectomy

Excludes: quadrant resection (85.22)

85.24 Excision of ectopic breast tissue
Excision of accessory nipple

85.25 Excision of nipple

Excludes: excision of accessory nipple (85.24)

85.3 Reduction mammoplasty and subcutaneous mammectomy

85.31 Unilateral reduction mammoplasty
Unilateral:
 amputative mammoplasty
 size reduction mammoplasty

85.32 Bilateral reduction mammoplasty
Amputative mammoplasty
Reduction mammoplasty (for gynecomastia)

85.33 Unilateral subcutaneous mammectomy with synchronous implant

Excludes: that without synchronous implant (85.34)

85.34 Other unilateral subcutaneous mammectomy
Removal of breast tissue with preservation of skin and nipple
Subcutaneous mammectomy NOS

85.35 Bilateral subcutaneous mammectomy with synchronous implant

Excludes: what without synchronous implant (85.36)

85.36 Other bilateral subcutaneous mammectomy

85.4 Mastectomy

85.41 Unilateral simple mastectomy
Mastectomy:
 NOS
 complete

85.42 Bilateral simple mastectomy
Bilateral complete mastectomy

85.43 Unilateral extended simple mastectomy
Extended simple mastectomy NOS
Modified radical mastectomy
Simple mastectomy with excision of regional lymph nodes

85.44 Bilateral extended simple mastectomy

85.45 Unilateral radical mastectomy
Excision of breast, pectoral muscles, and regional lymph nodes [axillary, clavicular, supraclavicular]
Radical mastectomy NOS

85.46 Bilateral radical mastectomy

85.47 Unilateral extended radical mastectomy
Excision of breast, muscles, and lymph nodes [axillary, clavicular, supraclavicular, internal mammary, and mediastinal]
Extended radical mastectomy NOS

85.48 Bilateral extended radical mastectomy

85.5 Augmentation mammoplasty

Excludes: that associated with subcutaneous mammectomy (85.33, 85.35)

85.50 Augmentation mammoplasty, not otherwise specified

85.51 Unilateral injection into breast for augmentation

85.52 Bilateral injection into breast for augmentation
Injection into breast for augmentation NOS

85.53 Unilateral breast implant

85.54 Bilateral breast implant
Breast implant NOS

85.6 Mastopexy

85.7 Total reconstruction of breast

85.8 Other repair and plastic operations on breast

Excludes: that for:
 augmentation (85.50–85.54)
 reconstruction (85.7)
 reduction (85.31–85.32)

85.81 Suture of laceration of breast

85.82 Split-thickness graft to breast

85.83 Full-thickness graft to breast

85.84 Pedicle graft to breast

85.85 Muscle flap graft to breast

85.86 Transposition of nipple

85.87 Other repair or reconstruction of nipple

85.89 Other mammoplasty

85.9 Other operations on the breast

85.91 Aspiration of breast

> Excludes: percutaneous biopsy of breast (85.11)

85.92 Injection of therapeutic agent into breast

> Excludes: that for augmentation of breast (85.51–85.52)

85.93 Revision of implant of breast

85.94 Removal of implant of breast

85.95 Insertion of breast tissue expander
Insertion (soft tissue) of tissue expander (one or more) under muscle or platysma to develop skin flaps for donor use

85.96 Removal of breast tissue expander(s)

85.99 Other

86 Operations on skin and subcutaneous tissue

Includes: operations on:
 hair follicles
 male perineum
 nails
 sebaceous glands
 subcutaneous fat pads
 sudoriferous glands
 superficial fossae

> Excludes: those on skin of:
> anus (49.01–49.99)
> breast (mastectomy site) (85.0–85.99)
> ear (18.01–18.9)
> eyebrow (08.01–08.99)
> eyelid (08.01–08.99)
> female perineum (71.01–71.9)
> lips (27.0–27.99)
> nose (21.00–21.99)
> penis (64.0–64.99)
> scrotum (61.0–61.99)
> vulva (71.01–71.9)

86.0 Incision of skin and subcutaneous tissue

86.01 Aspiration of skin and subcutaneous tissue
Aspiration of:
 abscess
 hematoma } of nail, skin, or subcutaneous tissue
 seroma

86.02 Injection or tattooing of skin lesion or defect
Injection } of filling material
Insertion
Pigmenting of skin

86.03 Incision of pilonidal sinus or cyst

> Excludes: marsupialization (86.21)

86.04 Other incision with drainage of skin and subcutaneous tissue

> Excludes: drainage of:
> fascial compartments of face and mouth (27.0)
> palmar or thenar space (82.04)
> pilonidal sinus or cyst (86.03)

86.05 Incision with removal of foreign body from skin and subcutaneous tissue
Removal of tissue expander(s) from skin or soft tissue other than breast tissue

> Excludes: removal of foreign body without incision (98.20–98.29)

86.06 Insertion of totally implantable infusion pump
Code also any associated catheterization

> Excludes: insertion of totally implantable vascular access device (86.07)

86.07 Insertion of totally implantable vascular access device [VAD] NOR
Totally implanted port

> Excludes: insertion of totally implantable infusion pump (86.06)

86.09 Other incision of skin and subcutaneous tissue NOR
Exploration:
 superficial fossa
 sinus tract, skin
Undercutting of hair follicle

> Excludes: that of fascial compartments of face and mouth (27.0)

86.1 Diagnostic procedures on skin and subcutaneous tissue

86.11 Biopsy of skin and subcutaneous tissue

86.19 Other diagnostic procedures on skin and subcutaneous tissue

> Excludes: microscopic examination of specimen from skin and subcutaneous tissue (91.61–91.79)

86.2 Excision or destruction of lesion or tissue of skin and subcutaneous tissue

86.21 Excision of pilonidal cyst or sinus
Marsupialization of cyst

> Excludes: incision of pilonidal cyst or sinus (86.03)

86.22 Excisional debridement of wound, infection, or burn
Removal by excision of:
 devitalized tissue
 necrosis
 slough

> Excludes: debridement of:
> abdominal wall (wound) (54.3)
> bone (77.60–77.69)
> muscle (83.45)
>   of hand (82.36)
> nail (bed) (fold) (86.27)
> nonexcisional debridement of wound, infection, or burn (86.28)
> open fracture site (79.60–79.69)
> pedicle or flap graft (86.75)

86.23 Removal of nail, nailbed, or nail fold

86.24 Chemosurgery of skin
Chemical peel of skin

86.25 Dermabrasion
That with laser

> Excludes: dermabrasion of wound to remove embedded debris (86.28)

86.26 Ligation of dermal appendage

> Excludes: excision of preauricular appendage (18.29)

86.27 Debridement of nail, nailbed, or nail fold
Removal of:
 necrosis
 slough

> Excludes: removal of nail, nailbed, or nail fold (86.23)

OPERATIONS ON THE INTEGUMENTARY SYSTEM (85-86)

86.28 Nonexcisional debridement of wound, infection, or burn
Debridement NOS
Removal of devitalized tissue, necrosis, and slough by such methods as:
  brushing
  irrigation (under pressure)
  scrubbing
  washing

86.3 Other local excision or destruction of lesion or tissue of skin and subcutaneous tissue NOR
Destruction of skin by:
  cauterization
  cryosurgery
  fulguration
  laser beam
That with Z-plasty

Excludes: adipectomy (86.83)
  biopsy of skin (86.11)
  wide or radical excision of skin (86.4)
  Z-plasty without excision (86.84)

86.4 Radical excision of skin lesion
Wide excision of skin lesion involving underlying or adjacent structure

Code also any lymph node dissection (40.3–40.5)

86.5 Suture of skin and subcutaneous tissue

86.51 Replantation of scalp

86.59 Suture of skin and subcutaneous tissue of other sites

86.6 Free skin graft
Includes: excision of skin for autogenous graft

Excludes: construction or reconstruction of:
  penis (64.43–64.44)
  trachea (31.75)
  vagina (70.61–70.62)

86.60 Free skin graft, not otherwise specified

86.61 Full-thickness skin graft to hand

Excludes: heterograft (86.65)
  homograft (86.66)

86.62 Other skin graft to hand

Excludes: heterograft (86.65)
  homograft (86.66)

86.63 Full-thickness skin graft to other sites

Excludes: heterograft (86.65)
  homograft (86.66)

86.64 Hair transplant

Excludes: hair follicle transplant to eyebrow or eyelash (08.63)

86.65 Heterograft to skin
Pigskin graft
Porcine graft

86.66 Homograft to skin
Graft to skin of:
  amnionic membrane } from donor
  skin

86.69 Other skin graft to other sites

Excludes: heterograft (86.65)
  homograft (86.66)

86.7 Pedicle grafts or flaps

Excludes: construction or reconstruction of:
  penis (64.43–64.44)
  trachea (31.75)
  vagina (70.61–70.62)

86.70 Pedicle or flap graft, not otherwise specified

86.71 Cutting and preparation of pedicle grafts or flaps
Elevation of pedicle from its bed
Flap design and raising
Partial cutting of pedicle or tube
Pedicle delay

Excludes: pollicization or digital transfer (82.61, 82.81)
  revision of pedicle (86.75)

86.72 Advancement of pedicle graft

86.73 Attachment of pedicle or flap graft to hand

Excludes: pollicization or digital transfer (82.61, 82.81)

86.74 Attachment of pedicle or flap graft to other sites
Attachment by: Attachment by:
  advanced flap   rotating flap
  double pedicled flap   sliding flap
  pedicle graft   tube graft

86.75 Revision of pedicle or flap graft
Debridement   } of pedicle or flap graft
Defatting

86.8 Other repair and reconstruction of skin and subcutaneous tissue

86.81 Repair for facial weakness

86.82 Facial rhytidectomy
Face lift

Excludes: rhytidectomy of eyelid (08.86–08.87)

86.83 Size reduction plastic operation
Reduction of adipose tissue of:
  abdominal wall (pendulous)
  arms (batwing)
  buttock
  thighs (trochanteric lipomatosis)

Excludes: breast (85.31–85.32)

86.84 Relaxation of scar or web contracture of skin
Z-plasty of skin

Excludes: Z-plasty with excision of lesion (86.3)

86.85 Correction of syndactyly

86.86 Onychoplasty

86.89 Other repair and reconstruction of skin and subcutaneous tissue

Excludes: mentoplasty (76.67–76.68)

86.9 Other operations on skin and subcutaneous tissue

86.91 Excision of skin for graft
Excision of skin with closure of donor site

Excludes: that with graft at same operative episode (86.60–86.69)

86.92 Electrolysis and other epilation of skin

Excludes: epilation of eyelid (08.91–08.93)

86.93 Insertion of tissue expander
Insertion (subcutaneous) (soft tissue) of expander (one or more) in scalp (subgaleal space), face, neck, trunk except breast, and upper and lower extremities for development of skin flaps for donor use

Excludes: *flap graft preparation (86.71)*
tissue expander, breast (85.95)

86.99 Other

Excludes: *removal of sutures from:*
   abdomen (97.83)
   head and neck (97.38)
   thorax (97.43)
   trunk NEC (97.84)
wound catheter:
   irrigation (96.58)
   replacement (97.15)

16. MISCELLANEOUS DIAGNOSTIC AND THERAPEUTIC PROCEDURES (87–99)

87 Diagnostic radiology

87.0 Soft tissue x-ray of face, head, and neck

Excludes: angiography (88.40–88.68)

- **87.01** Pneumoencephalogram
- **87.02** Other contrast radiogram of brain and skull
  - Pneumocisternogram
  - Pneumoventriculogram
  - Posterior fossa myelogram
- **87.03** Computerized axial tomography of head
  - C.A.T. scan of head
- **87.04** Other tomography of head
- **87.05** Contrast dacryocystogram
- **87.06** Contrast radiogram of nasopharynx
- **87.07** Contrast laryngogram
- **87.08** Cervical lymphangiogram
- **87.09** Other soft tissue x-ray of face, head, and neck
  - Noncontrast x-ray of:
    - adenoid
    - larynx
    - nasolacrimal duct
    - nasopharynx
    - salivary gland
    - thyroid region
    - uvula

Excludes: x-ray study of eye (95.14)

87.1 Other x-ray of face, head, and neck

Excludes: angiography (88.40–88.68)

- **87.11** Full-mouth x-ray of teeth
- **87.12** Other dental x-ray
  - Orthodontic cephalogram or cephalometrics
  - Panorex examination of mandible
  - Root canal x-ray
- **87.13** Temporomandibular contrast arthrogram
- **87.14** Contrast radiogram of orbit
- **87.15** Contrast radiogram of sinus
- **87.16** Other x-ray of facial bones
  - X-ray of:
    - frontal area
    - mandible
    - maxilla
    - nasal sinuses
    - nose
    - orbit
    - supraorbital area
    - symphysis menti
    - zygomaticomaxillary complex
- **87.17** Other x-ray of skull
  - Lateral projection ⎫
  - Sagittal projection ⎬ of skull
  - Tangential projection ⎭

87.2 X-ray of spine

- **87.21** Contrast myelogram
- **87.22** Other x-ray of cervical spine
- **87.23** Other x-ray of thoracic spine
- **87.24** Other x-ray of lumbosacral spine
  - Sacrococcygeal x-ray
- **87.29** Other x-ray of spine
  - Spinal x-ray NOS

87.3 Soft tissue x-ray of thorax

Excludes: angiocardiography (88.50–88.58)
angiography (88.40–88.68)

- **87.31** Endotracheal bronchogram
- **87.32** Other contrast bronchogram
  - Transcricoid bronchogram
- **87.33** Mediastinal pneumogram
- **87.34** Intrathoracic lymphangiogram
- **87.35** Contrast radiogram of mammary ducts
- **87.36** Xerography of breast
- **87.37** Other mammography
- **87.38** Sinogram of chest wall
  - Fistulogram of chest wall
- **87.39** Other soft tissue x-ray of chest wall

87.4 Other x-ray of thorax

Excludes: angiocardiography (88.50–88.58)
angiography (88.40–88.68)

- **87.41** Computerized axial tomography of thorax
  - C.A.T. scan ⎫
  - Crystal linea scan of x-ray beam ⎪
  - Electronic substraction ⎬ of thorax
  - Photoelectric response ⎪
  - Tomography with use of computer, x-rays, and camera ⎭
- **87.42** Other tomography of thorax
  - Cardiac tomogram
- **87.43** X-ray of ribs, sternum, and clavicle
  - Examination for:
    - cervical rib
    - fracture
- **87.44** Routine chest x-ray, so described
  - X-ray of chest NOS
- **87.49** Other chest x-ray
  - X-ray of:
    - bronchus NOS
    - diaphragm NOS
    - heart NOS
    - lung NOS
    - mediastinum NOS
    - trachea NOS

87.5 Biliary tract x-ray

- **87.51** Percutaneous hepatic cholangiogram
- **87.52** Intravenous cholangiogram
- **87.53** Intraoperative cholangiogram
- **87.54** Other cholangiogram
- **87.59** Other biliary tract x-ray
  - Cholecystogram

87.6 Other x-ray of digestive system

- **87.61** Barium swallow
- **87.62** Upper GI series
- **87.63** Small bowel series
- **87.64** Lower GI series
- **87.65** Other x-ray of intestine
- **87.66** Contrast pancreatogram
- **87.69** Other digestive tract x-ray

87.7 X-ray of urinary system

> Excludes: angiography of renal vessels (88.45, 88.65)

87.71 Computerized axial tomography of kidney
C.A.T scan of kidney

87.72 Other nephrotomogram

87.73 Intravenous pyelogram
Diuretic infusion pyelogram

87.74 Retrograde pyelogram

87.75 Percutaneous pyelogram

87.76 Retrograde cystourethrogram

87.77 Other cystogram

87.78 Ileal conduitogram

87.79 Other x-ray of the urinary system
KUB x-ray

87.8 X-ray of female genital organs

87.81 X-ray of gravid uterus ♀
Intrauterine cephalometry by x-ray

87.82 Gas contrast hysterosalpingogram ♀

87.83 Opaque dye contrast hysterosalpingogram ♀

87.84 Percutaneous hysterogram ♀

87.85 Other x-ray of fallopian tubes and uterus ♀

87.89 Other x-ray of female genital organs ♀

87.9 X-ray of male genital organs

87.91 Contrast seminal vesiculogram ♂

87.92 Other x-ray of prostate and seminal vesicles ♂

87.93 Contrast epididymogram ♂

87.94 Contrast vasogram ♂

87.95 Other x-ray of epididymis and vas deferens ♂

87.99 Other x-ray of male genital organs ♂

88 Other diagnostic radiology and related techniques

88.0 Soft tissue x-ray of abdomen

> Excludes: angiography (88.40–88.68)

88.01 Computerized axial tomography of abdomen
C.A.T. scan of abdomen

> Excludes: C.A.T. scan of kidney (87.71)

88.02 Other abdomen tomography

> Excludes: nephrotomogram (87.72)

88.03 Sinogram of abdominal wall
Fistulogram of abdominal wall

88.04 Abdominal lymphangiogram

88.09 Other soft tissue x-ray of abdominal wall

88.1 Other x-ray of abdomen

88.11 Pelvic opaque dye contrast radiography

88.12 Pelvic gas contrast radiography
Pelvic pneumoperitoneum

88.13 Other peritoneal pneumogram

88.14 Retroperitoneal fistulogram

88.15 Retroperitoneal pneumogram

88.16 Other retroperitoneal x-ray

88.19 Other x-ray of abdomen
Flat plate of abdomen

88.2 Skeletal x-ray of extremities and pelvis

> Excludes: contrast radiogram of joint (88.32)

88.21 Skeletal x-ray of shoulder and upper arm

88.22 Skeletal x-ray of elbow and forearm

88.23 Skeletal x-ray of wrist and hand

88.24 Skeletal x-ray of upper limb, not otherwise specified

88.25 Pelvimetry

88.26 Other skeletal x-ray of pelvis and hip

88.27 Skeletal x-ray of thigh, knee, and lower leg

88.28 Skeletal x-ray of ankle and foot

88.29 Skeletal x-ray of lower limb, not otherwise specified

88.3 Other x-ray

88.31 Skeletal series
X-ray of whole skeleton

88.32 Contrast arthrogram

> Excludes: that of temporomandibular joint (87.13)

88.33 Other skeletal x-ray

> Excludes: skeletal x-ray of:
> extremities and pelvis (88.21–88.29)
> face, head, and neck (87.11–87.17)
> spine (87.21–87.29)
> thorax (87.43)

88.34 Lymphangiogram of upper limb

88.35 Other soft tissue x-ray of upper limb

88.36 Lymphangiogram of lower limb

88.37 Other soft tissue x-ray of lower limb

> Excludes: femoral angiography (88.48, 88.66)

88.38 Other computerized axial tomography
C.A.T. scan NOS

> Excludes: C.A.T. scan of:
> abdomen (88.01)
> head (87.03)
> kidney (87.71)
> thorax (87.41)

88.39 X-ray, other and unspecified

88.4 Arteriography using contrast material
Includes: angiography of arteries
arterial puncture for injection of contrast material
radiography of arteries (by fluoroscopy)
retrograde arteriography

Note: The fourth-digit subclassification identifies the site to be viewed, not the site of injection.

> Excludes: arteriography using:
> radioisotopes or radionuclides (92.01–92.19)
> ultrasound (88.71–88.79)
> fluorescein angiography of eye (95.12)

88.40 Arteriography using contrast material, unspecified site

88.41 Arteriography of cerebral arteries
Angiography of:
basilar artery
carotid (internal)
posterior cerebral circulation
vertebral artery

88.42 Aortography
Arteriography of aorta and aortic arch

88.43 Arteriography of pulmonary arteries

MISCELLANEOUS DIAGNOSTIC & THERAPEUTIC PROCEDURES (87-99)

88.44 Arteriography of other intrathoracic vessels

> Excludes: angiocardiography (88.50–88.58)
> arteriography of coronary arteries (88.55–88.57)

88.45 Arteriography of renal arteries

88.46 Arteriography of placenta ♀
Placentogram using contrast material

88.47 Arteriography of other intra-abdominal arteries

88.48 Arteriography of femoral and other lower extremity arteries

88.49 Arteriography of other specified sites

88.5 Angiocardiography using contrast material
Includes: arterial puncture and insertion of arterial catheter for injection of contrast material
cineangiocardiography
selective angiocardiography

Code also synchronous cardiac catheterization (37.21–37.23)

> Excludes: angiography of pulmonary vessels (88.43, 88.62)

88.50 Angiocardiography, not otherwise specified

88.51 Angiocardiography of venae cavae
Inferior vena cavography
Phlebography of vena cava (inferior) (superior)

88.52 Angiocardiography of right heart structures [NOR]
Angiocardiography of:
pulmonary valve
right atrium
right ventricle (outflow tract)

> Excludes: that combined with left heart angiocardiography (88.54)

88.53 Angiocardiography of left heart structures [NOR]
Angiocardiography of:
aortic valve
left atrium
left ventricle (outflow tract)

> Excludes: that combined with right heart angiocardiography (88.54)

88.54 Combined right and left heart angiocardiography [NOR]

88.55 Coronary arteriography using a single catheter [NOR]
Coronary arteriography by Sones technique
Direct selective coronary arteriography using a single catheter

88.56 Coronary arteriography using two catheters [NOR]
Coronary arteriography by:
Judkins technique
Ricketts and Abrams technique
Direct selective coronary arteriography using two catheters

88.57 Other and unspecified coronary arteriography [NOR]
Coronary arteriography NOS

88.58 Negative-contrast cardiac roentgenography [NOR]
Cardiac roentgenography with injection of carbon dioxide

88.6 Phlebography
Includes: angiography of veins
radiography of veins (by fluoroscopy)
retrograde phlebography
venipuncture for injection of contrast material
venography using contrast material

The fourth-digit subclassification (88.60–88.67) identifies the site to be viewed, not the site of injection.

> Excludes: angiography using:
> radioisotopes or radionuclides (92.01–92.19)
> ultrasound (88.71–88.79)
> fluorescein angiography of eye (95.12)

88.60 Phlebography using contrast material, unspecified site

88.61 Phlebography of veins of head and neck using contrast material

88.62 Phlebography of pulmonary veins using contrast material

88.63 Phlebography of other intrathoracic veins using contrast material

88.64 Phlebography of the portal venous system using contrast material
Splenoportogram (by splenic arteriography)

88.65 Phlebography of other intra-abdominal veins using contrast material

88.66 Phlebography of femoral and other lower extremity veins using contrast material

88.67 Phlebography of other specified sites using contrast material

88.68 Impedance phlebography

88.7 Diagnostic ultrasound
Includes: echography
ultrasonic angiography
ultrasonography

88.71 Diagnostic ultrasound of head and neck
Determination of midline shift of brain
Echoencephalography

> Excludes: eye (95.13)

88.72 Diagnostic ultrasound of heart
Echocardiography

88.73 Diagnostic ultrasound of other sites of thorax
Aortic arch
Breast } ultrasonography
Lung

88.74 Diagnostic ultrasound of digestive system

88.75 Diagnostic ultrasound of urinary system

88.76 Diagnostic ultrasound of abdomen and retroperitoneum

88.77 Diagnostic ultrasound of peripheral vascular system
Deep vein thrombosis ultrasonic scanning

88.78 Diagnostic ultrasound of gravid uterus ♀
Intrauterine cephalometry:
echo
ultrasonic
Placental localization by ultrasound

88.79 Other diagnostic ultrasound
Ultrasonography of:
multiple sites
nongravid uterus
total body

88.8 Thermography

88.81 Cerebral thermography

88.82 Ocular thermography

88.83 Bone thermography
Osteoarticular thermography

88.84 Muscle thermography

88.85 Breast thermography

88.86 Blood vessel thermography
Deep vein thermography

88.89 Thermography of other sites
Lymph gland thermography
Thermography NOS

88.9 Other diagnostic imaging

88.90 Diagnostic imaging, not elsewhere classified

88.91 Magnetic resonance imaging of brain and brain stem

88.92 Magnetic resonance imaging of chest and myocardium for evaluation of hilar and mediastinal lymphadenopathy

88.93 Magnetic resonance imaging of spinal canal
Levels:
 cervical
 lumbar (lumbosacral)
 thoracic
Spinal cord
Spine

88.94 Magnetic resonance imaging of musculoskeletal
Bone marrow blood supply
Extremities (upper) (lower)

88.95 Magnetic resonance imaging of pelvis, prostate, and bladder

88.97 Magnetic resonance imaging of other and unspecified sites
Abdomen   Neck
Face   Eye orbit

88.98 Bone mineral density studies
Dual photon absorptiometry
Quantitative computed tomography (CT) studies
Radiographic densitometry
Single photon absorptiometry

89 Interview, evaluation, consultation, and examination

89.0 Diagnostic interview, consultation, and evaluation

> Excludes: psychiatric diagnostic interview (94.11–94.19)

89.01 Interview and evaluation, described as brief
Abbreviated history and evaluation

89.02 Interview and evaluation, described as limited
Interval history and evaluation

89.03 Interview and evaluation, described as comprehensive
History and evaluation of new problem

89.04 Other interview and evaluation

89.05 Diagnostic interview and evaluation, not otherwise specified

89.06 Consultation, described as limited
Consultation on a single organ system

89.07 Consultation, described as comprehensive

89.08 Other consultation

89.09 Consultation, not otherwise specified

89.1 Anatomic and physiologic measurements and manual examinations — nervous system and sense organs

> Excludes: ear examination (95.41–95.49)
> eye examination (95.01–95.26)
> the listed procedures when done as part of a general physical examination (89.7)

89.10 Intracarotid amobarbital test
Wada test

89.11 Tonometry

89.12 Nasal function study
Rhinomanometry

89.13 Neurologic examination

89.14 Electroencephalogram

> Excludes: that with polysomnogram (89.17)

89.15 Other nonoperative neurologic function tests

89.16 Transillumination of newborn skull

89.17 Polysomnogram
Sleep recording

89.18 Other sleep disorder function tests
Multiple sleep latency test [MSLT]

89.19 Video and radio-telemetered electroencephalographic monitoring
Radiographic } EEG Monitoring
Video

89.2 Anatomic and physiologic measurements and manual examinations — genitourinary system

> Excludes: the listed procedures when done as part of a general physical examination (89.7)

89.21 Urinary manometry
Manometry through:
 indwelling ureteral catheter
 nephrostomy
 pyelostomy
 ureterostomy

89.22 Cystometrogram

89.23 Urethral sphincter electromyogram

89.24 Uroflowmetry [UFR]

89.25 Urethral pressure profile [UPP]

89.26 Gynecological examination ♀
Pelvic examination

89.29 Other nonoperative genitourinary system measurements
Bioassay of urine
Renal clearance
Urine chemistry

89.3 Other anatomic and physiologic measurements and manual examinations

> Excludes: the listed procedures when done as part of a general physical examination (89.7)

89.31 Dental examination
Oral mucosal survey
Periodontal survey

89.32 Esophageal manometry

89.33 Distal examination of enterostomy stoma
Digital examination of colostomy stoma

89.34 Distal examination of rectum

89.35 Transillumination of nasal sinuses

89.36 Manual examination of breast

89.37 Vital capacity determination

89.38 Other nonoperative respiratory measurements
Plethysmography for measurement of respiratory function
Thoracic impedance plethysmography

MISCELLANEOUS DIAGNOSTIC & THERAPEUTIC PROCEDURES (87-99)

▲ **89.39 Other nonoperative measurements and examinations**
14 C-Urea breath test
Basal metabolic rate [BMR]
Gastric:
  analysis
  function NEC

Excludes: body measurement (93.07)
  cardiac tests (89.41–89.69)
  fundus photography (95.11)
  limb length measurement (93.06)

89.4 Cardiac stress tests and pacemaker checks

89.41 Cardiovascular stress test using treadmill

89.42 Masters' two-step stress test

89.43 Cardiovascular stress test using bicycle ergometer

89.44 Other cardiovascular stress test
Thallium stress test with or without transesophageal pacing

89.45 Artificial pacemaker rate check
Artificial pacemaker function check NOS

89.46 Artificial pacemaker artifact wave form check

89.47 Artificial pacemaker electrode impedance check

89.48 Artificial pacemaker voltage or amperage threshold check

89.5 Other nonoperative cardiac and vascular diagnostic procedures

Excludes: fetal EKG (75.32)

89.50 Ambulatory cardiac monitoring
Analog devices [Holter-type]

89.51 Rhythm electrocardiogram
Rhythm EKG (with one to three leads)

89.52 Electrocardiogram
ECG NOS
EKG (with 12 or more leads)

89.53 Vectorcardiogram (with ECG)

89.54 Electrographic monitoring
Telemetry

Excludes: ambulatory cardiac monitoring (89.50)
  electrographic monitoring during surgery — omit code

89.55 Phonocardiogram with ECG lead

89.56 Carotid pulse tracing with ECG lead

Excludes: oculoplethysmography (89.58)

89.57 Apexcardiogram (with ECG lead)

89.58 Plethysmogram

Excludes: plethysmography (for):
  measurement of respiratory function (89.38)
  thoracic impedance (89.38)

89.59 Other nonoperative cardiac and vascular measurements

89.6 Circulatory monitoring

Excludes: electrocardiographic monitoring during surgery — omit code

89.61 Systemic arterial pressure monitoring

89.62 Central venous pressure monitoring

89.63 Pulmonary artery pressure monitoring

Excludes: pulmonary artery wedge monitoring (89.64)

89.64 Pulmonary artery wedge monitoring
Pulmonary capillary wedge [PCW] monitoring
Swan-Ganz catheterization

89.65 Measurement of systemic arterial blood gases

89.66 Measurement of mixed venous blood gases

89.67 Monitoring of cardiac output by oxygen consumption technique
Fick method

89.68 Monitoring of cardiac output by other technique
Cardiac output monitor by thermodilution indicator

89.69 Monitoring of coronary blood flow
Coronary blood flow monitoring by coincidence counting technique

89.7 General physical examination

89.8 Autopsy

90 Microscopic examination—I

The following fourth-digit subclassification is for use with categories in section 90 to identify type of examination:

  1 bacterial smear
  2 culture
  3 culture and sensitivity
  4 parasitology
  5 toxicology
  6 cell block and Papanicolaou smear
  9 other microscopic examination

90.0 Microscopic examination of specimen from nervous system and of spinal fluid

90.1 Microscopic examination of specimen from endocrine gland, not elsewhere classified

90.2 Microscopic examination of specimen from eye

90.3 Microscopic examination of specimen from ear, nose, throat, and larynx

90.4 Microscopic examination of specimen from trachea, bronchus, pleura, lung, and other thoracic specimen, and of sputum

90.5 Microscopic examination of blood

90.6 Microscopic examination of specimen from spleen and of bone marrow

90.7 Microscopic examination of specimen from lymph node and of lymph

90.8 Microscopic examination of specimen from upper gastrointestinal tract and of vomitus

90.9 Microscopic examination of specimen from lower gastrointestinal tract and of stool

91 Microscopic examination—II

The following fourth-digit subclassification is for use with categories in section 91 to identify type of examination:

  1 bacterial smear
  2 culture
  3 culture and sensitivity
  4 parasitology

5 toxicology

6 cell block and Papanicolaou smear

9 other microscopic examination

91.0 Microscopic examination of specimen from liver, biliary tract, and pancreas

91.1 Microscopic examination of peritoneal and retroperitoneal specimen

91.2 Microscopic examination of specimen from kidney, ureter, perirenal and periureteral tissue

91.3 Microscopic examination of specimen from bladder, urethra, prostate, seminal vesicle, perivesical tissue, and of urine and semen

91.4 Microscopic examination of specimen from female genital tract ♀
Amnionic sac
Fetus

91.5 Microscopic examination of specimen from musculoskeletal system and of joint fluid
Microscopic examination of:
bone
bursa
cartilage
fascia
ligament
muscle
synovial membrane
tendon

91.6 Microscopic examination of specimen from skin and other integument
Microscopic examination of:
hair
nails
skin

Excludes: mucous membrane — code to organ site
that of operative wound (91.70–91.79)

91.7 Microscopic examination of specimen from operative wound

91.8 Microscopic examination of specimen from other site

91.9 Microscopic examination of specimen from unspecified site

92 Nuclear medicine

92.0 Radioisotope scan and function study

92.01 Thyroid scan and radioisotope function studies
Iodine-131 uptake
Protein-bound iodine
Radio-iodine uptake

92.02 Liver scan and radioisotope function study

92.03 Renal scan and radioisotope function study
Renal clearance study

92.04 Gastrointestinal scan and radioisotope function study
Radio-cobalt B_{12} Schilling test
Radio-iodinated triolein study

92.05 Cardiovascular and hematopoietic scan and radioisotope function study
Bone marrow
Cardiac output
Circulation time   } scan or function study
Radionuclide cardiac
   ventriculogram
Spleen

92.09 Other radioisotope function studies

92.1 Other radioisotope scan

92.11 Cerebral scan
Pituitary

92.12 Scan of other sites of head
Excludes: eye (95.16)

92.13 Parathyroid scan

92.14 Bone scan

92.15 Pulmonary scan

92.16 Scan of lymphatic system

92.17 Placental scan ♀

92.18 Total body scan

92.19 Scan of other sites

92.2 Therapeutic radiology and nuclear medicine

Excludes: that for:
ablation of pituitary gland (07.64–07.69)
destruction of chorioretinal lesion (14.26–14.27)

92.21 Superficial radiation
Contact radiation [up to 150 KVP]

92.22 Orthovoltage radiation
Deep radiation [200–300 KVP]

92.23 Radioisotopic teleradiotherapy
Teleradiotherapy using:
cobalt-60
iodine-125
radioactive cesium

92.24 Teleradiotherapy using photons
Megavoltage NOS
Supervoltage NOS
Use of:
betatron
linear accelerator

92.25 Teleradiotherapy using electrons
Beta particles

92.26 Teleradiotherapy of other particulate radiation
Neutrons   Protons NOS

92.27 Implantation or insertion of radioactive elements
Code also incision of site

92.28 Injection or instillation of radioisotopes
Intracavitary   } injection or instillation
Intravenous

92.29 Other radiotherapeutic procedure

93 Physical therapy, respiratory therapy, rehabilitation, and related procedures

93.0 Diagnostic physical therapy

93.01 Functional evaluation

93.02 Orthotic evaluation

93.03 Prosthetic evaluation

93.04 Manual testing of muscle function

93.05 Range of motion testing

93.06 Measurement of limb length

93.07 Body measurement
Girth measurement
Measurement of skull circumference

MISCELLANEOUS DIAGNOSTIC & THERAPEUTIC PROCEDURES (87-99)

93.08 Electromyography

> Excludes: eye EMG (95.25)
> that with polysomnogram (89.17)
> urethral sphincter EMG (89.23)

93.09 Other diagnostic physical therapy procedure

93.1 Physical therapy exercises

93.11 Assisting exercise

> Excludes: assisted exercise in pool (93.31)

93.12 Other active musculoskeletal exercise

93.13 Resistive exercise

93.14 Training in joint movements

93.15 Mobilization of spine

93.16 Mobilization of other joints

> Excludes: manipulation of temporomandibular joint (76.95)

93.17 Other passive musculoskeletal exercise

93.18 Breathing exercise

93.19 Exercise, not elsewhere classified

93.2 Other physical therapy musculoskeletal manipulation

93.21 Manual and mechanical traction

> Excludes: skeletal traction (93.43–93.44)
> skin traction (93.45–93.46)
> spinal traction (93.41–93.42)

93.22 Ambulation and gait training

93.23 Fitting of orthotic device

93.24 Training in use of prosthetic or orthotic device
Training in crutch walking

93.25 Forced extension of limb

93.26 Manual rupture of joint adhesions

93.27 Stretching of muscle or tendon

93.28 Stretching of fascia

93.29 Other forcible correction of deformity

93.3 Other physical therapy therapeutic procedures

93.31 Assisted exercise in pool

93.32 Whirlpool treatment

93.33 Other hydrotherapy

93.34 Diathermy

93.35 Other heat therapy
Acupuncture with smouldering moxa
Hot packs
Hyperthermia NEC
Infrared irradiation
Moxibustion
Paraffin bath

> Excludes: hyperthermia for treatment of cancer (99.85)

93.36 Cardiac retraining

93.37 Prenatal training
Training for natural childbirth

93.38 Combined physical therapy without mention of the components

93.39 Other physical therapy

93.4 Skeletal traction and other traction

93.41 Spinal traction using skull device
Traction using:
caliper tongs
Crutchfield tongs
halo device
Vinke tongs

> Excludes: insertion of tongs or halo traction device (02.94)

93.42 Other spinal traction
Cotrel's traction

> Excludes: cervical collar (93.52)

93.43 Intermittent skeletal traction

93.44 Other skeletal traction
Bryant's
Dunlop's
Lyman Smith   traction
Russell's

93.45 Thomas' splint traction

93.46 Other skin traction of limbs
Adhesive tape traction
Boot traction
Buck's traction
Gallows traction

93.5 Other immobilization, pressure, and attention to wound

> Excludes: wound cleansing (96.58–96.59)

93.51 Application of plaster jacket

> Excludes: Minerva jacket (93.52)

93.52 Application of neck support
Application of:
cervical collar,
Minerva jacket
molded neck support

93.53 Application of other cast

93.54 Application of splint
Plaster splint   Tray splint

> Excludes: periodontal splint (24.7)

93.55 Dental wiring

> Excludes: that for orthodontia (24.7)

93.56 Application of pressure dressing
Application of:
Gibney bandage
Robert Jones' bandage
Shanz dressing

93.57 Application of other wound dressing

93.58 Application of pressure trousers
Application of:
anti-shock trousers
MAST trousers
vasopneumatic device

93.59 Other immobilization, pressure, and attention to wound
Elastic stockings
Electronic gaiter
Intermittent pressure device
Oxygenation of wound (hyperbaric)
Velpeau dressing

93.6 Osteopathic manipulative treatment

93.61 Osteopathic manipulative treatment for general mobilization
General articulatory treatment

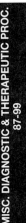

93.62 Osteopathic manipulative treatment using high-velocity, low-amplitude forces
    Thrusting forces

93.63 Osteopathic manipulative treatment using low-velocity, high-amplitude forces
    Springing forces

93.64 Osteopathic manipulative treatment using isotonic, isometric forces

93.65 Osteopathic manipulative treatment using indirect forces

93.66 Osteopathic manipulative treatment to move tissue fluids
    Lymphatic pump

93.67 Other specified osteopathic manipulative treatment

93.7 Speech and reading rehabilitation and rehabilitation of the blind

93.71 Dyslexia training

93.72 Dysphasia training

93.73 Esophageal speech training

93.74 Speech defect training

93.75 Other speech training and therapy

93.76 Training in use of lead dog for the blind

93.77 Training in braille or moon

93.78 Other rehabilitation for the blind

93.8 Other rehabilitation therapy

93.81 Recreational therapy
    Diversional therapy
    Play therapy

> *Excludes:* play psychotherapy (94.36)

93.82 Educational therapy
    Education of bed-bound children
    Special schooling for the handicapped

93.83 Occupational therapy
    Daily living activities therapy

> *Excludes:* training in activities of daily living for the blind (93.78)

93.84 Music therapy

93.85 Vocational rehabilitation
    Sheltered employment
    Vocational:
        assessment
        retraining
        training

93.89 Rehabilitation, not elsewhere classified

93.9 Respiratory therapy

> *Excludes:* insertion of airway (96.01–96.05)
> other continuous mechanical ventilation (96.70–96.72)

93.90 Continuous positive airway pressure [CPAP]

93.91 Intermittent positive pressure breathing [IPPB]

93.93 Nonmechanical methods of resuscitation
    Artificial respiration
    Manual resuscitation
    Mouth-to-mouth resuscitation

93.94 Respiratory medication administered by nebulizer
    Mist therapy

93.95 Hyperbaric oxygenation

> *Excludes:* oxygenation of wound (93.59)

93.96 Other oxygen enrichment
    Catalytic oxygen therapy
    Cytoreductive effect
    Oxygenators
    Oxygen therapy

> *Excludes:* oxygenation of wound (93.59)

93.97 Decompression chamber

93.98 Other control of atmospheric pressure and composition
    Antigen-free air conditioning
    Helium therapy

93.99 Other respiratory procedures
    Continuous negative pressure ventilation [CNP]
    Postural drainage

94 Procedures related to the psyche

94.0 Psychologic evaluation and testing

94.01 Administration of intelligence test
    Administration of:
        Stanford-Binet
        Wechsler Adult Intelligence Scale
        Wechsler Intelligence Scale for Children

94.02 Administration of psychologic test
    Administration of:
        Bender Visual - Motor Gestalt Test
        Benton Visual Retention Test
        Minnesota Multiphasic Personality Inventory
        Wechsler Memory Scale

94.03 Character analysis

94.08 Other psychologic evaluation and testing

94.09 Psychologic mental status determination, not otherwise specified

94.1 Psychiatric interviews, consultations, and evaluations

94.11 Psychiatric mental status determination
    Clinical psychiatric mental status determination
    Evaluation for criminal responsibility
    Evaluation for testimentary capacity
    Medicolegal mental status determination
    Mental status determination NOS

94.12 Routine psychiatric visit, not otherwise specified

94.13 Psychiatric commitment evaluation
    Pre-commitment interview

94.19 Other psychiatric interview and evaluation
    Follow-up psychiatric interview NOS

94.2 Psychiatric somatotherapy

94.21 Narcoanalysis
    Narcosynthesis

94.22 Lithium therapy

94.23 Neuroleptic therapy

94.24 Chemical shock therapy

94.25 Other psychiatric drug therapy

94.26 Subconvulsive electroshock therapy

94.27 Other electroshock therapy
    Electroconvulsive therapy (ECT)
    EST

94.29 Other psychiatric somatotherapy

MISCELLANEOUS DIAGNOSTIC & THERAPEUTIC PROCEDURES (87-99)

94.3 Individual psychotherapy

    94.31 Psychoanalysis

    94.32 Hypnotherapy
        Hypnodrome
        Hypnosis

    94.33 Behavior therapy
        Aversion therapy
        Behavior modification
        Desensitization therapy
        Extinction therapy
        Relaxation training
        Token economy

    94.34 Individual therapy for psychosexual dysfunction

        Excludes: that performed in group setting (94.41)

    94.35 Crisis intervention

    94.36 Play psychotherapy

    94.37 Exploratory verbal psychotherapy

    94.38 Supportive verbal psychotherapy

    94.39 Other individual psychotherapy
        Biofeedback

94.4 Other psychotherapy and counselling

    94.41 Group therapy for psychosexual dysfunction

    94.42 Family therapy

    94.43 Psychodrama

    94.44 Other group therapy

    94.45 Drug addiction counselling

    94.46 Alcoholism counselling

    94.49 Other counselling

94.5 Referral for psychologic rehabilitation

    94.51 Referral for psychotherapy

    94.52 Referral for psychiatric aftercare
        That in:
            halfway house
            outpatient (clinic) facility

    94.53 Referral for alcoholism rehabilitation

    94.54 Referral for drug addiction rehabilitation

    94.55 Referral for vocational rehabilitation

    94.59 Referral for other psychologic rehabilitation

94.6 Alcohol and drug rehabilitation and detoxification

    94.61 Alcohol rehabilitation NOR

    94.62 Alcohol detoxification

    94.63 Alcohol rehabilitation and detoxification NOR

    94.64 Drug rehabilitation NOR

    94.65 Drug detoxification

    94.66 Drug rehabilitation and detoxification NOR

    94.67 Combined alcohol and drug rehabilitation NOR

    94.68 Combined alcohol and drug detoxification

    94.69 Combined alcohol and drug rehabilitation and detoxification NOR

95 Ophthalmologic and otologic diagnosis and treatment

95.0 General and subjective eye examination

    95.01 Limited eye examination
        Eye examination with prescription of spectacles

    95.02 Comprehensive eye examination
        Eye examination covering all aspects of the visual system

    95.03 Extended ophthalmologic work-up
        Examination (for):
            glaucoma
            neuro-ophthalmology
            retinal disease

    95.04 Eye examination under anesthesia

        Code also type of examination

    95.05 Visual field study

    95.06 Color vision study

    95.07 Dark adaptation study

    95.09 Eye examination, not otherwise specified
        Vision check NOS

95.1 Examinations of form and structure of eye

    95.11 Fundus photography

    95.12 Fluorescein angiography or angioscopy of eye

    95.13 Ultrasound study of eye

    95.14 X-ray study of eye

    95.15 Ocular motility study

    95.16 P^{32} and other tracer studies of eye

95.2 Objective functional tests of eye

    Excludes: that with polysomnogram (89.17)

    95.21 Electroretinogram [ERG]

    95.22 Electro-oculogram [EOG]

    95.23 Visual evoked potential [VEP]

    95.24 Electronystagmogram [ENG]

    95.25 Electromyogram of eye [EMG]

    95.26 Tonography, provocative tests, and other glaucoma testing

95.3 Special vision services

    95.31 Fitting and dispensing of spectacles

    95.32 Prescription, fitting, and dispensing of contact lens

    95.33 Dispensing of other low vision aids

    95.34 Ocular prosthetics

    95.35 Orthoptic training

    95.36 Ophthalmologic counselling and instruction
        Counselling in:
            adaptation to visual loss
            use of low vision aids

95.4 Nonoperative procedures related to hearing

    95.41 Audiometry
        Békésy 5-tone audiometry
        Impedance audiometry
        Stapedial reflex response
        Subjective audiometry
        Tympanogram

    95.42 Clinical test of hearing
        Tuning fork test
        Whispered speech test

95.43 Audiological evaluation
  Audiological evaluation by:
    Bárány noise machine
    blindfold test
    delayed feedback
    masking
    Weber lateralization

95.44 Clinical vestibular function tests
  Thermal test of vestibular function

95.45 Rotation tests
  Bárány chair

95.46 Other auditory and vestibular function tests

95.47 Hearing examination, not otherwise specified

95.48 Fitting of hearing aid
  Excludes: *implantation of electromagnetic hearing device (20.95)*

95.49 Other nonoperative procedures related to hearing
  Adjustment (external components) of cochlear prosthetic device

96 Nonoperative intubation and irrigation

96.0 Nonoperative intubation of gastrointestinal and respiratory tracts

96.01 Insertion of nasopharyngeal airway

96.02 Insertion of oropharyngeal airway

96.03 Insertion of esophageal obturator airway

96.04 Insertion of endotracheal tube

96.05 Other intubation of respiratory tract

96.06 Insertion of Sengstaken tube
  Esophageal tamponade

96.07 Insertion of other (naso-) gastric tube
  Intubation for decompression
  Excludes: *that for enteral infusion of nutritional substance (96.6)*

96.08 Insertion of (naso-) intestinal tube
  Miller-Abbott tube (for decompression)

96.09 Insertion of rectal tube
  Replacement of rectal tube

96.1 Other nonoperative insertion
  Excludes: *nasolacrimal intubation (09.44)*

96.11 Packing of external auditory canal

96.14 Vaginal packing ♀

96.15 Insertion of vaginal mold ♀

96.16 Other vaginal dilation ♀

96.17 Insertion of vaginal diaphragm ♀

96.18 Insertion of other vaginal pessary ♀

96.19 Rectal packing

96.2 Nonoperative dilation and manipulation

96.21 Dilation of frontonasal duct

96.22 Dilation of rectum

96.23 Dilation of anal sphincter

96.24 Dilation and manipulation of enterostomy stoma

96.25 Therapeutic distention of bladder
  Intermittent distention of bladder

96.26 Manual reduction of rectal prolapse

96.27 Manual reduction of hernia

96.28 Manual reduction of enterostomy prolapse

96.3 Nonoperative alimentary tract irrigation, cleaning, and local instillation

96.31 Gastric cooling
  Gastric hypothermia

96.32 Gastric freezing

96.33 Gastric lavage

96.34 Other irrigation of (naso-) gastric tube

96.35 Gastric gavage

96.36 Irrigation of gastrostomy or enterostomy

96.37 Proctoclysis

96.38 Removal of impacted feces
  Removal of impaction:
    by flushing
    manually

96.39 Other transanal enema
  Rectal irrigation

96.4 Nonoperative irrigation, cleaning, and local instillation of other digestive and genitourinary organs

96.41 Irrigation of cholecystostomy and other biliary tube

96.42 Irrigation of pancreatic tube

96.43 Digestive tract instillation, except gastric gavage

96.44 Vaginal douche ♀

96.45 Irrigation of nephrostomy and pyelostomy

96.46 Irrigation of ureterostomy and ureteral catheter

96.47 Irrigation of cystostomy

96.48 Irrigation of other indwelling urinary catheter

96.49 Other genitourinary instillation
  Insertion of prostaglandin suppository

96.5 Other nonoperative irrigation and cleaning

96.51 Irrigation of eye
  Irrigation of cornea
  Excludes: *irrigation with removal of foreign body (98.21)*

96.52 Irrigation of ear
  Irrigation with removal of cerumen

96.53 Irrigation of nasal passages

96.54 Dental scaling, polishing, and debridement
  Dental prophylaxis
  Plaque removal

96.55 Tracheostomy toilette

96.56 Other lavage of bronchus and trachea

96.57 Irrigation of vascular catheter

96.58 Irrigation of wound catheter

96.59 Other irrigation of wound
  Wound cleaning NOS
  Excludes: *debridement (86.22, 86.27–86.28)*

96.6 Enteral infusion of concentrated-nutritional substances

MISCELLANEOUS DIAGNOSTIC & THERAPEUTIC PROCEDURES (87-99)

▲ **96.7 Other continuous mechanical ventilation**
Includes: Endotracheal respiratory assistance
Intermittent mandatory ventilation [IMV]
Positive end expiratory pressure [PEEP]
Pressure support ventilation [PSV]
That by tracheostomy
Weaning of an intubated (endotracheal tube) patient

Excludes: *bi-level airway pressure (93.90)*
continuous negative pressure ventilation [CNP]
(iron lung) (cuirass) (93.99)
continuous positive airway pressure [CPAP]
(93.90)
intermittent positive pressure breathing [IPPB]
(93.91)
that by face mask (93.90–93.99)
that by nasal cannula (93.90–93.99)
that by nasal catheter (93.90–93.99)

Code also any associated:
endotracheal tube insertion (96.04)
tracheostomy (31.1–31.29)

Endotracheal Intubation

To calculate the number of hours (duration) of continuous mechanical ventilation during a hospitalization, begin the count from the start of the (endotracheal) intubation. The duration ends with (endotracheal) extubation.

If a patient is intubated prior to admission, begin counting the duration from the time of the admission. If a patient is transferred (discharged) while intubated, the duration would end at the time of transfer (discharge).

For patients who begin on (endotracheal) intubation and subsequently have a tracheostomy performed for mechanical ventilation, the duration begins with the (endotracheal) intubation and ends when the mechanical ventilation is turned off (after the weaning period).

Tracheostomy

To calculate the number of hours of continuous mechanical ventilation during a hospitalization, begin counting the duration when mechanical ventilation is started. The duration ends when the mechanical ventilator is turned off (after the weaning period).

If a patient has received a tracheostomy prior to admission and is on mechanical ventilation at the time of admission, begin counting the duration from the time of admission. If a patient is transferred (discharged) while still on mechanical ventilation via tracheostomy, the duration would end at the time of the transfer (discharge).

96.70 Continuous mechanical ventilation of unspecified duration NOR
Mechanical ventilation NOS

96.71 Continuous mechanical ventilation for less than 96 consecutive hours NOR

96.72 Continuous mechanical ventilation for 96 consecutive hours or more NOR

97 Replacement and removal of therapeutic appliances

97.0 Nonoperative replacement of gastrointestinal appliance

97.01 Replacement of (naso-) gastric or esophagostomy tube

97.02 Replacement of gastrostomy tube

97.03 Replacement of tube or enterostomy device of small intestine

97.04 Replacement of tube or enterostomy device of large intestine

97.05 Replacement of stent (tube) in biliary or pancreatic duct

97.1 Nonoperative replacement of musculoskeletal and integumentary system appliance

97.11 Replacement of cast on upper limb

97.12 Replacement of cast on lower limb

97.13 Replacement of other cast

97.14 Replacement of other device for musculoskeletal immobilization

97.15 Replacement of wound catheter

97.16 Replacement of wound packing or drain

Excludes: *repacking of:*
dental wound (97.22)
vulvar wound (97.26)

97.2 Other nonoperative replacement

97.21 Replacement of nasal packing

97.22 Replacement of dental packing

97.23 Replacement of tracheostomy tube

97.24 Replacement and refitting of vaginal diaphragm ♀

97.25 Replacement of other vaginal pessary ♀

97.26 Replacement of vaginal or vulvar packing or drain ♀

97.29 Other nonoperative replacements

97.3 Nonoperative removal of therapeutic device from head and neck

97.31 Removal of eye prosthesis

Excludes: *removal of ocular implant (16.71)*
removal of orbital implant (16.72)

97.32 Removal of nasal packing

97.33 Removal of dental wiring

97.34 Removal of dental packing

97.35 Removal of dental prosthesis

97.36 Removal of other external mandibular fixation device

97.37 Removal of tracheostomy tube

97.38 Removal of sutures from head and neck

97.39 Removal of other therapeutic device from head and neck

Excludes: *removal of skull tongs (02.94)*

97.4 Nonoperative removal of therapeutic device from thorax

97.41 Removal of thoracotomy tube or pleural cavity drain

97.42 Removal of mediastinal drain

97.43 Removal of sutures from thorax

97.49 Removal of other device from thorax

97.5 Nonoperative removal of therapeutic device from digestive system

97.51 Removal of gastrostomy tube

97.52 Removal of tube from small intestine

97.53 Removal of tube from large intestine or appendix

97.54 Removal of cholecystostomy tube

97.55 Removal of T-tube, other bile duct tube, or liver tube

97.56 Removal of pancreatic tube or drain

97.59 Removal of other device from digestive system
Removal of rectal packing

97.6 Nonoperative removal of therapeutic device from urinary system

97.61 Removal of pyelostomy and nephrostomy tube

97.62 Removal of ureterostomy tube and ureteral catheter

97.63 Removal of cystostomy tube

97.64 Removal of other urinary drainage device
Removal of indwelling urinary catheter

97.65 Removal of urethral stent

97.69 Removal of other device from urinary system

97.7 Nonoperative removal of therapeutic device from genital system

97.71 Removal of intrauterine contraceptive device ♀

97.72 Removal of intrauterine pack ♀

97.73 Removal of vaginal diaphragm ♀

97.74 Removal of other vaginal pessary ♀

97.75 Removal of vaginal or vulvar packing ♀

97.79 Removal of other device from genital tract
Removal of sutures

97.8 Other nonoperative removal of therapeutic device

97.81 Removal of retroperitoneal drainage device

97.82 Removal of peritoneal drainage device

97.83 Removal of abdominal wall sutures

97.84 Removal of sutures from trunk, not elsewhere classified

97.85 Removal of packing from trunk, not elsewhere classified

97.86 Removal of other device from abdomen

97.87 Removal of other device from trunk

97.88 Removal of external immobilization device
Removal of:
brace
cast
splint

97.89 Removal of other therapeutic device

98 Nonoperative removal of foreign body or calculus

98.0 Removal of intraluminal foreign body from digestive system without incision

Excludes: *removal of therapeutic device (97.51–97.59)*

98.01 Removal of intraluminal foreign body from mouth without incision

98.02 Removal of intraluminal foreign body from esophagus without incision

98.03 Removal of intraluminal foreign body from stomach and small intestine without incision

98.04 Removal of intraluminal foreign body from large intestine without incision

98.05 Removal of intraluminal foreign body from rectum and anus without incision

98.1 Removal of intraluminal foreign body from other sites without incision

Excludes: *removal of therapeutic device (97.31–97.49 97.61–97.89)*

98.11 Removal of intraluminal foreign body from ear without incision

98.12 Removal of intraluminal foreign body from nose without incision

98.13 Removal of intraluminal foreign body from pharynx without incision

98.14 Removal of intraluminal foreign body from larynx without incision

98.15 Removal of intraluminal foreign body from trachea and bronchus without incision

98.16 Removal of intraluminal foreign body from uterus without incision ♀

Excludes: *removal of intrauterine contraceptive device (97.71)*

98.17 Removal of intraluminal foreign body from vagina without incision ♀

98.18 Removal of intraluminal foreign body from artificial stoma without incision

98.19 Removal of intraluminal foreign body from urethra without incision

98.2 Removal of other foreign body without incision

Excludes: *removal of intraluminal foreign body (98.01–98.19)*

98.20 Removal of foreign body, not otherwise specified

98.21 Removal of superficial foreign body from eye without incision

98.22 Removal of other foreign body without incision from head and neck
Removal of embedded foreign body from eyelid or conjunctiva without incision

98.23 Removal of foreign body from vulva without incision ♀

98.24 Removal of foreign body from scrotum or penis without incision ♂

98.25 Removal of other foreign body without incision from trunk except scrotum, penis, or vulva

98.26 Removal of foreign body from hand without incision

98.27 Removal of foreign body without incision from upper limb, except hand

98.28 Removal of foreign body from foot without incision

98.29 Removal of foreign body without incision from lower limb, except foot

98.5 Extracorporeal shockwave lithotripsy [ESWL]
Lithotriptor tank procedure
Disintegration of stones by extracorporeal induced shockwaves
That with insertion of stent

98.51 Extracorporeal shockwave lithotripsy [ESWL] of the kidney, ureter and/or bladder NOR

Extracorporeal shockwave lithotripsy [ESWL] of the gallbladder and/or bile duct

Extracorporeal shockwave lithotripsy of other sites

99 Other nonoperative procedures

99.0 Transfusion of blood and blood components

Use additional code for that done via catheter or cutdown (38.92–38.94)

99.01 Exchange transfusion
Transfusion:
exsanguination
replacement

99.02 Autotransfusion of whole blood

99.03 Other transfusion of whole blood
Transfusion:
NOS
blood NOS

99.04 Transfusion of packed cells

99.05 Transfusion of platelets
Transfusion of thrombocytes

99.06 Transfusion of coagulation factors
Transfusion of antihemophilic factor

MISCELLANEOUS DIAGNOSTIC & THERAPEUTIC PROCEDURES (87-99)

99.07 Transfusion of other serum
Transfusion of plasma

Excludes: injection [transfusion] of:
antivenin (99.16)
gamma globulin (99.14)

99.08 Transfusion of blood expander
Transfusion of Dextran

99.09 Transfusion of other substance
Transfusion of:
blood surrogate
granulocytes

Excludes: transplantation [transfusion] of bone marrow (41.0)

99.1 Injection or infusion of therapeutic or prophylactic substance

Includes: injection or infusion given:
hypodermically
intramuscularly   acting locally or systemically
intravenously

99.11 Injection of rh immune globulin
Injection of:
Anti-D (Rhesus) globulin
RhoGAM

99.12 Immunization for allergy
Desensitization

99.13 Immunization for autoimmune disease

99.14 Injection of gamma globulin
Injection of immune sera

99.15 Parenteral infusion of concentrated nutritional substances
Hyperalimentation
Total parenteral nutrition [TPN]
Peripheral parenteral nutrition [PPN]

99.16 Injection of antidote
Injection of:
antivenin
heavy metal antagonist

99.17 Injection of insulin

99.18 Injection or infusion of electrolytes

99.19 Injection of anticoagulant

99.2 Injection or infusion of other therapeutic or prophylactic substance

Includes: injection or infusion given:
hypodermically
intramuscularly   acting locally or systemically
intravenously

Use additional code for:
injection (into):
breast (85.92)
bursa (82.94, 83.96)
intraperitoneal (cavity) (54.97)
intrathecal (03.92)
joint (76.96, 81.92)
kidney (55.96)
liver (50.94)
orbit (16.91)
other sites — see Alphabetic Index
perfusion:
NOS (39.97)
intestine (46.95, 46.96)
kidney (55.95)
liver (50.93)
total body (39.96)

99.21 Injection of antibiotic

99.22 Injection of other anti-infective

99.23 Injection of steroid
Injection of cortisone
Subdermal implantation of progesterone

99.24 Injection of other hormone

▲ **99.25 Injection or infusion of cancer chemotherapeutic substance**
Injection or infusion of antineoplastic agent

Excludes: immunotherapy, antineoplastic (99.28)
injection of radioisotopes (92.28)
injection or infusion of biological response modifier [BRM] as an antineoplastic agent (99.28)

99.26 Injection of tranquilizer

99.27 Iontophoresis

● **99.28 Injection or infusion of biological response modifier [BRM] as an antineoplastic agent**
Immunotherapy, antineoplastic

99.29 Injection or infusion of other therapeutic or prophylactic substance

Excludes: immunization (99.31–99.59)
injection of sclerosing agent into:
esophageal varices (42.33)
hemorrhoids (49.42)
veins (39.92)

99.3 Prophylactic vaccination and inoculation against certain bacterial diseases

99.31 Vaccination against cholera

99.32 Vaccination against typhoid and paratyphoid fever
Administration of TAB vaccine

99.33 Vaccination against tuberculosis
Administration of BCG vaccine

99.34 Vaccination against plague

99.35 Vaccination against tularemia

99.36 Administration of diphtheria toxoid

Excludes: administration of:
diphtheria antitoxin (99.58)
diphtheria-tetanus-pertussis, combined (99.39)

99.37 Vaccination against pertussis

Excludes: administration of diphtheria-tetanus-pertussis, combined (99.39)

99.38 Administration of tetanus toxoid

Excludes: administration of:
diphtheria-tetanus-pertussis, combined (99.39)
tetanus antitoxin (99.56)

99.39 Administration of diphtheria-tetanus-pertussis, combined

99.4 Prophylactic vaccination and inoculation against certain viral diseases

99.41 Administration of poliomyelitis vaccine

99.42 Vaccination against smallpox

99.43 Vaccination against yellow fever

99.44 Vaccination against rabies

99.45 Vaccination against measles

Excludes: administration of measles-mumps-rubella vaccine (99.48)

99.46 Vaccination against mumps

Excludes: administration of measles-mumps-rubella vaccine (99.48)

99.47 Vaccination against rubella

> Excludes: administration of measles-mumps-rubella vaccine (99.48)

99.48 Administration of measles-mumps-rubella vaccine

99.5 Other vaccination and inoculation

99.51 Prophylactic vaccination against the common cold

99.52 Prophylactic vaccination against influenza

99.53 Prophylactic vaccination against arthropod-borne viral encephalitis

99.54 Prophylactic vaccination against other arthropod-borne viral diseases

99.55 Prophylactic administration of vaccine against other diseases
Vaccination against:
  anthrax
  brucellosis
  Rocky Mountain spotted fever
  Staphylococcus
  Streptococcus
  typhus

99.56 Administration of tetanus antitoxin

99.57 Administration of botulism antitoxin

99.58 Administration of other antitoxins
Administration of:
  diphtheria antitoxin
  gas gangrene antitoxin
  scarlet fever antitoxin

99.59 Other vaccination and inoculation
Vaccination NOS

> Excludes: injection of:
>   gamma globulin (99.14)
>   Rh immune globulin (99.11)
> immunization for:
>   allergy (99.12)
>   autoimmune disease (99.13)

99.6 Conversion of cardiac rhythm

> Excludes: open chest cardiac:
>   electric stimulation (37.91)
>   massage (37.91)

99.60 Cardiopulmonary resuscitation, not otherwise specified

99.61 Atrial cardioversion

99.62 Other electric countershock of heart
Cardioversion:
  NOS
  External
Conversion to sinus rhythm
Defibrillation
External electrode stimulation

99.63 Closed chest cardiac massage
Cardiac massage NOS
Manual external cardiac massage

99.64 Carotid sinus stimulation

99.69 Other conversion of cardiac rhythm

99.7 Therapeutic apheresis

99.71 Therapeutic plasmapheresis

99.72 Therapeutic leukopheresis
Therapeutic leukocytapheresis

99.73 Therapeutic erythrocytapheresis
Therapeutic erythropheresis

99.74 Therapeutic plateletpheresis

▲**99.79 Other**
Apheresis (harvest) of stem cells

99.8 Miscellaneous physical procedures

99.81 Hypothermia (central) (local)

> Excludes: gastric cooling (96.31)
> gastric freezing (96.32)
> that incidental to open heart surgery (39.62)

99.82 Ultraviolet light therapy
Actinotherapy

99.83 Other phototherapy
Phototherapy of the newborn

> Excludes: extracorporeal photochemotherapy (99.88)
> photocoagulation of retinal lesion (14.23–14.25, 14.33–14.35, 14.53–14.55)

99.84 Isolation
Isolation after contact with infectious disease
Protection of individual from his surroundings
Protection of surroundings from individual

99.85 Hyperthermia for treatment of cancer
Hyperthermia (adjunct therapy) induced by microwave, ultrasound, low energy radiofrequency, probes (interstitial), or other means in the treatment of cancer

Code also any concurrent chemotherapy or radiation therapy

99.86 Non-invasive placement of bone growth stimulator
Transcutaneous (surface) placement of pads or patches for stimulation to aid bone healing

> Excludes: insertion of invasive or semi-invasive bone growth stimulators (device) (percutaneous electrodes) (78.90–78.99)

99.88 Therapeutic photopheresis
Extracorporeal photochemotherapy
Extracorporeal photopheresis

> Excludes: other phototherapy (99.83)
> ultraviolet light therapy (99.82)

99.9 Other miscellaneous procedures

99.91 Acupuncture for anesthesia

99.92 Other acupuncture

> Excludes: that with smouldering moxa (93.35)

99.93 Rectal massage (for levator spasm)

99.94 Prostatic massage ♂

99.95 Stretching of foreskin ♂

99.96 Collection of sperm for artificial insemination ♂

99.97 Fitting of denture

99.98 Extraction of milk from lactating breast ♀

99.99 Other

ICD-9-CM PROCEDURE CLASSIFICATION

Alphabetic Index

A

Abbe operation
  construction of vagina 70.61
  intestinal anastomosis — *see* Anastomosis, intestine
Abdominocentesis 54.91
Abdominohysterectomy 68.4
Abdominoplasty 86.83
Abdominoscopy 54.21
Abdominouterotomy 68.0
  obstetrical 74.99
Abduction, arytenoid 31.69
Ablation
  biliary tract (lesion) by ERCP 51.64
  inner ear (cryosurgery) (ultrasound) 20.79
    by injection 20.72
  lesion
    esophagus 42.39
      endoscopic 42.33
    heart (ventricular) 37.33
      by cardiac catheter 37.34
    intestine
      large 45.49
        endoscopic 45.43
    large intestine 45.49
      endoscopic 45.43
  pituitary 07.69
    by
      Cobalt-60 07.68
      implantation (strontium-yttrium) (Y) NEC 07.68
        transfrontal approach 07.64
        transphenoidal approach 07.65
      proton beam (Bragg peak) 07.68
Abortion, therapeutic 69.51
  by
    aspiration curettage 69.51
    dilation and curettage 69.01
    hysterectomy — *see* Hysterectomy
    hysterotomy 74.91
    insertion
      laminaria 69.93
      prostaglandin suppository 96.49
    intra-amniotic injection (saline) 75.0
Abrasion
  corneal epithelium 11.41
    for smear or culture 11.21
  epicardial surface 36.3
  pleural 34.6
  skin 86.25
Abscission, cornea 11.49
Absorptiometry
  photon (dual) (single) 88.98
Aburel operation (intra-amniotic injection for abortion) 75.0
Accouchement force 73.99
Acetabulectomy 77.85
Acetabuloplasty NEC 81.40
  with prosthetic implant 81.52
Achillorrhaphy 83.64
  delayed 83.62
Achillotenotomy 83.11
  plastic 83.85
Achillotomy 83.11
  plastic 83.85
Acid peel, skin 86.24
Acromionectomy 77.81
Acromioplasty 81.83
  for recurrent dislocation of shoulder 81.82
  partial replacement 81.81
  total replacement 81.80
Actinotherapy 99.82
Activities of daily living (ADL)
  therapy 93.83
  training for the blind 93.78
Acupuncture 99.92
  with smouldering moxa 93.35
  for anesthesia 99.91
Adams operation
  advancement of round ligament 69.22
  crushing of nasal septum 21.88
  excision of palmar fascia 82.35
Adenectomy — *see also* Excision, by site
  prostate NEC 60.69
  retropubic 60.4
Adenoidectomy (without tonsillectomy) 28.6
  with tonsillectomy 28.3
Adhesiolysis — *see also* Lysis, adhesions
  for collapse of lung 33.39
  middle ear 20.23
Adipectomy 86.83
Adjustment
  cardiac pacemaker program (reprogramming) — omit code
  cochlear prosthetic device (external components) 95.49
  dental 99.97
  occlusal 24.8
  spectacles 95.31
Administration (of) — *see also* Injection
  antitoxins NEC 99.58
    botulism 99.57
    diphtheria 99.58
    gas gangrene 99.58
    scarlet fever 99.58
    tetanus 99.56
  Bender Visual-Motor Gestalt test 94.02
  Benton Visual Retention test 94.02
  intelligence test or scale (Stanford-Binet) (Wechsler) (adult) (children) 94.01
  Minnesota Multiphasic Personality Inventory (MMPI) 94.02
  MMPI (Minnesota Multiphasic Personality Inventory) 94.02
  psychologic test 94.02
  Stanford-Binet test 94.01
  toxoid
    diphtheria 99.36
      with tetanus and pertussis, combined (DTP) 99.39
    tetanus 99.38
      with diphtheria and pertussis, combined (DTP) 99.39
  vaccine — *see also* Vaccination
    BCG 99.33
    measles-mumps-rubella (MMP) 99.48
    poliomyelitis 99.41
    TAB 99.32
  Wechsler
    Intelligence Scale (adult) (children) 94.01
    Memory Scale 94.02
Adrenalectomy (unilateral) 07.22
  with partial removal of remaining gland 07.29
  bilateral 07.3
    partial 07.29
    subtotal 07.29
  complete 07.3
  partial NEC 07.29
  remaining gland 07.3
  subtotal NEC 07.29
  total 07.3
Adrenalorrhaphy 07.44
Adrenalotomy (with drainage) 07.41
Advancement
  extraocular muscle 15.12
    multiple (with resection or recession) 15.3
  eyelid muscle 08.59
  eye muscle 15.12
    multiple (with resection or recession) 15.3
  graft — *see* Graft
  leaflet (heart) 35.10
  pedicle (flap) 86.72
  profundus tendon (Wagner) 82.51
  round ligament 69.22
  tendon 83.71
    hand 82.51
      profundus (Wagner) 82.51
  Wagner (profundus tendon) 82.51
Albee operation
  bone peg, femoral neck 78.05
  graft for slipping patella 78.06
  sliding inlay graft, tibia 78.07
Albert operation (arthrodesis of knee) 81.22
Aldridge (-Studdiford) **operation** (urethral sling) 59.5
Alexander operation
  prostatectomy
    perineal 60.62
    suprapubic 60.3
  shortening of round ligaments 69.22
Alexander-Adams operation (shortening of round ligaments) 69.22
Alimentation, parenteral 99.29
Allograft — *see* Graft
Almoor operation (extrapetrosal drainage) 20.22
Altemeier operation (perineal rectal pull-through) 48.49
Alveolectomy (interradicular) (intraseptal) (radical) (simple) (with graft) (with implant) 24.5
Alveoloplasty (with graft or implant) 24.5
Alveolotomy (apical) 24.0
Ambulatory cardiac monitoring (ACM) 89.50
Ammon operation (dacryocystotomy) 09.53
Amniocentesis (transuterine) (diagnostic) 75.1
  with intra-amniotic injection of saline 75.0
Amniography 87.81
Amnioscopy, internal 75.31
Amniotomy 73.09
  to induce labor 73.01
Amputation (cineplastic) (closed flap) (guillotine) (kineplastic) (open) 84.91
  abdominopelvic 84.19
  above-elbow 84.07
  above-knee (AK) 84.17
  ankle (disarticulation) 84.13
    through malleoli of tibia and fibula 84.14

arm NEC 84.00
   through
      carpals 84.03
      elbow (disarticulation) 84.06
      forearm 84.05
      humerus 84.07
      shoulder (disarticulation) 84.08
      wrist (disarticulation) 84.04
   upper 84.07
Batch-Spittler-McFaddin (knee disarticulation) 84.16
below-knee (BK) NEC 84.15
   conversion into above-knee amputation 84.17
Boyd (hip disarticulation) 84.18
Callander's (knee disarticulation) 84.16
carpals 84.03
cervix 67.4
Chopart's (midtarsal) 84.12
clitoris 71.4
Dieffenbach (hip disarticulation) 84.18
Dupuytren's (shoulder disarticulation) 84.08
ear, external 18.39
elbow (disarticulation) 84.06
finger, except thumb 84.01
   thumb 84.02
foot (middle) 84.12
forearm 84.05
forefoot 84.12
forequarter 84.09
Gordon-Taylor (hindquarter) 84.19
Gritti-Stokes (knee disarticulation) 84.16
Guyon (ankle) 84.13
hallux 84.11
hand 84.03
Hey's (foot) 84.12
hindquarter 84.19
hip (disarticulation) 84.18
humerus 84.07
interscapulothoracic 84.09
interthoracoscapular 84.09
King-Steelquist (hindquarter) 84.19
Kirk (thigh) 84.17
knee (disarticulation) 84.16
Kutler (revision of current traumatic amputation of finger) 84.01
Larry (shoulder disarticulation) 84.08
leg NEC 84.10
   above knee (AK) 84.17
   below knee (BK) 84.15
   through
      ankle (disarticulation) 84.13
      femur (AK) 84.17
      foot 84.12
      hip (disarticulation) 84.18
      tibia and fibula (BK) 84.15
Lisfranc
   foot 84.12
   shoulder (disarticulation) 84.08
Littlewood (forequarter) 84.09
lower limb NEC (see also Amputation leg) 84.10
Mazet (knee disarticulation) 84.16
metacarpal 84.03
metatarsal 84.11
   head (bunionectomy) 77.59
metatarsophalangeal (joint) 84.11
midtarsal 84.12
nose 21.4
penis (circle) (complete) (flap) (partial) (radical) 64.3

Pirogoff's (ankle amputation through malleoli of tibia and fibula) 84.14
ray, finger 84.01
root (tooth) (apex) 23.73
   with root canal therapy 23.72
shoulder (disarticulation) 84.08
Sorondo-Ferre (hindquarter) 84.19
S.P. Rogers (knee disarticulation) 84.16
supracondylar, above-knee 84.17
supramalleolar, foot 84.14
Syme's (ankle amputation through malleoli of tibia and fibula) 84.14
thigh 84.17
thumb 84.02
toe (through metatarsophalangeal joint) 84.11
transcarpal 84.03
transmetatarsal 84.12
upper limb NEC (see also Amputation, arm) 84.00
wrist (disarticulation) 84.04
Amygdalohippocampotomy 01.39
Amygdalotomy 01.39
Analysis
   character 94.03
   gastric 89.39
   psychologic 94.31
   transactional
      group 94.44
      individual 94.39
Anastomosis
   accessory-facial nerve 04.72
   accessory-hypoglossal nerve 04.73
   anus (with formation of endorectal ileal pouch) 45.95
   aorta (descending)-pulmonary (artery) 39.0
   aorta-renal artery 39.24
   aorta-subclavian artery 39.22
   aortoceliac 39.26
   aorto(ilio)femoral 39.25
   aortomesenteric 39.26
   appendix 47.99
   arteriovenous NEC 39.29
      for renal dialysis 39.27
   artery (suture of distal to proximal end) 39.31
      with
         bypass graft 39.29
            extracranial-intracranial [EC-IC] 39.28
         excision or resection of vessel — see Arteriectomy, with anastomosis, by site
         revision
   bile ducts 51.39
   bladder NEC 57.88
      with
         isolated segment of intestine 57.87 [45.50]
            colon (sigmoid) 57.87 [45.52]
            ileum 57.87 [45.51]
            open loop of ileum 57.87 [45.51]
         to intestine 57.88
            ileum 57.87 [45.51]
   bowel — (see also Anastomosis, intestine) 45.90
   bronchotracheal 33.48
   bronchus 33.48
   carotid-subclavian artery 39.22
   caval-mesenteric vein 39.1
   caval-pulmonary artery 39.21
   cervicoesophageal 42.59
   colohypopharyngeal (intrathoracic) 42.55

      antesternal or antethoracic 42.65
   common bile duct 51.39
   common pulmonary trunk and left atrium (posterior wall) 35.82
   cystic bile duct 51.39
   cystocolic 57.88
   epididymis to vas deferens 63.83
   esophagocolic (intrathoracic) NEC 42.56
      with interposition 42.55
      antesternal or antethoracic NEC 42.66
         with interposition 42.65
   esophagocologastric (intrathoracic) 42.55
      antesternal or antethoracic 42.65
   esophagoduodenal (intrathoracic) NEC 42.54
      with interposition 42.53
   esophagoenteric (intrathoracic) NEC (see also Anastomosis, esophagus, to intestinalsegment) 42.54
      antesternal or antethoracic NEC (see also Anastomosis, esophagus, antesternal, tointestinal segment) 42.64
   esophagoesophageal (intrathoracic) 42.51
      antesternal or antethoracic 42.61
   esophagogastric (intrathoracic) 42.52
      antesternal or antethoracic 42.62
   esophagus (intrapleural) (intrathoracic) (retrosternal) NEC 42.59
      with
         gastrectomy (partial) 43.5
            complete or total 43.99
         interposition (of) NEC 42.58
            colon 42.55
            jejunum 42.53
            small bowel 42.53
      antesternal or antethoracic NEC 42.69
         with
            interposition (of) NEC 42.68
               colon 42.65
               jejunal loop 42.63
               small bowel 42.63
            rubber tube 42.68
      to intestinal segment NEC 42.64
         with interposition 42.68
         colon 42.66
            with interposition 42.65
         small bowel NEC 42.64
            with interposition 42.63
      to intestinal segment (intrathoracic) NEC 42.54
         with interposition 42.58
         antesternal or antethoracic NEC 42.64
            with interposition 42.68
         colon (intrathoracic) NEC 42.56
            with interposition 42.55
            antesternal or antethoracic 42.66
               with interposition 42.65
         small bowel NEC 42.54
            with interposition 42.53
            antesternal or antethoracic 42.64
               with interposition 42.63
   facial-accessory nerve 04.72
   facial-hypoglossal nerve 04.71
   fallopian tube 66.73
   gallbladder 51.35
      to
         hepatic ducts 51.31
         intestine 51.32
         pancreas 51.33
         stomach 51.34
   hepatic duct 51.39

hypoglossal-accessory nerve 04.73
hypoglossal-facial nerve 04.71
ileal loop to bladder 57.87 [45.51]
ileoanal 45.95
ileorectal 45.93
inferior vena cava and portal vein 39.1
internal mammary artery (to)
    coronary artery (single vessel) 36.15
        double vessel 36.16
    myocardium 36.2
intestine 45.90
    large-to-anus 45.95
    large-to-large 45.94
    large-to-rectum 45.94
    large-to-small 45.93
    small-to-anus 45.95
    small-to-large 45.93
    small-to-rectal stump 45.92
    small-to-small 45.91
intrahepatic 51.79
intrathoracic vessel NEC 39.23
kidney (pelvis) 55.86
lacrimal sac to conjunctiva 09.82
left-to-right (systemic-pulmonary artery) 39.0
lymphatic (channel) (peripheral) 40.9
mesenteric-caval 39.1
mesocaval 39.1
nasolacrimal 09.81
nerve (cranial) (peripheral) NEC 04.74
    accessory-facial 04.72
    accessory-hypoglossal 04.73
    hypoglossal-facial 04.71
pancreas (duct) (to) 52.96
    bile duct 51.39
    gall bladder 51.53
    intestine 52.96
    jejunum 52.96
    stomach 52.96
pleurothecal (with valve) 03.79
portacaval 39.1
portal vein to inferior vena cava 39.1
pulmonary-aortic (Pott's) 39.0
pulmonary artery and superior vena cava 39.21
pulmonary-innominate artery (Blalock) 39.0
pulmonary-subclavian artery (Blalock-Taussig) 39.0
pulmonary vein and azygos vein 39.23
pyeloileocutaneous 56.51
pyeloureterovesical 55.86
rectum, rectal NEC 48.74
    stump to small intestine 45.92
renal (pelvis) 55.86
    vein and splenic vein 39.1
renoportal 39.1
salpingothecal (with valve) 03.79
splenic to renal veins 39.1
▸ splenorenal (venous) 39.1
▸   arterial 39.26
subarachnoid-peritoneal (with valve) 03.71
    subarachnoid-ureteral (with valve) 03.72
subclavian-aortic 39.22
superior vena cava to pulmonary artery 39.21
systemic-pulmonary artery 39.0
thoracic artery (to)
    coronary artery (single) 36.15
        double 36.16
    myocardium 36.2
ureter (to) NEC 56.79

bladder 56.74
colon 56.71
ileal pouch (bladder) 56.51
ileum 56.71
intestine 56.71
skin 56.61
ureterocalyceal 55.86
ureterocolic 56.71
ureterovesical 56.74
urethra (end-to-end) 58.44
vas deferens 63.82
veins (suture of proximal to distal end) (with bypass graft) 39.29
    with excision or resection of vessel — see Phlebectomy, with anastomosis, by site
    mesenteric to vena cava 39.1
    portal to inferior vena cava 39.1
    revision 39.49
    splenic and renal 39.1
ventricle, ventricular (intracerebral) (with valve) (see also Shunt, ventricular) 02.2
ventriculoatrial (with valve) 02.32
ventriculocaval (with valve) 02.32
ventriculomastoid (with valve) 02.31
ventriculopleural (with valve) 02.33
vesicle — see Anastomosis, bladder

Anderson operation (tibial lengthening) 78.37
Anel operation (dilation of lacrimal duct) 09.42
Anesthesia, spinal — omit code
Aneurysmectomy 38.60
    with
        anastomosis 38.30
            abdominal
                artery 38.36
                vein 38.37
            aorta (arch) (ascending) (descending) 38.34
            head and neck NEC 38.32
            intracranial NEC 38.31
            lower limb
                artery 38.38
                vein 38.39
            thoracic NEC 38.35
            upper limb (artery) (vein) 38.33
        graft replacement (interposition) 38.40
            abdominal
                aorta 38.44
                artery 38.46
                vein 38.47
            aorta (arch) (ascending) (descending thoracic)
                abdominal 38.44
                thoracic 38.45
                thoracoabdominal 38.45 [38.44]
            head and neck NEC 38.42
            intracranial NEC 38.41
            lower limb
                artery 38.48
                vein 38.49
            thoracic NEC 38.45
            upper limb (artery) (vein) 38.43
    abdominal
        artery 38.66
        vein 38.67
    aorta (arch) (ascending) (descending) 38.64
    atrial, auricular 37.32
    head and neck NEC 38.62
    heart 37.32

    intracranial NEC 38.61
    lower limb
        artery 38.68
        vein 38.69
    sinus of Valsalva 35.39
    thoracic NEC 38.65
    upper limb (artery) (vein) 38.63
    ventricle (myocardium) 37.32
Aneurysmoplasty — see Aneurysmorrhaphy
Aneurysmorrhaphy NEC 39.52
    by or with
        anastomosis — see Aneurysmectomy, with anastomosis, by site
        clipping 39.51
        coagulation 39.52
        electrocoagulation 39.52
        excision or resection — see also Aneurysmectomy, by site
        with
            anastomosis — see Aneurysmectomy, with anastomosis, by site
            graft replacement — see Aneurysmectomy, with graft replacement, by site
        filipuncture 39.52
        graft replacement — Aneurysmectomy, with graft replacement, by site
        methyl methacrylate 39.52
        suture 39.52
        wiring 39.52
        wrapping 39.52
    Matas' 39.52
Aneurysmotomy — see Aneurysmectomy
Angiectomy
    with
        anastomosis 38.30
            abdominal
                artery 38.36
                vein 38.37
            aorta (arch) (ascending) (descending) 38.34
            head and neck NEC 38.32
            intracranial NEC 38.31
            lower limb
                artery 38.38
                vein 38.39
            thoracic vessel NEC 38.35
            upper limb (artery) (vein) 38.33
        graft replacement (interposition) 38.40
            abdominal
                aorta 38.44
                artery 38.46
                vein 38.47
            aorta (arch) (ascending) (descending thoracic)
                abdominal 38.44
                thoracic 38.45
                thoracoabdominal 38.45 [38.44]
            head and neck NEC 38.42
            intracranial NEC 38.41
            lower limb
                artery 38.48
                vein 38.49
            thoracic vessel NEC 38.45
            upper limb (artery) (vein) 38.43
Angiocardiography (selective) 88.50
    carbon dioxide (negative contrast) 88.58
    combined right and left heart 88.54
    left heart (aortic valve) (atrium) (ventricle) (ventricular outflow tract) 88.53
        combined with right heart 88.54

right heart (atrium) (pulmonary valve) (ventricle) (ventricular outflow tract) 88.52
    combined with left heart 88.54
vena cava (inferior) (superior) 88.51
Angiography (arterial) (*see also* Arteriography) 88.40
  by radioisotope — *see* Scan, radioisotope, by site
  by ultrasound — *see* Ultrasonography, by site
  basilar 88.41
  brachial 88.49
  carotid (internal) 88.41
  celiac 88.47
  cerebral (posterior circulation) 88.41
  coronary NEC 88.57
  eye (fluorescein) 95.12
  femoral 88.48
  heart 88.50
  intra-abdominal NEC 88.47
  intracranial 88.41
  intrathoracic vessels NEC 88.44
  lower extremity NEC 88.48
  neck 88.41
  placenta 88.46
  pulmonary 88.43
  renal 88.45
  specified artery NEC 88.49
  transfemoral 88.48
  upper extremity NEC 88.49
  veins — *see* Phlebography
  vertebral 88.41
Angioplasty (laser) — *see also* Repair, blood vessel
  balloon (percutaneous transluminal) NEC 39.59
    coronary artery (single vessel) 36.01
      with thrombolytic agent infusion 36.02
      multiple vessels 36.05
    other sites (femoropopliteal) (iliac) (renal) (vertebral) 39.59
  coronary 36.09
    open chest approach 36.03
    percutaneous transluminal (balloon) (single vessel) 36.01
      with thrombolytic agent infusion 36.02
      multiple vessels 36.05
  percutaneous transluminal (balloon) (single vessel) 39.59
    coronary (balloon) (single vessel) 36.01
      with thrombolytic agent infusion 36.02
      multiple vessels 36.05
    femoropopliteal 39.59
    iliac 39.59
    renal 39.59
    vertebral 39.59
  specified site NEC 39.59
Angiorrhaphy 39.30
  artery 39.31
  vein 39.32
Angioscopy, percutaneous 38.22
  eye (fluorescein) 95.12
Angiotomy 38.00
  abdominal
    artery 38.06
    vein 38.07
  aorta (arch) (ascending) (descending) 38.04

  head and neck NEC 38.02
  intracranial NEC 38.01
  lower limb
    artery 38.08
    vein 38.09
  thoracic NEC 38.05
  upper limb (artery) (vein) 38.03
Angiotripsy 39.98
Ankylosis, production of — *see* Arthrodesis
Annuloplasty (heart) (posteromedial) 35.33
Anoplasty 49.79
  with hemorrhoidectomy 49.46
Anoscopy 49.21
Antibiogram — *see* Examination, microscopic
Antiembolic filter, vena cava 38.7
Antiphobic treatment 94.39
Antrectomy
  mastoid 20.49
  maxillary 22.39
    radical 22.31
  pyloric 43.6
Antrostomy — *see* Antrotomy
Antrotomy (exploratory) (nasal sinus) 22.2
  Caldwell-Luc (maxillary sinus) 22.39
    with removal of membrane lining 22.31
  intranasal 22.2
    with external approach (Caldwell-Luc) 22.39
      radical 22.31
  maxillary (simple) 22.2
    with Caldwell-Luc approach 22.39
      with removal of membrane lining 22.31
    external (Caldwell-Luc approach) 22.39
      with removal of membrane lining 22.31
    radical (with removal of membrane lining) 22.31
Antrum window operation — *see* Antrotomy, maxillary
Aorticopulmonary window operation 39.59
Aortogram, aortography (abdominal) (retrograde) (selective) (translumbar) 88.42
Aortoplasty (aortic valve) (gusset type) 35.11
Aortotomy 38.04
Apexcardiogram (with ECG lead) 89.57
Apheresis, therapeutic — *see* category 99.7
Apicectomy
  lung 32.3
  petrous pyramid 20.59
  tooth (root) 23.73
    with root canal therapy 23.72
Apicoectomy 23.73
  with root canal therapy 23.72
Apicolysis (lung) 33.39
Apicostomy, alveolar 24.0
Aponeurectomy 83.42
  hand 82.33
Aponeurorrhaphy (*see also* Suture, tendon) 83.64
  hand (*see also* Suture, tendon, hand) 82.45
Aponeurotomy 83.13
  hand 82.11
Appendectomy (with drainage) 47.0
  incidental 47.1
Appendicectomy (with drainage) 47.0
  incidental 47.1
Appendicocecostomy 47.91

Appendicoenterostomy 47.91
Appendicolysis 54.5
  with appendectomy 47.0
Appendicostomy 47.91
  closure 47.92
Appendicotomy 47.2
Application
  anti-shock trousers 93.58
  arch bars (orthodontic) 24.7
    for immobilization (fracture) 93.55
  Barton's tongs (skull) (with synchronous skeletal traction) 02.94
  bone growth stimulator (surface) (transcutaneous 99.86
  Bryant's traction 93.44
    with reduction of fracture or dislocation — *see* Reduction, fracture and Reduction, dislocation
  Buck's traction 93.46
  caliper tongs (skull) (with synchronous skeletal traction) 02.94
  cast (fiberglass) (plaster) (plastic) NEC 93.53
    with reduction of fracture or dislocation — *see* Reduction, fracture and Reduction, dislocation
    spica 93.51
  cervical collar 93.52
    with reduction of fracture or dislocation — *see* Reduction, fracture and Reduction, dislocation
  clamp, cerebral aneurysm (Crutchfield) (Silverstone) 39.51
  croupette, croup tent 93.94
  crown (artificial) 23.41
  Crutchfield tongs (skull) (with synchronous skeletal traction) 02.94
  Dunlop's traction 93.44
    with reduction of fracture or dislocation — *see* Reduction, fracture and Reduction, dislocation
  elastic stockings 93.59
  electronic gaiter 93.59
  external, fixator device (bone) 78.10
    carpal, metacarpal 78.14
    clavicle 78.11
    femur 78.15
    fibula 78.17
    humerus 78.12
    patella 78.16
    pelvic 78.19
    phalanges (foot) (hand) 78.19
    radius 78.13
    scapula 78.11
    specified site NEC 78.19
    tarsal, metatarsal 78.18
    thorax (ribs) (sternum) 78.11
    tibia 78.17
    ulna 78.13
    vertebrae 78.19
  forceps, with delivery — *see* Delivery, forceps
  graft — *see* Graft
  gravity (G-) suit 93.59
  intermittent pressure device 93.59
  Jewett extension brace 93.59
  Jobst pumping unit (reduction of edema) 93.59
  Lyman Smith traction 93.44
    with reduction of fracture or dislocation — *see* Reduction, fracture and Reduction, dislocation
  MAST (military anti-shock trousers) 93.58

Minerva jacket 93.52
minifixator device (bone) — see category 78.1
neck support (molded) 93.52
obturator (orthodontic) 24.7
orthodontic appliance (obturator) (wiring) 24.7
pelvic sling 93.44
    with reduction of fracture or dislocation — see Reduction, fracture and Reduction, dislocation
periodontal splint (orthodontic) 24.7
plaster jacket 93.51
    Minerva 93.52
pressure
    dressing (bandage) (Gibney) (Robert Jones') (Shanz) 93.56
    trousers (anti-shock) (MAST) 93.58
prosthesis for missing ear 18.71
Russell's traction 93.44
    with reduction of fracture or dislocation — see Reduction, fracture and Reduction, dislocation
splint, for immobilization (plaster) (pneumatic) (tray) 93.54
    with fracture reduction — see Reduction, fracture
Thomas collar 93.52
    with reduction of fracture or dislocation — see Reduction, fracture and Reduction, dislocation
traction
    with reduction of fracture or dislocation — see Reduction, fracture and Reduction, dislocation
    adhesive tape (skin) 93.46
    boot 93.46
    Bryant's 93.44
    Buck's 93.46
    Cotrel's 93.42
    Dunlop's 93.44
    gallows 93.46
    Lyman Smith 93.44
    Russell's 93.44
    skeletal NEC 93.44
        intermittent 93.43
    skin, limbs NEC 93.46
    spinal NEC 93.42
        with skull device (halo) (caliper) (Crutchfield) (Gardner-Wells) (Vinke) (tongs) 93.41
            with synchronous insertion 02.94
    Thomas' splint 93.45
Unna's paste boot 93.53
vasopneumatic device 93.58
Velpeau dressing 93.49
Vinke tongs (skull) (with synchronous skeletal traction) 02.94
wound dressing NEC 93.57

Arc lamp — see Photocoagulation
Arrest
    bone growth (epiphyseal) 78.20
        by stapling — see Stapling, epiphyseal plate
        femur 78.25
        fibula 78.27
        humerus 78.22
        radius 78.23
        tibia 78.27
        ulna 78.23
    cardiac, induced (anoxic) (circulatory) 39.63
    circulatory, induced (anoxic) 39.63

hemorrhage — see Control, hemorrhage
Arslan operation (fenestration of inner ear) 20.61
Arteriectomy 38.60
    with
        anastomosis 38.30
            abdominal 38.36
            aorta (arch) (ascending) (descending) 38.34
            head and neck NEC 38.32
            intracranial NEC 38.31
            lower limb 38.38
            thoracic NEC 38.35
            upper limb 38.33
        graft replacement (interposition) 38.40
            abdominal
                aorta 38.44
            aorta (arch) (ascending) (descending thoracic
                abdominal 38.44
                thoracic 38.45
                thoracoabdominal 38.45 [38.44]
            head and neck NEC 38.42
            intracranial NEC 38.41
            lower limb 38.48
            thoracic NEC 38.45
            upper limb 38.43
    abdominal 38.66
    aorta (arch) (ascending) (descending) 38.64
    head and neck NEC 38.62
    intracranial NEC 38.61
    lower limb 38.68
    thoracic NEC 38.65
    upper limb 38.63
Arteriography (contrast) (fluoroscopic) (retrograde) 88.40
    by
        radioisotope — see Scan, radioisotope
        ultrasound (Doppler) — see Ultrasonography, by site
    aorta (arch) (ascending) (descending) 88.42
    basilar 88.41
    brachial 88.49
    carotid (internal) 88.41
    cerebral (posterior circulation) 88.41
    coronary (direct) (selective) NEC 88.57
        double catheter technique (Judkins) (Ricketts and Abrams) 88.56
        single catheter technique (Sones) 88.55
    Doppler (ultrasonic) — see Ultrasonography, by site
    femoral 88.48
    head and neck 88.41
    intra-abdominal NEC 88.47
    intrathoracic NEC 88.44
    lower extremity 88.48
    placenta 88.46
    pulmonary 88.43
    radioisotope — see Scan, radioisotope
    renal 88.45
    specified site NEC 88.49
    superior mesenteric artery 88.47
    transfemoral 88.48
    ultrasound — see Ultrasonography, by site
    upper extremity 88.49
Arterioplasty — see Repair, artery
Arteriorrhaphy 39.31
Arteriotomy 38.00
    abdominal 38.06

aorta (arch) (ascending) (descending) 38.04
head and neck NEC 38.02
intracranial NEC 38.01
lower limb 38.08
thoracic NEC 38.05
upper limb 38.03
Arteriovenostomy 39.29
    for renal dialysis 39.27
Arthrectomy 80.90
    ankle 80.97
    elbow 80.92
    foot and toe 80.98
    hand and finger 80.94
    hip 80.94
    intervertebral disc 80.5
    knee 80.96
        semilunar cartilage 80.6
    shoulder 80.91
    specified site NEC 80.99
    spine NEC 80.99
    wrist 80.93
Arthrocentesis 81.91
    for arthrography — see Arthrogram
Arthrodesis (compression) (extra-articular) (intra-articular) (with bone graft) (with fixation device) 81.20
    ankle 81.11
    carporadial 81.25
    cricoarytenoid 31.69
    elbow 81.24
    finger 81.28
    foot NEC 81.17
    hip 81.21
    interphalangeal
        finger 81.28
        toe NEC 77.58
            claw toe repair 77.57
            hammer toe repair 77.56
    ischiofemoral 81.21
    knee 81.22
    lumbosacral, lumbar NEC 81.08
        anterior (interbody), anterolateral technique 81.06
        lateral transverse process technique 81.07
        posterior (interbody), postero-lateral technique) 81.08
    McKeever (metatarsophalangeal) 81.16
    metacarpocarpal 81.26
    metacarpophalangeal 81.27
    metatarsophalangeal 81.16
    midtarsal 81.14
    pantalar 81.11
    sacroiliac 81.08
    shoulder 81.23
    specified joint NEC 81.29
    spinal (see also Fusion, spinal) 81.00
    subtalar 81.13
    tarsometatarsal 81.15
    tibiotalar 81.11
    toe NEC 77.58
        claw toe repair 77.57
        hammer toe repair 77.56
    triple 81.12
    wrist 81.26
Arthroendoscopy — see Arthroscopy
Arthrogram, arthrography 88.32
    temporomandibular 87.13
Arthrolysis 93.26
Arthroplasty (with fixation device) (with traction) 81.96

Arthroscopy   ICD–9–CM   Astragalectomy

ankle 81.49
carpals 81.75
  with prosthetic implant 81.74
carpocarpal, carpometacarpal 81.75
  with prosthetic implant 81.74
Carroll and Taber (proximal
    interphalangeal joint) 81.72
cup (partial hip) 81.52
Curtis (interphalangeal joint) 81.72
elbow 81.85
  with prosthetic replacement (total)
    81.84
femoral head NEC 81.40
  with prosthetic implant 81.52
finger(s) 81.72
  with prosthetic implant 81.71
foot (metatarsal) with joint replacement
    81.57
Fowler (metacarpophalangeal joint) 81.72
hand (metacarpophalangeal)
    (interphalangeal) 81.72
  with prosthetic implant 81.71
hip (with bone graft) 81.40
  cup (partial hip) 81.52
  femoral head NEC 81.40
    with prosthetic implant 81.52
      with total replacement 81.51
    partial replacement 81.52
    total replacement 81.51
interphalangeal joint 81.72
  with prosthetic implant 81.71
Kessler (carpometacarpal joint) 81.74
knee (see also Repair, knee) 81.47
  prosthetic replacement
    (bicompartmental) (hemijoint)
    (partial) (total)
    (tricompartmental)
    (unicompartmental) 81.54
  revision 81.55
metacarpophalangeal joint 81.72
  with prosthetic implant 81.71
shoulder 81.83
  for recurrent dislocation 81.82
  prosthetic replacement (partial) 81.81
    total 81.80
temporomandibular 76.5
toe NEC 77.58
  with prosthetic replacement 81.57
  for hallux valgus repair 77.59
wrist 81.75
  with prosthetic implant 81.74
    total replacement 81.73
Arthroscopy 80.20
  ankle 80.27
  elbow 80.22
  finger 80.24
  foot 80.28
  hand 80.24
  hip 80.25
  knee 80.26
  shoulder 80.21
  specified site NEC 80.29
  toe 80.28
  wrist 80.23
Arthrostomy (see also Arthrotomy) 80.10
Arthrotomy 80.10
  as operative approach — omit code
  with
    arthrography — see Arthrogram
    arthroscopy — see Arthroscopy
    injection of drug 81.92
    removal of prothesis (see also Removal,
      prosthesis, joint structures) 80.00

ankle 80.17
elbow 80.12
foot and toe 80.18
hand and finger 80.14
hip 80.15
knee 80.16
shoulder 80.11
specified site NEC 80.19
spine 80.19
wrist 80.13
Artificial
  insemination 69.92
  kidney 39.95
  rupture of membranes 73.09
Arytenoidectomy 30.29
Arytenoidopexy 31.69
Asai operation (larynx) 31.75
Aspiration
  abscess — see Aspiration, by site
  anterior chamber, eye (therapeutic) 12.91
    diagnostic 12.21
  aqueous (eye) (humor) (therapeutic) 12.91
    diagnostic 12.21
  ascites 54.91
  Bartholin's gland (cyst) (percutaneous)
    71.21
  biopsy — see Biopsy, by site
  bladder (catheter) 57.0
    percutaneous (needle) 57.11
  bone marrow (for biopsy) 41.31
    from donor for transplant 41.91
    stem cell 99.79
  branchial cleft cyst 29.0
  breast 85.91
  bronchus 96.05
    with lavage 96.56
  bursa (percutaneous) 83.94
    hand 82.92
  calculus, bladder 57.0
  cataract 13.3
    with
      phacoemulsification 13.41
      phacofragmentation 13.43
        posterior route 13.42
  chest 34.91
  cisternal 01.01
  cranial (puncture) 01.09
  craniobuccal pouch 07.72
  craniopharyngioma 07.72
  cul-de-sac (abscess) 70.0
  curettage, uterus 69.59
    after abortion or delivery 69.52
    diagnostic 69.59
    to terminate pregnancy 69.51
  cyst — see Aspiration, by site
  diverticulum, pharynx 29.0
  endotracheal 96.04
    with lavage 96.56
  extradural 01.09
  eye (anterior chamber) (therapeutic) 12.91
    diagnostic 12.21
  fallopian tube 66.91
  fascia 83.95
    hand 82.93
  gallbladder (percutaneous) 51.01
  hematoma — see also Aspiration, by site
    obstetrical 75.92
      incisional 75.91
  hydrocele, tunica vaginalis 61.91
  hygroma — see Aspiration, by site
  hyphema 12.91
  hypophysis 07.72

intracranial space (epidural) (extradural)
    (subarachnoid) (subdural)
    (ventricular) 01.09
  through previously implanted catheter
    or reservoir (Ommaya)
    (Rickham) 01.02
joint 81.91
  for arthrography — see Arthrogram
kidney (cyst) (pelvis) (percutaneous)
    (therapeutic) 55.92
  diagnostic 55.23
liver (percutaneous) 50.91
lung (percutaneous) (puncture) (needle)
    (trocar) 33.93
middle ear 20.09
  with intubation 20.01
muscle 83.95
  hand 82.93
nail 86.01
nasal sinus 22.00
  by puncture 22.01
  through natural ostium 22.02
nasotracheal 96.04
  with lavage 96.56
orbit, diagnostic 16.22
ovary 65.91
percutaneous — see Aspiration, by site
pericardium (wound) 37.0
pituitary gland 07.72
pleural cavity 34.91
prostate (percutaneous) 60.91
Rathke's pouch 07.72
seminal vesicles 60.71
seroma — see Aspiration, by site
skin 86.01
soft tissue NEC 83.95
  hand 82.93
spermatocele 63.91
spinal (puncture) 03.31
spleen (cyst) 41.1
stem cell 99.79
subarachnoid space (cerebral) 01.09
subcutaneous tissue 86.01
subdural space (cerebral) 01.09
tendon 83.95
  hand 82.93
testis 62.91
thymus 07.92
thyroid (field) (gland) 06.01
  postoperative 06.02
trachea 96.04
  with lavage 96.56
  percutaneous 31.99
tunica vaginalis (hydrocele) (percutaneous)
    61.91
vitreous (and replacement) 14.72
  diagnostic 14.11
Assessment
  fitness to testify 94.11
  mental status 94.11
  nutritional status 89.39
  personality 94.03
  temperament 94.02
  vocational 93.85
Assistance
  cardiac — see also Resuscitation, cardiac
    extracorporeal circulation 39.61
  endotracheal respiratory - see category 96.7
  hepatic, extracorporeal 50.92
  respiratory (endotracheal) (mechanical) -
    see ventilation, mechanical
Astragalectomy 77.98

Asymmetrogammagram — *see* Scan, radioisotope
Atherectomy
 coronary — *see* angioplasty
 peripheral 39.59
Atriocommissuropexy (mitral valve) 35.12
Atrioplasty NEC 37.99
 combined with repair of valvular and ventricular septal defects — *see* Repair, endocardialcushion defect
 septum (heart) NEC 35.71
Atrioseptopexy (*see also* Repair, atrial septal defect) 35.71
Atrioseptoplasty (*see also* Repair, atrial septal defect) 35.71
Atrioseptostomy (balloon) 34.51
Atriotomy 37.11
Atrioventriculostomy (cerebral-heart) 02.32
Attachment
 eye muscle
  orbicularis oculi to eyebrow 08.36
  rectus to frontalis 15.9
 pedicle (flap) graft 86.74
  hand 86.73

 lip 27.57
 mouth 27.57
 pharyngeal flap (for cleft palate repair) 27.62
  secondary or subsequent 27.63
 retina — *see* Reattachment, retina
Atticoantrostomy (ear) 20.49
Atticoantrotomy (ear) 20.49
Atticotomy (ear) 20.23
Audiometry (Bekesy 5-tone) (impedance) (stapedial reflex response) (subjective) 95.41
Augmentation
 bladder 57.87
 breast — *see* Mammoplasty, augmentation
 buttock ("fanny-lift") 86.89
 chin 76.68
 genioplasty 76.68
 mammoplasty — *see* Mammoplasty, augmentation
 outflow tract (pulmonary valve) (gusset type) 35.26
  in total repair of tetralogy of Fallot 35.81

 vocal cord(s) 31.0
Auriculectomy 18.39
Autograft — *see* Graft
Autopsy 89.8
Autotransfusion (whole blood) 99.02
Autotransplant, autotransplantation — *see also* Reimplantation adrenal tissue (heterotopic)(orthotopic) 07.45
 kidney 55.61
 lung 33.5
 ovary 65.72
 pancreatic tissue 52.81
 parathyroid tissue (heterotopic) (orthotopic) 06.95
 thyroid tissue (heterotopic) (orthotopic) 06.94
 tooth 23.5
Avulsion, nerve (cranial) (peripheral) NEC 04.07
 acoustic 04.01
 phrenic 33.31
 sympathetic 05.29
Azygography 88.63

B

Bacterial smear — *see* Examination, microscopic
Baffes operation (interatrial transposition of venous return) 35.91
Baffle, atrial or interatrial 35.91
Balanoplasty 64.49
Baldy-Webster operation (uterine suspension) 69.22
Ball operation
    herniorrhaphy — *see* Repair, hernia, inguinal
    undercutting 49.02
Ballistocardiography 89.59
Balloon
    angioplasty — *see* Angioplasty, balloon
    pump, intra-aortic 37.61
    systostomy (atrial) 35.41
Bandage 93.57
    elastic 93.56
Banding, pulmonary artery 38.85
Bankhart operation (capsular repair into glenoid, for shoulder dislocation) 81.82
Bardenheurer operation (ligation of innominate artery) 38.85
Barium swallow 87.61
Barkan operation (goniotomy) 12.52
    with goniopuncture 12.53
Barr operation (transfer of tibialis posterior tendon) 83.75
Barsky operation (closure of cleft hand) 82.82
Basal metabolic rate 89.39
Basiotripsy 73.8
Bassett operation (vulvectomy with inguinal lymph node dissection) 71.5 [40.3]
Bassini operation — *see* Repair, hernia, inguinal
Batch-Spittler-McFaddin operation (knee disarticulation) 84.16
Beck operation
    aorta-coronary sinus shunt 36.3
    epicardial poudrage 36.3
Beck-Jianu operation (permanent gastrostomy) 43.19
Behavior modification 94.33
Bell-Beuttner operation (subtotal abdominal hysterectomy) 68.3
Belsey operation (esophagogastric sphincter) 44.65
Benenenti operation (rotation of bulbous urethra) 58.49
Berke operation (levator resection of eyelid) 08.33
Bicuspidization of heart valve 35.10
    aortic 35.11
    mitral 35.12
Bicycle dynamometer 93.01
Biesenberger operation (size reduction of breast, bilateral) 85.32
    unilateral 85.31
Bifurcation, bone (*see also* Osteotomy) 77.30
Bigelow operation (litholapaxy) 57.0
Bililite therapy (ultraviolet) 99.82
Billroth I operation (partial gastrectomy with gastroduodenostomy) 43.6
Billroth II operation (partial gastrectomy with gastrojejunostomy) 43.7
Binnie operation (hepatopexy) 50.69
Biofeedback, psychotherapy 94.39
Biopsy
    abdominal wall 54.22
    adenoid 28.11
    adrenal gland NEC 07.11
        closed 07.11
        open 07.12
        percutaneous (aspiration) (needle) 07.11
    alveolus 24.12
    anus 49.23
    appendix 45.26
    artery (any site) 38.21
    aspiration — *see* Biopsy, by site
    bile ducts 51.14
        closed (endoscopic) 51.14
        open 51.13
        percutaneous (needle) 51.12
    bladder 57.33
        closed 57.33
        open 57.34
        transurethral 57.33
    blood vessel (any site) 38.21
    bone 77.40
        carpal, metacarpal 77.44
        clavicle 77.41
        facial 76.11
        femur 77.45
        fibula 77.47
        humerus 77.42
        marrow 41.31
        patella 77.46
        pelvic 77.49
        phalanges (foot) (hand) 77.49
        radius 77.43
        scapula 77.41
        specified site NEC 77.49
        tarsal, metatarsal 77.48
        thorax (ribs) (sternum) 77.41
        tibia 77.47
        ulna 77.43
        vertebrae 77.49
    bowel — *see* Biopsy, intestine
    brain NEC 01.13
        closed 01.13
        open 01.14
        percutaneous (needle) 01.13
    breast 85.11
        blind 85.11
        closed 85.11
        open 85.12
        percutaneous (needle) (Vimm-Silverman) 85.11
    bronchus NEC 33.24
        brush 33.24
        closed (endoscopic) 33.24
        open 33.25
        washings 33.24
    bursa 83.21
    cardioesophageal (junction) 44.14
        closed (endoscopic) 44.14
        open 44.15
    cecum 45.25
        brush 45.25
        closed (endoscopic) 45.25
        open 45.26
    cerebral meninges NEC 01.11
        closed 01.11
        open 01.12
        percutaneous (needle) 01.11
    cervix (punch) 67.12
        conization (sharp) 67.2
    chest wall 34.23
    clitoris 71.11
    colon 45.25
        brush 45.25
        closed (endoscopic) 45.25
        open 45.26
    conjunctiva 10.21
    cornea 11.22
    cul-de-sac 70.23
    diaphragm 34.27
    duodenum 45.14
        brush 45.14
        closed (endoscopic) 45.14
        open 45.15
    ear (external) 18.12
        middle or inner ear 20.32
    endocervix 67.11
    endometrium NEC 68.16
        by
            aspiration curettage 69.59
            dilation and curettage 69.09
        closed (endoscopic) 68.16
        open 68.13
    epididymis 63.01
    esophagus 42.24
        closed (endoscopic) 42.24
        open 42.25
    extraocular muscle or tendon 15.01
    eye 16.23
        muscle (oblique) (rectus) 15.01
    eyelid 08.11
    fallopian tube 66.11
    fascia 83.21
    fetus 75.33
    gallbladder 51.12
        closed (endoscopic) 51.14
        open 51.13
        percutaneous (needle) 51.12
    ganglion (cranial) (peripheral) NEC 04.11
        closed 04.11
        open 04.12
        percutaneous (needle) 04.11
        sympathetic nerve 05.11
    gum 24.11
    heart 37.25
    hypophysis (*see also* Biopsy, pituitary gland) 07.15
    ileum 45.14
        brush 45.14
        closed (endoscopic) 45.14
        open 45.15
    intestine NEC 45.27
        large 45.25
            brush 45.25
            closed (endoscopic) 45.25
            open 45.26
        small 45.14
            brush 45.14
            closed (endoscopic) 45.14
            open 45.15
    intra-abdominal mass 54.24
        closed 54.24
        percutaneous (needle) 54.24
    iris 12.22
    jejunum 45.14
        brush 45.14
        closed (endoscopic) 45.14

open 45.15
joint structure (aspiration) 80.30
   ankle 80.37
   elbow 80.32
   foot and toe 80.38
   hand and finger 80.34
   hip 80.35
   knee 80.36
   shoulder 80.31
   specified site NEC 80.39
   spine 80.39
   wrist 80.33
kidney 55.23
   closed 55.23
   open 55.24
   percutaneous (aspiration) (needle) 55.23
labia 71.11
lacrimal
   gland 09.11
   sac 09.12
larynx 31.43
   brush 31.43
   closed (endoscopic) 31.43
   open 31.45
lip 27.23
liver 50.11
   closed 50.11
   open 50.12
   percutaneous (aspiration) (needle) 50.11
lung NEC 33.27
   brush 33.24
   closed (percutaneous) (needle) 33.26
      brush 33.24
      endoscopic 33.27
         brush 33.24
   endoscopic 33.27
   open 33.28
   transbronchial 33.27
lymphatic structure (channel) (node) (vessel) 40.11
mediastinum NEC 34.25
   closed 34.25
   open 34.26
   percutaneous (needle) 34.25
meninges (cerebral) NEC 01.11
   closed 01.11
   open 01.12
   percutaneous (needle) 01.11
   spinal 03.32
mesentery 54.23
mouth NEC 27.24
muscle 83.21
   extraocular 15.01
   ocular 15.01
nasopharynx 29.12
nerve (cranial) (peripheral) NEC 04.11
   closed 04.11
   open 04.12
   percutaneous (needle) 04.11
   sympathetic 05.11
nose, nasal 21.22
   sinus 22.11
      closed (endoscopic) (needle) 22.11
      open 22.12
ocular muscle or tendon 15.01
omentum 54.23
orbit 16.23
   by aspiration 16.22
ovary 65.12
   by aspiration 65.11
palate (bony) 27.21
   soft 27.22
pancreas 52.11
   closed (endoscopic) 52.11
   open 52.12
   percutaneous (aspiration) (needle) 52.11
pancreatic duct 52.14
   closed (endoscopic) 52.14
parathyroid gland 06.13
penis 64.11
perianal tissue 49.22
pericardium 37.24
periprostatic 60.15
perirectal tissue 48.26
perirenal tissue 59.21
peritoneal implant 54.23
peritoneum 54.23
periurethral tissue 58.24
perivesical tissue 59.21
pharynx, pharyngeal 29.12
pineal gland 07.17
pituitary gland 07.15
   transfrontal approach 07.13
   transsphenoidal approach 07.14
pleura, pleural 34.24
prostate NEC 60.11
   closed (transurethral) 60.11
   open 60.12
   percutaneous (needle) 60.11
   transrectal 60.11
rectum 48.24
   brush 48.24
   closed (endoscopic) 48.24
   open 48.25
salivary gland or duct 26.11
   closed (needle) 26.11
   open 26.12
scrotum 61.11
seminal vesicle NEC 60.13
   closed 60.13
   open 60.14
   percutaneous (needle) 60.13
sigmoid colon 45.25
   brush 45.25
   closed (endoscopic) 45.25
   open 45.26
sinus, nasal 22.11
   closed (endoscopic) (needle) 22.11
   open 22.12
skin (punch) 86.11
skull 01.15
soft palate 27.22
soft tissue NEC 83.21
spermatic cord 63.01
sphincter of Oddi 51.14
   closed (endoscopic) 51.14
   open 51.13
spinal cord (meninges) 03.32
spleen 41.32
   closed 41.32
   open 41.33
   percutaneous (aspiration) (needle) 41.32
stomach 44.14
   brush 44.14
   closed (endoscopic) 44.14
   open 44.15
subcutaneous tissue (punch) 86.11
supraglottic mass 29.12
sympathetic nerve 05.11
tendon 83.21
   extraocular 15.01
   ocular 15.01
testis NEC 62.11
   closed 62.11
   open 62.12
   percutaneous (needle) 62.11
thymus 07.16
thyroid gland NEC 06.11
   closed 06.11
   open 06.12
   percutaneous (aspiration) (needle) 06.11
tongue 25.01
   closed (needle) 25.01
   open 25.02
tonsil 28.11
trachea 31.44
   brush 31.44
   closed (endoscopic) 31.44
   open 31.45
tunica vaginalis 61.11
umbilicus 54.22
ureter 56.33
   closed (percutaneous) 56.32
      endoscopic 56.33
   open 56.34
   transurethral 56.33
urethra 58.23
uterus, uterine (endometrial) 68.16
   by
      aspiration curettage 69.59
      dilation and curettage 69.09
   closed (endoscopic) 68.16
   ligaments 68.15
      closed (endoscopic) 68.15
      open 68.14
   open 68.13
uvula 27.22
vagina 70.24
vas deferens 63.01
vein (any site) 38.21
vulva 71.11
Bischoff operation (ureteroneocystostomy) 56.74
Bisection — *see also* Excision
   hysterectomy 68.3
   ovary 65.29
   stapes foot plate 19.19
      with incus replacement 19.11
Bishoff operation (spinal myelotomy) 03.29
Blalock operation (systemic-pulmonary anastomosis) 39.0
Blalock-Hanlon operation (creation of atrial septal defect) 35.42
Blalock-Taussig operation (subclavian-pulmonary anastomosis) 39.0
Blascovic operation (resection and advancement of levator palpebrae superioris) 08.33
Blepharectomy 08.20
Blepharoplasty (*see also* Reconstruction, eyelid) 08.70
   extensive 08.44
Blepharorrhaphy 08.52
   division or severing 08.02
Blepharotomy 08.09
Blind rehabilitation therapy NEC 93.78
Block
   caudal — *see* Injection, spinal
   celiac ganglion or plexus 05.31
   dissection
      breast
         bilateral 85.46
         unilateral 85.45
      bronchus 32.6
      larynx 30.3
      lymph nodes 40.50

neck 40.40
vulva 71.5
epidural, spinal — *see* Injection, spinal
gasserian ganglion 04.81
intercostal nerves 04.81
intrathecal — *see* Injection, spinal
nerve (cranial) (peripheral) NEC 04.81
paravertebral stellate ganglion 05.31
peripheral nerve 04.81
spinal nerve root (intrathecal) — *see* Injection, spinal
stellate (ganglion) 05.31
subarachnoid, spinal — *see* Injection, spinal
sympathetic nerve 05.31
trigeminal nerve 04.81

Blood
flow study, Doppler-type (ultrasound) — *see* Ultrasonography
patch, spine (epidural) 03.95

Blount operation
femoral shortening (with blade plate) 78.25
by epiphyseal stapling 78.25

Boari operation (bladder flap) 56.74
Bobb operation (cholelithotomy) 51.04
Bone
age studies 88.33
mineral density study 88.98

Bonney operation (abdominal hysterectomy) 68.4
Borthen operation (iridotasis) 12.63
Bost operation
plantar dissection 80.48
radiocarpal fusion 81.26

Bosworth operation
arthroplasty for acromioclavicular separation 81.83
fusion of posterior lumbar and lumbosacral spine 81.08
for pseudarthrosis 81.09
resection of radial head ligaments (for tennis elbow) 80.92
shelf procedure, hip 81.40

Bottle repair of hydrocele, tunica vaginalis 61.2
Boyd operation (hip disarticulation) 84.18
Brauer operation (cardiolysis) 37.10
Breech extraction — *see* Extraction, breech
Bricker operation (ileoureterostomy) 56.51
Brisement (force) 93.26
Bristow operation (repair of shoulder dislocation) 81.82
Brock operation (pulmonary valvotomy) 35.03
Brockman operation (soft tissue release for clubfoot) 83.84
Bronchogram, bronchography 87.32
endotracheal 87.31
transcricoid 87.32

Bronchoplasty 33.48
Bronchorrhaphy 33.41
Bronchoscopy NEC 33.23
with biopsy 33.24
lung 33.27
brush 33.24
fiberoptic 33.22
with biopsy 33.24
lung 33.27
brush 33.24

through tracheostomy 33.21
with biopsy 33.24
lung 33.27
brush 33.24

Bronchospirometry 89.38
Bronchostomy 33.0
closure 33.42
Bronchotomy 33.0
Browne (-Denis) operation (hypospadias repair) 58.45
Brunschwig operation (temporary gastrostomy) 43.19
Buckling, scleral 14.49
with
air tamponade 14.49
implant (silicone) (vitreous) 14.41
resection of sclera 14.49
vitrectomy 14.49
vitreous implant (silicone) 14.41

Bunionectomy (radical) 77.59
with
arthrodesis 77.52
osteotomy of first metatarsal 77.51
resection of joint with prosthetic implant 77.59
soft tissue correction NEC 77.53

Bunnell operation (tendon transfer) 82.56
Burgess operation (amputation of ankle) 84.14
Burn dressing 93.57
Burr holes 01.24
Bursectomy 83.5
hand 82.31
Bursocentesis 83.94
hand 92.92
Bursotomy 83.03
hand 82.03
Burying of fimbriae in uterine wall 66.97
Bypass
aortocoronary (catheter stent) (with prosthesis) (with saphenous vein graft) (with veingraft) 36.10
one coronary vessel 36.11
two coronary vessels 36.12
three coronary vessels 36.13
four coronary vessels 36.14
arterial (graft) (mandril grown graft) (vein graft) NEC 39.29
carotid-cerebral 39.28
carotid-vertebral 39.28
extracranial-intracranial [EC-IC] 39.28
intra-abdominal NEC 39.26
intrathoracic NEC 39.23
peripheral NEC 39.29
cardiopulmonary 39.61
open 39.61
percutaneous (closed) 39.66
coronary (*see also* Bypass, aortocoronary) 36.10
carotid-cerebral 39.28
carotid-vertebral 39.28
extracranial-intracranial [EC-IC] 39.28
gastric 44.39
high 44.31
Printen and Mason 44.31
gastroduodenostomy (Jaboulay's) 44.39
gastroenterostomy 44.39
gastrogastrostomy 44.39
heart-lung (complete) (partial) 39.61
open 39.61

percutaneous (closed) 39.66
high gastric 44.31
ileo-jejunal 45.91
internal mammary-coronary artery (single) 36.15
double vessel 36.16
jejunal-ileum 45.91
pulmonary 39.61
open 39.61
percutaneous (closed) 39.66
shunt
intestine
large-to-large 45.94
small-to-large 45.93
small-to-small 45.91
stomach 44.39
high gastric 44.31
terminal ileum 45.93
vascular (arterial) (graft) (mandril grown graft) (vein graft) NEC 39.29
aorta-carotid-brachial 39.22
aorta-iliac-femoral 39.25
aorta-renal 39.24
aorta-subclavian-carotid 39.22
aortic-superior mesenteric 39.26
aortocarotid 39.22
aortoceliac 39.26
aortocoronary (*see also* Bypass, aortocoronary) 36.10
aortofemoral 39.25
aortofemoral-popliteal 39.25
aortoiliac 39.25
to popliteal 39.25
aortoiliofemoral 39.25
aortomesenteric 39.26
aortopopliteal 39.25
aortorenal 39.24
aortosubclavian 39.22
axillary-brachial 39.29
axillary-femoral (superficial) 39.29
axillofemoral (superficial) 39.29
carotid to subclavian artery 39.22
carotid-cerebral 39.28
carotid-vertebral 39.28
common hepatic-common iliac-renal 39.26
coronary (*see also* Bypass, aortocoronary) 36.10
extracranial-intracranial [EC-IC] 39.28
femoral-femoral 39.29
femoroperoneal 39.29
femoropopliteal (reversed saphenous vein) (saphenous) 39.29
femorotibial (anterior) (posterior) 39.29
iliofemoral 39.25
ilioiliac 39.26
internal mammary-coronary artery (single) 36.15
double vessel 36.16
intra-abdominal (arterial) NEC 39.26
venous NEC 39.1
intrathoracic NEC 39.23
peripheral artery NEC 39.29
popliteal-tibial 39.29
renal artery 39.24
splenorenal (venous) 39.1
arterial 39.26
subclavian-axillary 39.29
subclavian-carotid 39.22
subclavian-subclavian 39.22
Y graft to renal arteries 39.24

C

Caldwell operation (sulcus extension) 24.91
Caldwell-Luc operation (maxillary sinusotomy) 22.39
 with removal of membrane lining 22.31
Calibration, urethra 89.29
Calicectomy (renal) 55.4
Callander operation (knee disarticulation) 84.16
Caloric test, vestibular function 95.44
Calycectomy (renal) 55.4
Calyco-ileoneocystostomy 55.86
Calycotomy (renal) 55.11
Campbell operation
 bone block, ankle 81.11
 fasciotomy (iliac crest) 83.14
 reconstruction of anterior cruciate ligament 81.45
Campimetry 95.05
Canaliculodacryocystorhinostomy 09.81
Canaliculoplasty 09.73
Canaliculorhinostomy 09.81
Canaloplasty, external auditory meatus 18.6
Cannulation — *see also* Insertion, catheter
 ampulla of Vater 51.99
 antrum 22.01
 arteriovenous 39.93
 artery 38.91
 caval-mesenteric vein 39.1
 cisternal chyli 40.61
 Eustachian tube 20.8
 lacrimal apparatus 09.42
 lymphatic duct, left (thoracic) 40.61
 nasal sinus (by puncture) 22.01
  through natural ostium 22.02
 pancreatic duct 52.92
  by retrograde endoscopy (ERP) 52.93
 renoportal 39.1
 sinus (nasal) (by puncture) 22.01
  through natural ostium 22.02
 ▸ splenorenal (venous) 39.1
 ▸ arterial 39.26
 thoracic duct (cervical approach) (thoracic approach) 40.61
Cannulization — *see* Cannulation
Canthocystostomy 09.82
Canthoplasty 08.59
Canthorrhaphy 08.52
 division or severing 08.02
Canthotomy 08.51
Capsulectomy
 joint (*see also* Arthrectomy) 80.90
 kidney 55.91
 lens 13.65
  with extraction of lens 13.51
 ovary 65.29
Capsulo-iridectomy 13.65
Capsuloplasty — *see* Arthroplasty
 with arthroplasty — *see* Arthroplasty
 ankle 81.94
 foot 81.94
 lower extremity NEC 81.95
 upper extremity 81.93
Capsulotomy
 joint (*see also* Division, joint capsule) 80.40
  for claw toe repair 77.57
 lens 13.64

 with
  discission of lens 13.2
  removal of foreign body 13.02
   by magnet extraction 13.01
Cardiac
 mapping 37.27
 massage (external) (closed chest) 99.63
  open chest 37.91
 retraining 93.36
Cardiectomy (stomach) 43.5
Cardiocentesis 37.0
Cardiography (*see also* Angiocardiography) 88.50
Cardiolysis 37.10
Cardiomyopexy 36.3
Cardiomyotomy 42.7
Cardio-omentopexy 36.3
Cardiopericardiopexy 36.3
Cardioplasty (stomach and esophagus) 44.65
 stomach alone 44.66
Cardioplegia 39.63
Cardiopneumopexy 36.3
Cardiorrhaphy 37.4
Cardioschisis 37.12
Cardiosplenopexy 36.3
Cardiotomy (exploratory) 37.11
Cardiovalvulotomy — *see* Valvulotomy, heart
Cardioversion (external) 99.62
 atrial 99.61
Carotid pulse tracing with ECG lead 89.56
Carpectomy (partial) 77.84
 total 77.94
Carroll and Taber arthroplasty (proximal interphalangeal joint) 81.72
Casting (for immobilization) NEC 93.53
 with fracture-reduction — *see* Reduction, fracture
Castration
 female (oophorectomy, bilateral) 65.51
 male 62.41
C.A.T. (computerized axial tomography) (*see also* Scan, C.A.T.) 88.38
Catheterization — *see also* Insertion, catheter
 arteriovenous 39.93
 artery 38.91
 bladder, indwelling 57.94
  percutaneous (cystostomy) 57.17
  suprapubic NEC 57.18
 bronchus 96.05
  with lavage 96.56
 cardiac (right) 37.21
  combined left and right 37.23
  left 37.22
   combined with right heart 37.23
  right 37.21
   combined with left heart 37.23
 Eustachian tube 20.8
  combined left and right 37.23
  left 37.22
   combined with right heart 37.23
  right 37.21
   combined with left heart 37.23
 hepatic vein 38.93
 inferior vena cava 38.93
 lacrimonasal duct 09.44

 laryngeal 96.05
 nasolacrimal duct 09.44
 pancreatic cyst 52.01
 renal vein 38.93
 Swan-Ganz (pulmonary) 89.64
 transtracheal for oxygenation 31.99
 umbilical vein 38.92
 ureter (to kidney) 59.8
  for retrograde pyelogram 87.74
 urethra, indwelling 57.94
 vein NEC 38.93
  for renal dialysis 38.95
Cattell operation (herniorrhaphy) 53.51
Cauterization — *see also* Destruction, lesion, by site
 anus NEC 49.39
  endoscopic 49.31
 Bartholin's gland 71.24
 broad ligament 69.19
 bronchus 32.09
  endoscopic 32.01
 canaliculi 09.73
 cervix 67.32
 chalazion 08.25
 choroid plexus 02.14
 conjunctiva 10.33
  lesion 10.32
 cornea (fistula) (ulcer) 11.42
 ear, external 18.29
 endometrial implant — *see* Excision, lesion, by site
 entropion 08.41
 esophagus 42.39
  endoscopic 42.33
 eyelid 08.25
  for entropion or ectropion 08.41
 fallopian tube 66.61
  by endoscopy (hysteroscopy) (laparoscopy) 66.29
 hemorrhoids 49.43
 iris 12.41
 lacrimal
  gland 09.21
  punctum 09.72
   for eversion 09.71
  sac 09.6
 larynx 30.09
 liver 50.29
 lung 32.39
  endoscopic 32.28
 meibomian gland 08.25
 nose, for epistaxis (with packing) 21.03
 ovary 65.29
 palate (bony) 27.31
 pannus (superficial) 11.42
 pharynx 29.39
 punctum, lacrimal 09.72
  for eversion 09.71
 rectum 48.32
  radical 48.31
 round ligament 69.19
 sclera 12.84
  with iridectomy 12.62
 skin 86.3
 subcutaneous tissue 86.3
 tonsillar fossa 28.7
 urethra 58.3
  endoscopic 58.31
 uterosacral ligament 69.19
 uterotubal ostia 66.61

uterus 68.29
vagina 70.33
vocal cords 30.09
vulva 71.3
Cavernoscopy 34.21
Cavernostomy 33.1
Cavernotomy, kidney 55.39
Cavography (inferior vena cava) 88.51
Cecectomy (with resection of terminal ileum) 45.72
Cecil operation (urethral reconstruction) 58.46
Cecocolopficopexy 46.63
Cecocolostomy 45.94
Cecofixation 46.64
Ceco-ileostomy 45.93
Cecopexy 46.64
Cecoplication 46.62
Cecorrhaphy 46.75
Cecosigmoidostomy 45.94
Cecostomy (tube) (see also Colostomy) 46.10
Cecotomy 45.03
Celiocentesis 54.91
Celioscopy 54.21
Celiotomy, exploratory 54.11
Cell block and Papanicolaou smear — see Examination, microscopic
Cephalogram 87.17
 dental 87.12
 orthodontic 87.12
Cephalometry, cephalometrics 87.17
 echo 88.78
 orthodontic 87.12
 ultrasound (sonar) 88.78
 x-ray 87.81
Cephalotomy, fetus 73.8
Cerclage
 anus 49.72
 cervix 67.5
 isthmus uteri (cervix) 67.5
 retinal reattachment (see also Buckling, scleral) 14.49
 sclera (see also Buckling, scleral) 14.49
Cervicectomy (with synchronous colporrhaphy) 67.4
Cervicoplasty 67.69
Cesarean section 74.99
 classical 74.0
 corporeal 74.0
 extraperitoneal 74.2
 fundal 74.0
 laparotrachelotomy 74.1
 Latzko 74.2
 low cervical 74.1
 lower uterine segment 74.1
 peritoneal exclusion 74.4
 specified type NEC 74.4
 supravesical 74.4
 transperitoneal 74.4
  classical 74.0
  low cervical 74.1
 upper uterine segment 74.0
 vaginal 74.4
 Waters 74.2
Chandler operation (hip fusion) 81.21
Change — see also Replacement
 cast NEC 97.13
  lower limb 97.12
  upper limb 97.11
 cystostomy catheter or tube 59.94
 gastrostomy tube 97.02
 length
  bone — see either category 78.2 Shortening, bone or category 78.3 Lengthening, bone
  muscle 83.85
   hand 82.55
  tendon 83.85
   hand 82.55
 nephrostomy catheter or tube 55.93
 pyelostomy catheter or tube 55.94
 tracheostomy tube 97.23
 ureterostomy catheter or tube 57.95
 urethral catheter, indwelling 57.95
Character analysis, psychologic 94.03
Charles operation (correction of lymphedema) 40.9
Charnley operation (compression arthrodesis)
 ankle 81.11
 hip 81.21
 knee 81.22
Cheatie-Henry operation — see Repair, hernia, femoral
Check
 pacemaker, artificial (cardiac) (function) (rate) 89.45
  amperage threshold 89.48
  artifact wave form 89.46
  electrode impedance 89.47
  voltage threshold 89.48
 vision NEC 95.09
Cheiloplasty 27.59
Cheilorrhaphy 27.51
Cheilostomatoplasty 27.59
Cheilotomy 27.0
Chemical peel, skin 86.24
Chemocauterization — see also Destruction, lesion, by site
 corneal epithelium 11.41
 palate 27.31
Chemodectomy 39.8
Chemolysis
 nerve (peripheral) 04.2
 spinal canal structure 03.8
Chemoneurolysis 04.2
Chemonucleolysis (nucleus pulposus) 80.52
Chemopallidectomy 01.42
Chemopeel (skin) 86.24
Chemosurgery
 esophagus 42.39
  endoscopic 42.33
 Moh's 86.24
 skin (superficial) 86.24
 stomach 43.49
  endoscopic 43.41
Chemothalamectomy 01.41
Chemotherapy
 Antabuse 94.25
 for cancer NEC 99.25
 lithium 94.22
 methadone 94.25
 palate (bony) 27.31
Chevalier-Jackson operation (partial laryngectomy) 30.29
Child operation (radical subtotal pancreatectomy) 52.53
Cholangiocholangiostomy 51.39
Cholangiocholecystocholedochectomy 51.22
Cholangio-enterostomy 51.39
Cholangiogastrostomy 51.39
Cholangiogram 87.54
 endoscopic retrograde (ERC) 51.11
 intraoperative 87.53
 intravenous 87.52
 percutaneous hepatic 87.51
 transhepatic 87.53
Cholangiography (see also Cholangiogram) 87.54
Cholangiojejunostomy (intrahepatic) 51.39
Cholangiopancreatography, endoscopic retrograde (ERCP) 51.10
Cholangiostomy 51.59
Cholangiotomy 51.59
Cholecystectomy (total) 51.22
 laparoscopic 51.23
Cholecystenterorrhaphy 51.91
Cholecystocecostomy 51.32
Cholecystocholangiogram 87.59
Cholecystocolostomy 51.32
Cholecystoduodenostomy 51.32
Cholecystoenterostomy (Winiwater) 51.32
Cholecystogastrostomy 51.34
Cholecystogram 87.59
Cholecystoileostomy 51.32
Cholecystojejunostomy (Roux-en-Y) (with jejunojejunostomy) 51.32
Cholecystopancreatostomy 51.33
Cholecystopexy 51.99
Cholecystorrhaphy 51.91
Cholecystostomy NEC 51.03
 by trocar 51.02
Cholecystotomy 51.04
Choledochectomy 51.63
Choledochoduodenostomy 51.36
Choledochoenterostomy 51.36
Choledochojejunostomy 51.36
Choledocholithotomy 51.41
 endoscopic 51.88
Choledocholithotripsy 51.41
 endoscopic 51.88
Choledochopancreatostomy 51.39
Choledochoplasty 51.72
Choledochorrhaphy 51.71
Choledochoscopy 51.11
Choledochostomy 51.51
Choledochotomy 51.51
Cholelithotomy 51.04
Chondrectomy 80.90
 ankle 80.97
 elbow 80.92
 foot and toe 80.98
 hand and finger 80.94
 hip 80.95
 intervertebral cartilage — see category 80.5
 knee (semilunar cartilage) 80.6
 nasal (submucous) 21.5
 semilunar cartilage (knee) 80.6
 shoulder 80.91
 specified site NEC 80.99
 spine 80.5
 wrist 80.93
Chondroplasty — see Arthroplasty
Chondrosternoplasty (for pectus excavatum repair) 34.74
Chondrotomy (see also Division, cartilage) 80.40
 nasal 21.1

Chopart operation (midtarsal amputation) 84.12
Chordectomy, vocal 30.22
Chordotomy (spinothalmic) (anterior) (posterior) NEC 03.29
    percutaneous 03.21
    stereotactic 03.21
Ciliarotomy 12.55
Ciliectomy (ciliary body) 12.44
    eyelid margin 08.20
Cinch, cinching
    for scleral buckling (see also Buckling, scleral) 14.49
    ocular muscle (oblique) (rectus) 15.22
        multiple (two or more muscles) 15.4
Cineangiocardiography (see also angiocardiography) 88.50
Cineplasty, cineplastic prosthesis
    amputation — see Amputation
    arm 84.44
    biceps 84.44
    extremity 88.40
        lower 84.48
        upper 84.44
    leg 84.48
Cineradiograph — see Radiography
Cingulumotomy (brain) (percutaneous radiofrequency) 01.32
Circumcision (male) 64.0
    female 71.4
Clagett operation (closure of chest wall following open flap drainage) 34.72
Clamp and cautery, hemorrhoids 49.43
Clamping
    aneurysm (cerebral) 39.51
    blood vessel — see Ligation, blood vessel
    ventricular shunt 02.43
Clavicotomy 77.31
    fetal 73.8
Claviculectomy (partial) 77.81
    total 77.91
Clayton operation (resection of metatarsal heads and bases of phalanges) 77.88
Cleaning, wound 96.59
Clearance
    bladder (transurethral) 57.0
    pelvic
        female 68.8
            male 57.71
    prescalene fat pad 40.21
    renal pelvis (transurethral) 56.0
    ureter (transurethral) 56.0
Cleidotomy 77.31
    fetal 73.8
Clipping
    aneurysm (basilar) (carotid) (cerebellar) (cerebellopontine) (communicating artery)(vertebral) 39.51
    arteriovenous fistula 39.53
    frenulum, frenum
        labia (lips) 27.91
        linguae (tongue) 25.91
    tip of uvula 27.72
Clitoridectomy 71.4
Clitoridotomy 71.4
Clivogram 87.02
Closure — see also Repair
    abdominal wall 54.63
        delayed (granulating wound) 54.62
        secondary 54.61
        tertiary 54.62
    amputation stump, secondary 84.3
    aortopulmonary fenestration (fistula) 39.59
    appendicostomy 47.92
    artificial opening
        bile duct 51.79
        bladder 57.82
        bronchus 33.42
        common duct 51.72
        esophagus 42.83
        gallbladder 51.92
        hepatic duct 51.79
        intestine 46.50
            large 46.52
            small 46.51
        kidney 55.82
        larynx 31.62
        rectum 48.72
        stomach 44.62
        thorax 34.72
        trachea 31.72
        ureter 56.83
        urethra 58.42
    atrial septal defect — (see also Repair, atrial septal defect) 35.71
        with umbrella device (King-Mills type) 35.52
        combined with repair of valvular and ventricular septal defects — see Repair, endocardialcushion defect
    bronchostomy 33.42
    cecostomy 46.52
    cholecystostomy 51.92
    cleft hand 82.82
    colostomy 46.52
    cystostomy 57.82
    diastema (alveolar) (dental) 24.8
    disrupted abdominal wall (postoperative) 54.61
    duodenostomy 46.51
    encephalocele 02.12
    endocardial cushion defect (see also Repair, endocardial cushion defect) 35.73
    enterostomy 46.50
    esophagostomy 42.83
    fenestration
        aorticopulmonary 39.59
        septal, heart (see also Repair, heart, septum) 35.70
    filtering bleb, corneoscleral (postglaucoma) 12.66
    fistula
        abdominothoracic 34.83
        anorectal 48.73
        anovaginal 70.73
        antrobuccal 22.71
        anus 49.73
        aorticopulmonary (fenestration) 39.59
        aortoduodenal 39.59
        appendix 47.92
        biliary tract 51.79
        bladder NEC 57.84
        branchial cleft 29.52
        bronchocutaneous 33.42
        bronchoesophageal 33.42
        bronchomediastinal 34.73
        bronchopleural 34.73
        bronchopleurocutaneous 34.73
        bronchopleuromediastinal 34.73
        bronchovisceral 33.42
        bronchus 33.42
        cecosigmoidal 46.76
        cerebrospinal fluid 02.12
        cervicoaural 18.79
        cervicosigmoidal 67.62
        cervicovesical 57.84
        cervix 67.62
        cholecystocolic 51.93
        cholecystoduodenal 51.93
        cholecystoenteric 51.93
        cholecystogastric 51.93
        cholecystojejunal 51.93
        cisterna chyli 40.63
        colon 46.76
        colovaginal 70.72
        common duct 51.72
        cornea 11.49
            with lamellar graft (homograft) 11.62
                autograft 11.61
        diaphragm 34.83
        duodenum 46.72
        ear, middle 19.9
        ear drum 19.4
        enterocolic 46.74
        enterocutaneous 46.74
        enterouterine 69.42
        enterovaginal 70.74
        enterovesical 57.83
        esophagobronchial 33.42
        esophagocutaneous 42.84
        esophagopleurocutaneous 34.73
        esophagotracheal 31.73
        esophagus NEC 42.84
        fecal 46.79
        gallbladder 51.93
        gastric NEC 44.63
        gastrocolic 44.63
        gastroenterocolic 44.63
        gastroesophageal 42.84
        gastrojejunal 44.63
        gastrojejunocolic 44.63
        heart valve — see Repair, heart, valve
        hepatic duct 51.79
        hepatopleural 34.73
        hepatopulmonary 34.73
        ileorectal 46.74
        ileosigmoidal 46.74
        ileovesical 57.83
        ileum 46.74
        in ano 49.73
        intestine 46.79
            large 46.76
            small NEC 46.74
        intestinocolonic 46.74
        intestinoureteral 56.84
        intestinouterine 69.42
        intestinovaginal 70.74
        intestinovesical 57.83
        jejunum 46.74
        kidney 55.83
        lacrimal 09.99
        laryngotracheal 31.62
        larynx 31.62
        lymphatic duct, left (thoracic) 40.63
        mastoid (antrum) 19.9
        mediastinobronchial 34.73
        mediastinocutaneous 34.73
        mouth (external) 27.53
        nasal 21.82
            sinus 22.71
        nasolabial 21.82
        nasopharyngeal 21.82
        oroantral 22.71
        oronasal 21.82
        oval window (ear) 20.93
        pancreaticoduodenal 52.95
        perilymph 20.93
        perineorectal 48.73
        perineosigmoidal 46.76

perineourethroscrotal 58.43
perineum 71.72
perirectal 48.93
pharyngoesophageal 29.53
pharynx NEC 29.53
pleura, pleural NEC 34.93
pleurocutaneous 34.73
pleuropericardial 37.4
pleuroperitoneal 34.83
pulmonoperitoneal 34.83
rectolabial 48.73
rectoureteral 56.84
rectourethral 54.43
rectovaginal 70.73
rectovesical 57.83
rectovesicovaginal 57.83
rectovulvar 48.73
rectum NEC 48.73
renal 55.83
reno-intestinal 55.83
round window 20.93
salivary (gland) (duct) 26.42
scrotum 61.42
sigmoidovaginal 70.74
sigmoidovesical 57.83
splenocolic 41.95
stomach NEC 44.63
thoracic duct 40.63
thoracoabdominal 34.83
thoracogastric 34.83
thoracointestinal 34.83
thorax NEC 34.71
trachea NEC 31.73
tracheoesophageal 31.73
tympanic membrane (see also Tympanoplasty) 19.4
umbilicourinary 57.51
ureter 56.84
ureterocervical 56.84
ureterorectal 56.84
ureterosigmoidal 56.84
ureterovaginal 56.84
ureterovesical 56.84
urethra 58.43
urethroperineal 58.43
urethroperineovesical 57.84
urethrorectal 58.43
urethroscrotal 58.43
urethrovaginal 58.43
uteroenteric 69.42
uterointestinal 69.42
uterorectal 69.42
uteroureteric 56.84
uterovaginal 69.42
uterovesical 57.84
vagina 70.75
vaginocutaneous 70.75
vaginoenteric 70.74
vaginoperineal 70.75
vaginovesical 57.84
vesicocervicovaginal 57.84
vesicocolic 57.83
vesicocutaneous 57.84
vesicoenteric 57.83
vesicometrorectal 57.83
vesicoperineal 57.84
vesicorectal 57.83
vesicosigmoidal 57.83
vesicosigmoidovaginal 57.83
vesicoureteral 56.84
vesicoureterovaginal 56.84
vesicourethral 57.84
vesicourethrorectal 57.83
vesicouterine 57.84
vesicovaginal 57.84
vulva 71.72
vulvorectal 48.73

foramen ovale (patent) 35.71
  with
    prosthesis (open heart technique) 35.51
      closed heart technique 35.52
    tissue graft 35.61
gastroduodenostomy 44.5
gastrojejunostomy 44.5
gastrostomy 44.62
ileostomy 46.51
jejunostomy 46.51
laceration — see also Suture, by site
  liver 50.61
laparotomy, delayed 54.62
meningocele (spinal) 03.51
  cerebral 02.12
myelomeningocele 03.52
nephrostomy 55.82
palmar cleft 82.82
patent ductus arteriosus 38.85
pelviostomy 55.82
peptic ulcer (bleeding) (perforated) 44.40
perforation
  ear drum (see also Tympanoplasty) 19.4
  esophagus 42.82
  nasal septum 21.88
  tympanic membrane (see also Tympanoplasty) 19.4
proctostomy 48.72
punctum, lacrimal (papilla) 09.91
pyelostomy 55.82
rectostomy 48.72
septum defect (heart) (see also Repair, heart, septum) 35.70
sigmoidostomy 46.52
skin (V-Y type) 86.59
stoma
  bile duct 51.79
  bladder 57.82
  bronchus 33.42
  common duct 51.72
  esophagus 42.83
  gallbladder 51.92
  hepatic duct 51.79
  intestine 46.50
    large 46.52
    small 46.51
  kidney 55.82
  larynx 31.62
  rectum 48.72
  stomach 44.62
  thorax 34.72
  trachea 31.72
  ureter 56.83
  urethra 58.42
thoracostomy 34.72
tracheostomy 31.72
ulcer (bleeding) (peptic) (perforated) 44.40
  duodenum 44.42
  gastric 44.41
  intestine (perforated) 46.79
  skin 86.59
  stomach 44.41
ureterostomy 56.83
urethrostomy 58.42
▶ vagina 70.8
vesicostomy 57.82
wound — see also Suture, by site
  with graft — see Graft

Coagulation, electrocoagulation — see also Destruction, lesion, by site
  aneurysm (cerebral) (peripheral vessel) 39.52
    arteriovenous fistula 39.53
  brain tissue (incremental) (radiofrequency) 01.59
  broad ligament 69.19
  cervix 67.32
  ear
    external 18.29
    inner 20.79
    middle 20.51
  fallopian tube 66.61
  gasserian ganglion 04.05
  nose, for epistaxis (with packing) 21.03
  ovary 65.29
  pharynx (by diathermy) 29.39
  prostatic bed 60.94
  rectum (polyp) 48.32
    radical 48.31
  retina (for)
    destruction of lesion 14.21
    reattachment 14.51
    repair of tear 14.31
  round ligament 69.19
  semicircular canals 20.79
  spinal cord (lesion) 03.4
  urethrovesical junction, transurethral 57.49
  uterosacral ligament 69.19
  uterus 68.29
  vaginal 70.33
  vulva 71.3

Coating, aneurysm of brain 39.52
Cobalt-60 therapy (treatment) 92.23
Coccygectomy (partial) 77.89
  total 77.99
Coccygotomy 77.39
'Cocked hat' procedure (metacarpal lengthening and transfer of local flap) 82.69
Cockett operation (varicose vein) 38.5
  lower limb 38.59
  upper limb 38.53
Cody tack (perforation of footplate) 19.0
Coffey operation (uterine suspension) (Meig's modification) 69.22
Cole operation (anterior tarsal wedge osteotomy) 77.28
Colectomy (partial) (segmental) (subtotal) 45.79
  cecum (with terminal ileum) 45.72
  left (Hartmann) (lower) (radical) 45.75
  multiple segmental 45.71
  right (radical) 45.73
  sigmoid 45.76
  terminal ileum with cecum 45.72
  total 45.8
  transverse 45.74
Collapse, lung, surgical 33.39
  by
    destruction of phrenic nerve 33.31
    pneumoperitoneum 33.33
    pneumothorax, artificially-induced 33.32
    thoracoplasty 33.34
Collection, sperm for artificial insemination 99.96
Collis-Nissen operation (hiatal hernia repair with esophagogastroplasty) 53.80
Colocentesis 45.03
Colocolostomy 45.94
  proximal to distal segment 45.79
Colocystoplasty 57.87 [45.52]
Colofixation 46.64

Coloileotomy 45.00
Colonna operation
    adductor tenotomy (first stage) 83.12
    hip arthroplasty (second stage) 81.40
    reconstruction of hip (second stage) 81.40
Colonoscopy 45.23
    with biopsy 45.25
        rectum 48.24
    fiberoptic (flexible) 45.23
    intraoperative 45.21
    through stoma (artificial) 45.22
    transabdominal 45.21
Colopexy 46.63
Coloplication 46.64
Coloproctostomy 45.94
Colorectosigmoidostomy 45.94
Colorectostomy 45.94
Colorrhaphy 46.75
Coloscopy — *see* Colonoscopy
Colosigmoidostomy 45.94
Colostomy (ileo-ascending) (ileo-transverse) (perineal) (transverse) 46.10
    with anterior rectal resection 48.62
    delayed opening 46.14
    loop 46.03
    permanent (magnetic) 46.13
    temporary 46.11
Colotomy 45.03
Colpectomy 70.4
Colpoceliocentesis 70.0
Colpocentesis 70.0
Colpocleisis (complete) (partial) 70.8
Colpohysterectomy 68.5
Colpoperineoplasty 70.79
    with repair of urethrocele 70.50
Colpoperineorrhaphy 70.71
    following delivery 75.69
Colpopexy 70.77
Colpoplasty 70.79
Colpopoiesis 70.61
Colporrhaphy 70.71
    anterior (cystocele repair) 70.51
    for repair of
        cystocele 70.51
            with rectocele 70.50
        enterocele 70.92
        rectocele 70.52
            with cystocele 70.50
        urethrocele 70.51
    posterior (rectocele repair) 70.52
Colposcopy 70.21
Colpotomy 70.14
    for pelvic peritoneal drainage 70.12
Commando operation (radical glossectomy) 25.4
Commissurotomy
    closed heart technique — *see* Valvulotomy, heart
    open heart technique — *see* Valvuloplasty, heart
Compression, trigeminal nerve 04.02
Conchectomy 21.69
Conchotomy 21.1
Conduction study, nerve 89.15
Conduitogram, ileum 87.78
Condylectomy — *see category* 77.8
    mandible 76.5
Condylotomy NEC (*see also* Division, joint capsule) 80.40
    mandible (open) 76.62

closed 76.61
Conization
    cervix (knife) (sharp) (biopsy) 67.2
    by
        cryosurgery 67.33
        electroconization 67.32
Conjunctivocystorhinostomy 09.82
    with insertion of tube or stent 09.83
Conjunctivodacryocystorhinostomy (CDCR) 09.82
    with insertion of tube or stent 09.83
Conjunctivodacryocystostomy 09.82
    with insertion of tube or stent 09.83
Conjunctivoplasty 10.49
Conjunctivorhinostomy 09.82
    with insertion of tube or stent 09.83
Constriction of globe, for scleral buckling (*see also* Buckling, scleral) 14.49
Construction
    auricle, ear (with graft) (with implant) 18.71
    ear
        auricle (with graft) (with implant) 18.71
        meatus (osseous) (skin-lined) 18.6
    endorectal ileal pouch (J-pouch) (H-pouch) (S-pouch) (with anastomosis to anus) 45.95
    esophagus, artificial — *see* Anastomosis, esophagus
    ileal bladder (open) 56.51
        closed 57.87 [45.51]
    ileal conduit 56.51
    larynx, artificial 31.75
    patent meatus (ear) 18.6
    penis (rib graft) (skin graft) (myocutaneous flap) 64.43
    pharyngeal valve, artificial 31.75
    urethra 58.46
    vagina, artificial 70.61
    venous valves (peripheral) 39.59
Consultation 89.09
    comprehensive 89.07
    limited (single organ system) 89.06
    specified type NEC 89.08
Continuous positive airway pressure (CPAP) 93.90
Control
    atmospheric pressure and composition NEC 93.98
        antigen-free air conditioning 93.98
        decompression chamber 93.97
        mountain sanatorium 93.98
    epistaxis 21.00
    by
        cauterization (and packing) 21.03
        coagulation (with packing) 21.03
        electrocoagulation (with packing) 21.03
        excision of nasal mucosa with grafting 21.07
        ligation of artery 21.09
            ethmoidal 21.04
            external carotid 21.06
            maxillary (transantral) 21.05
        packing (nasal) (anterior) 21.01
            posterior (and anterior) 21.02
        specified means NEC 21.09
    hemorrhage 39.98
        abdominal cavity 54.19
        adenoids (postoperative) 28.7

        anus (postoperative) 49.95
        bladder (postoperative) 57.93
        chest 34.09
        colon 45.49
            endoscopic 45.43
        duodenum (ulcer) 44.49
        by
            embolization (transcatheter) 44.44
            suture (ligation) 44.42
        endoscopic 44.43
        esophagus 42.39
            endoscopic 42.33
        gastric (ulcer) 44.49
        by
            embolization (transcatheter) 44.44
            suture (ligation 44.41
        endoscopic 44.43
        intrapleural 34.09
            postoperative (recurrent) 34.03
        laparotomy site 54.12
        nose (*see also* Control, epistaxis) 21.00
        peptic (ulcer) 44.49
        by
            embolization (transcatheter) 44.44
            suture (ligation) 44.40
        endoscopic 44.43
        pleura, pleural cavity 34.09
            postoperative (recurrent) 34.03
        postoperative NEC 39.98
        postvascular surgery 39.41
        prostrate 60.94
        specified site NEC 39.98
        stomach — *see* Control, hemorrhage, gastric
        thorax NEC 34.09
            postoperative (recurrent) 34.03
        thyroid (postoperative) 06.02
        tonsils (postoperative) 28.7
Conversion
    anastomosis — *see* Revision, anastomosis
    cardiac rhythm NEC 99.69
        to sinus rhythm 99.62
    gastrostomy to jejunostomy (endoscopic) 46.32
    obstetrical position — *see* Version
Cooling, gastric 96.31
Cordectomy, vocal 30.22
Cordopexy, vocal 31.69
Cordotomy
    spinal (bilateral) NEC 03.29
        percutaneous 03.21
    vocal 31.3
Corectomy 12.12
Corelysis 12.35
Coreoplasty 12.35
Corneoconjunctivoplasty 11.53
Correction — *see also* Repair
    atresia
        esophageal 42.85
            by magnetic forces 42.99
        external meatus (ear) 18.6
        nasopharynx, nasopharyngeal 29.4
        rectum 48.0
        tricuspid 35.94
    atrial septal defect (*see also* Repair, atrial septal defect) 35.71
        combined with repair of valvular and ventricular septal defects — *see* Repair endocardialcushion defect
    blepharoptosis (*see also* Repair, blepharoptosis) 08.36

bunionette (with osteotomy) 77.54
chordee 64.42
claw toe 77.57
cleft
    lip 27.54
    palate 27.62
clubfoot NEC 83.84
coarctation of aorta
    with
        anastomosis 38.34
        graft replacement 38.44
cornea NEC 11.59
    refractive NEC 11.79
        epikeratophakia 11.76
        keratomeleusis 11.71
        keratophakia 11.72
        radial keratotomy 11.75
esophageal atresia 42.85
    by magnetic forces 42.99
everted lacrimal punctum 09.71
eyelid
    ptosis (see also Repair, blepharoptosis) 08.36
    retraction 08.38
fetal defect 75.36
forcible, of musculoskeletal deformity NEC 93.29
hammer toe 77.56
hydraulic pressure, open surgery for
    penile inflatable prosthesis 64.99
    urinary artificial sphincter 58.99
intestinal malrotation 46.80
    large 46.82
    small 46.81
inverted uterus — see Repair, inverted uterus
lymphedema (of limb) 40.9
    excision with graft 40.9
    obliteration of lymphatics 40.9
    transplantation of autogenous lymphatics 40.9
nasopharyngeal atresia 29.4
overlapping toes 77.58
palate (cleft) 27.62
prognathism NEC 76.64
prominent ear 18.5
punctum (everted) 09.71
spinal pseudoarthrosis 81.09
syndactyly 86.85
tetralogy of Fallot
    one-stage 35.81
    partial — see specific procedure
    total 35.81
total anomalous pulmonary venous connection
    one-stage 35.82
    partial — see specific procedure
    total 35.82
transposition, great arteries, total 35.84
tricuspid atresia 35.94
truncus arteriosus
    one-stage 35.83
    partial — see specific procedure
    total 35.83
ureteropelvic junction 55.87
ventricular septal defect (see also Repair, ventricular septal defect) 35.72
    combined with repair of valvular and atrial septal defects — see Repair, endocardialcushion defect

Costectomy 77.91
    with lung excision — see Excision, lung
    associated with thoracic operation — omit code

Costochondrectomy 77.91
    associated with thoracic operation — omit code

Costosternoplasty (pectus excavatum repair) 34.74

Costotomy 77.31

Costotransversectomy 77.91
    associated with thoracic operation — omit code

Counseling (for) NEC 94.49
    alcoholism 94.46
    drug addiction 94.45
    employers 94.49
    family (medical) (social) 94.49
    marriage 94.49
    ophthalmologic (with instruction) 95.36
    pastoral 94.49

Countershock, cardiac NEC 99.62

Coventry operation (tibial wedge osteotomy) 77.27

CPAP (continuous positive airway pressure) 93.90

Craniectomy 01.25
    linear (opening of cranial suture) 02.01
    reopening of site 01.23
    strip (opening of cranial suture) 02.01

Cranioclasis, fetal 73.8

Cranioplasty 02.06
    with synchronous repair of encephalocele 02.12

Craniotomy 01.24
    as operative approach — omit code
    fetal 73.8
    for decompression of fracture 02.02
    reopening of site 01.23

Craterization, bone (see also Excision, lesion, bone) 77.60

Crawford operation (tarso-frontalis sling of eyelid) 08.32

Creation — see also Formation
    cardiac pacemaker pocket
        with initial insertion of pacemaker — omit code
        new site (skin) (subcutaneous) 37.79
    conduit
        ileal (urinary) 56.51
        left ventricle and aorta 35.93
        right atrium and pulmonary artery 35.94
        right ventricle and pulmonary (distal) artery 35.92
        in repair of
            pulmonary artery atresia 35.92
            transposition of great vessels 35.92
            truncus arteriosus 35.83
    endorectal ileal pouch (J-pouch) (H-pouch) (S-pouch) (with anastomosis to anus) 45.95
    esophagogastric sphincteric competence NEC 44.66
    Hartmann pouch — see Colectomy, by site
    interatrial fistula 35.42
    pericardial window 37.12
    pleural window, for drainage 34.09
    shunt — see also Shunt
        arteriovenous fistula, for dialysis 39.93
        left-to-right (systemic to pulmonary circulation) 39.0
    subcutaneous tunnel for esophageal anastomosis 42.86
        with anastomosis — see Anastomosis, esophagus, antesternal
    syndactyly (finger) (toe) 86.89
    tracheoesophageal fistula 31.95
    window
        pericardial 37.12
        pleura, for drainage 34.09

Crede maneuver 73.59

Cricoidectomy 30.29

Cricothyreotomy (for assistance in breathing) 31.1

Cricothyroidectomy 30.29

Cricothyrostomy 31.1

Cricothyrotomy (for assistance in breathing) 31.1

Cricotomy (for assistance in breathing) 31.1

Cricotracheotomy (for assistance in breathing) 31.1

Crisis intervention 94.35

Croupette, croup tent 93.94

Crown, dental (ceramic) (gold) 23.41

Crushing
    bone — see category 78.4
    calculus
        bile (hepatic) passage 51.49
            endoscopic 51.88
        bladder (urinary) 52.09
            endoscopic 52.94
        fallopian tube (see also Ligation, fallopian tube) 66.39
    ganglion — see Crushing, nerve
    hemorrhoids 49.45
    nasal septum 21.88
    nerve (cranial) (peripheral) NEC 04.03
        acoustic 04.01
        auditory 04.01
        phrenic 04.03
            for collapse of lung 33.31
        sympathetic 05.0
        trigeminal 04.02
        vestibular 04.01
    vas deferens 63.71

Cryoablation — see Ablation

Cryoconization, cervix 67.33

Cryodestruction — see Destruction, lesion, by site

Cryoextraction, lens (see also Extraction, cataract, intracapsular) 13.19

Cryohypophysectomy (complete) (total) (see also Hypophysectomy) 07.69

Cryoleucotomy 01.32

Cryopexy, retinal — see Cryotherapy, retina

Cryoretinopexy (for)
    reattachment 14.52
    repair of tear or defect 14.32

Cryosurgery — see Cryotherapy

Cryothalamectomy 01.41

Cryotherapy — see also Destruction, lesion, by site
    bladder 57.59
    brain 01.59
    cataract 13.19
    cervix 67.33
    choroid — see Cryotherapy, retina
    ciliary body 12.72
    corneal lesion (ulcer) 11.43
        to reshape cornea 11.79
    ear
        external 18.29
        inner 20.79
    esophagus 42.39
        endoscopic 42.33

eyelid 08.25
hemorrhoids 49.44
iris 12.41
nasal turbinates 21.61
palate (bony) 27.31
retina (for)
    destruction of lesion 14.22
    reattachment 14.52
    repair of tear 14.32
skin 86.3
stomach 43.49
    endoscopic 43.41
subcutaneous tissue 86.3
turbinates (nasal) 21.61
warts 86.3
    genital 71.3

Cryptectomy (anus) 49.39
    endoscopic 49.31
Cryptorchidectomy (unilateral) 62.3
    bilateral 62.41
Cryptotomy (anus) 49.39
    endoscopic 49.31
Cuirass 93.99
Culdocentesis 70.0
Culdoplasty 70.92
Culdoscopy (exploration) (removal of foreign body or lesion) 70.22
Culdotomy 70.12
Culp-Deweerd operation (spiral flap pyeloplasty) 55.87
Culp-Scardino operation (ureteral flap pyeloplasty) 55.87
Culture (and sensitivity) — *see* Examination, microscopic
Curettage (with packing) (with secondary closure) — *see also* Dilation and curettage
    adenoids 28.6
    anus 49.39
        endoscopic 49.31
    bladder 57.59
        transurethral 57.49
    bone (*see also* Excision, lesion, bone) 77.60
    brain 01.59
    bursa 83.39
        hand 82.29
    cartilage (*see also* Excision, lesion, joint) 80.80
    cerebral meninges 01.51
    chalazion 08.25
    conjunctiva (trachoma follicles) 10.33
    corneal epithelium 11.41
        for smear or culture 11.21

ear, external 18.29
eyelid 08.25
joint (*see also* Excision, lesion, joint) 80.80
meninges (cerebral) 01.51
    spinal 03.4
muscle 83.32
    hand 82.22
nerve (peripheral) 04.07
    sympathetic 05.29
sclera 12.84
skin 86.3
spinal cord (meninges) 03.4
subgingival 24.31
tendon 83.39
    hand 82.29
    sheath 83.31
        hand 82.21
uterus (with dilation) 69.09
    aspiration (diagnostic) NEC 69.59
        after abortion or delivery 69.52
        to terminate pregnancy 69.51
    following delivery or abortion 69.02

Curette evacuation, lens 13.2
Curtis operation (interphalangeal joint arthroplasty) 81.72
Cutaneolipectomy 86.83
Cutdown, venous 38.94
Cutting
    nerve (cranial) (peripheral) NEC 04.03
        acoustic 04.01
        auditory 04.01
        root, spinal 03.1
        sympathetic 05.0
        trigeminal 04.02
        vestibular 04.01
    pedicle (flap) graft 86.71
    pylorus (with wedge resection) 43.3
    spinal nerve root 03.1
    ureterovesical orifice 56.1
    urethral sphincter 58.5
CVP (central venous pressure monitoring) 89.62
Cyclectomy (ciliary body) 12.44
    eyelid margin 08.20
Cyclicotomy 12.55
Cycloanemization 12.74
Cyclocryotherapy 12.72
Cyclodialysis (initial) (subsequent) 12.55
Cyclodiathermy (penetrating) (surface) 12.71
Cycloelectrolysis 12.71
Cyclophotocoagulation 12.73

Cyclotomy 12.55
Cystectomy — *see also* Excision, lesion, by site
    gallbladder — *see* Cholecystectomy
    urinary (partial) (subtotal) 57.6
        complete (with urethrectomy) 57.79
        radical 57.71
            with pelvic exenteration (female) 68.8
        total (with urethrectomy) 57.79
Cystocolostomy 57.88
Cystogram, cystography NEC 87.77
Cystolitholapaxy 57.0
Cystolithotomy 57.19
Cystometrogram 89.22
Cystopexy NEC 57.89
Cystoplasty NEC 57.89
Cystoproctostomy 57.88
Cystoprostatectomy, radical 57.71
Cystopyelography 87.74
Cystorrhaphy 57.81
Cystoscopy (transurethral) 57.32
    with biopsy 57.33
    for
        control of hemorrhage
            bladder 57.93
            prostate 60.94
        retrograde pyelography 87.74
    ileal conduit 56.35
    through stoma (artificial) 57.31
Cystostomy
    closed (suprapubic) (percutaneous) 57.17
    open (suprapubic) 57.18
    percutaneous (closed) (suprapubic) 57.17
    suprapubic
        closed 57.17
        open 57.18
Cystotomy (open) (for removal of calculi) 57.19
Cystourethrogram (retrograde) (voiding) 87.76
    levator muscle sling 59.71
    retropubic suspension 59.5
    suprapubic suspension 59.4
Cystourethroplasty 57.85
Cystourethroscopy 57.32
    with biopsy
        bladder 57.33
        ureter 56.33
Cytology — *see* Examination, microscopic

D

Dacryoadenectomy 09.20
   partial 09.22
   total 09.23
Dacryoadenotomy 09.0
Dacryocystectomy (complete) (partial) 09.6
Dacryocystogram 87.05
Dacryocystorhinostomy (DCR) (by intubation) (external)(intranasal) 09.81
Dacryocystostomy 09.53
Dacryocystosyringotomy 09.53
Dacryocystotomy 09.53
Dahlman operation (excision of esophageal diverticulum) 42.31
Dana operation (posterior rhizotomy) 03.1
Danforth operation (fetal) 73.8
Darrach operation (ulnar resection) 77.83
Davis operation (intubated ureterotomy) 56.2
de Grandmont operation (tarsectomy) 08.35
Deaf training 95.49
Debridement
   abdominal wall 54.3
   bone (*see also* Excision, lesion, bone) 77.60
      fracture — *see* Debridement, open fracture
   brain 01.59
   burn (skin) 86.28
      excisional 86.22
      nonexcisional 86.28
   cerebral meninges 01.51
   dental 96.54
   flap graft 86.75
   graft (flap) (pedicle) 86.75
   heart valve (calcified) — *see* Valvuloplasty, heart
   infection (skin) 86.28
      excisional 86.22
      nail bed or fold 86.27
      nonexcisional 86.28
   joint — *see* Excision, lesion, joint
   meninges (cerebral) 01.51
      spinal 03.4
   muscle 83.45
      hand 82.36
   nail 86.27
   nerve (peripheral) 04.07
   open fracture (compound) 79.60
      arm NEC 79.62
      carpal, metacarpal 79.63
      facial bone 76.2
      femur 79.65
      fibula 79.66
      foot NEC 79.67
      hand NEC 79.63
      humerus 79.61
      leg NEC 79.66
      phalanges
         foot 79.68
         hand 79.64
      radius 79.62
      specified site NEC 79.69
      tarsal, metatarsal 79.67
      tibia 79.66
      ulna 79.62
   patella 77.66
   pedicle graft 86.75
   skin or subcutaneous tissue (burn) (infection) (wound) 86.28
      excisional 86.22

      graft 86.75
      nail, nail bed, or nail fold 86.27
      nonexcisional 86.28
      pacemaker pocket 37.79
   skull 01.25
      compound fracture 02.02
   spinal cord (meninges) 03.4
   wound (skin) 86.28
      excisional 86.22
      nonexcisional 86.28
Decapitation, fetal 73.8
Decapsulation, kidney 55.91
Declotting — *see also* Removal, thrombus
   arteriovenous cannula or shunt 39.49
Decompression
   anus (imperforate) 48.0
   biliary tract 51.49
      by intubation 51.43
         endoscopic 51.87
         percutaneous 51.98
   brain 01.24
   carpal tunnel 04.43
   cauda equina 03.09
   chamber 93.97
   colon 96.08
      by incision 45.03
      endoscopic (balloon) 46.85
   common bile duct 51.42
      by intubation 51.43
         endoscopic 51.87
         percutaneous 51.98
   cranial 01.24
      for skull fracture 02.02
   endolymphatic sac 20.79
   ganglion (peripheral) NEC 04.49
      cranial NEC 04.42
   gastric 96.07
   heart 37.0
   intestine 96.08
      by incision 45.00
      endoscopic (balloon) 46.85
   intracranial 01.24
   labyrinth 20.79
   laminectomy 03.09
   laminotomy 03.09
   median nerve 04.43
   muscle 83.02
      hand 82.02
   nerve (peripheral) NEC 04.49
      auditory 04.42
      cranial NEC 04.42
      median 04.43
      trigeminal (root) 04.41
   orbit (*see also* Orbitotomy) 16.09
   pancreatic duct 52.92
      endoscopic 52.93
   pericardium 37.0
   rectum 48.0
   skull fracture 02.02
   spinal cord (canal) 03.09
   tarsal tunnel 04.44
   tendon (sheath) 83.01
      hand 82.01
   thoracic outlet
      by
         myotomy (division of scalenus anticus muscle) 83.19
         tenotomy 83.13
   trigeminal (nerve root) 04.41
Decortication

   arterial 39.7
   brain 01.51
   cerebral meninges 01.51
   heart 37.31
   kidney 55.91
   lung (partial) (total) 34.51
   nasal turbinates — *see* Turbinectomy
   nose 21.89
   ovary 65.29
   periarterial 39.7
   pericardium 37.31
   ventricle, heart (complete) 37.31
Deepening
   alveolar ridge 24.5
   buccolabial sulcus 24.91
   lingual sulcus 24.91
Defatting, flap or pedicle graft 86.75
Defibrillation, electric (external) (internal) 99.62
Delaying of pedicle graft 86.71
Delivery (with)
   assisted spontaneous 73.59
   breech extraction (assisted) 72.52
      partial 72.52
         with forceps to aftercoming head 72.51
      total 72.54
         with forceps to aftercoming head 72.53
      unassisted (spontaneous delivery) — omit code
   cesarean section — *see* Cesarean section
   Crede maneuver 73.59
   De Lee maneuver 72.4
   forceps 72.9
      application to aftercoming head (Piper) 72.6
      with breech extraction
         partial 72.51
         total 72.53
      Barton's 72.4
      failed 73.3
      high 72.39
         with episiotomy 72.31
      low (outlet) 72.0
         with episiotomy 72.1
      mid 72.29
         with episiotomy 72.21
      outlet (low) 72.0
         with episiotomy 72.1
      rotation of fetal head 72.4
      trial 73.3
   instrumental NEC 72.9
      specified NEC 72.8
   key-in-lock rotation 72.4
   Kielland rotation 72.4
   Malstrom's extraction 72.79
      with episiotomy 72.71
   manually assisted (spontaneous) 73.59
   spontaneous (unassisted) 73.59
      assisted 73.59
   vacuum extraction 72.79
      with episiotomy 72.71
Delorme operation
   pericardiectomy 37.31
   proctopexy 48.76
   repair of prolapsed rectum 48.76
   thoracoplasty 33.34
Denervation
   aortic body 39.8

carotid body 39.8
facet, percutaneous (radiofrequency) 03.96
ovarian 65.94
paracervical uterine 69.3
uterosacral 69.3

Denker operation (radical maxillary antrotomy) 22.31

Dennis-Barco operation — see Repair, hernia, femoral

Denonvillier operation (limited rhinoplasty) 21.86

Densitometry, bone (serial) (radiographic) 88.98

Depilation, skin 86.92

Derlacki operation (tympanoplasty) 19.4

Dermabrasion (laser) 86.25
for wound debridement 86.28

Derotation — see Reduction, torsion

Desensitization
allergy 99.12
psychologic 94.33

Desmotomy (see also Division, ligament) 80.40

Destruction
breast 85.20
chorioretinopathy (see also Destruction, lesion, choroid) 14.29
ciliary body 12.74
epithelial downgrowth, anterior chamber 12.93
fallopian tube 66.39
  with
    crushing (and ligation) 66.31
      by endoscopy (laparoscopy) 66.21
    division (and ligation) 66.32
      by endoscopy (culdoscopy) (hysteroscopy) (laparoscopy) (peritoneoscopy) 66.22
  ligation 66.39
    with
      crushing 66.31
        by endoscopy (laparoscopy) 66.21
      division 66.32
        by endoscopy (culdoscopy) (hysteroscopy) (laparoscopy) (peritoneoscopy) 66.22
  unilateral 66.92
fetus 73.8
hemorrhoids 49.49
  by
    cryotherapy 49.44
    sclerotherapy 49.42
inner ear (NEC) 20.79
  by injection 20.72
intervertebral disc (NOS) 80.50
  by injection 80.52
  by other specified method 80.59
  herniated (nucleus pulposus) 80.51
lacrimal sac 09.6
lesion (local)
  anus 49.39
    endoscopic 49.31
  Bartholin's gland 71.24
    by
      aspiration 71.21
      excision 71.24
      incision 71.22
      marsupialization 71.23

biliary ducts 51.69
  endoscopic 51.64
bladder 57.59
  transurethral 57.49
bone — see Excision, lesion, bone
bowel — see Destruction, lesion, intestine
brain (transtemporal approach) NEC 01.59
breast NEC 85.20
bronchus NEC 32.09
  endoscopic 32.01
cerebral NEC 01.59
  meninges 01.51
cervix 67.39
  by
    cauterization 67.32
    cryosurgery, cryoconization 67.33
    electroconization 67.32
choroid 14.29
  by
    cryotherapy 14.22
    diathermy 14.21
    implantation of radiation source 14.27
    photocoagulation 14.25
      laser 14.24
      xenon arc 14.23
    radiation therapy 14.26
ciliary body (nonexcisional) 12.43
  by excision 12.44
conjunctiva 10.32
  by excision 10.31
cornea NEC 11.49
  by
    cryotherapy 11.43
    electrocauterization 11.42
    thermocauterization 11.42
cul-de-sac 70.32
duodenum NEC 45.32
  by excision 45.31
  endoscopic 45.30
  endoscopic 45.30
esophagus (chemosurgery) (cryosurgery) (electroresection) (fulguration) NEC 42.39
  by excision 42.32
    endoscopic 42.33
  endoscopic 42.33
eye NEC 16.93
eyebrow 08.25
eyelid 08.25
  excisional — see Excision, lesion, eyelid
heart 37.33
  by catheter ablation 37.34
intestine (large) 45.49
  by excision 45.41
    endoscopic 45.43
      polypectomy 45.42
  endoscopic 45.43
    polypectomy 45.42
  small 45.34
    by excision 45.33
intranasal 21.31
iris (nonexcisional) NEC 12.41
  by excision 12.42
kidney 55.39
  by marsupialization 55.31
lacrimal sac 09.6
larynx 30.09
liver 50.29
lung 32.29
  endoscopic 32.28
meninges (cerebral) 01.51

spinal 03.4
nerve (peripheral) 04.07
  sympathetic 05.29
neuroma 04.07
  acoustic
    by craniotomy 04.01
    by radiosurgery 04.07
  cranial 04.07
  Morton's 04.07
  peripheral
    Morton's 04.07
nose 21.30
  intranasal 21.31
  specified NEC 21.32
ovary
  by
    aspiration 65.91
    excision 65.29
  cyst by rupture (manual) 65.93
palate (bony) (local) 27.31
  wide 27.32
pancreas 52.22
  by marsupialization 52.3
  endoscopic 52.21
pancreatic duct 52.22
  endoscopic 52.21
penis 64.2
pharynx (excisional) 29.39
rectum (local) 48.32
  by
    cryosurgery 58.34
    electrocoagulation 48.32
    excision 48.35
    fulguration 48.32
    laser (Argon) 48.33
  radical 48.31
retina 14.29
  by
    cryotherapy 14.22
    diathermy 14.21
    implantation of radiation source 14.27
    photocoagulation 14.25
      laser 14.24
      xenon arc 14.23
    radiation therapy 14.26
salivary gland NEC 26.29
  by marsupialization 26.21
sclera 12.84
scrotum 61.3
skin NEC 86.3
sphincter of Oddi 51.69
  endoscopic 51.64
spinal cord (meninges) 03.4
spleen 41.42
  by marsupialization 41.41
stomach NEC 43.49
  by excision 43.42
    endoscopic 43.41
  endoscopic 43.41
subcutaneous tissue NEC 86.3
testis 62.2
tongue 25.1
urethra (excisional) 58.39
  endoscopic 58.31
uterus 68.29
nerve (cranial) (peripheral) (by radiofrequency) 04.2
  sympathetic, by injection of neurolytic agent 05.32
neuroma 04.07
  acoustic
    by craniotomy 04.01
    by radiosurgery 04.07
  cranial 04.07
  Morton's 04.07

peripheral
- Morton's 04.07
- unilateral 66.92
- semicircular canals, by injection 20.72
- vestibule, by injection 20.72

Detachment, uterosacral ligaments 69.3

Determination
- mental status (clinical) (medico-legal) (psychiatric) NEC 94.11
- psychologic NEC 94.09
- vital capacity (pulmonary) 89.37

Detorsion
- intestine (twisted) (volvulus) 46.80
  - large 46.82
    - endoscopic (balloon) 46.85
  - small 46.81
- kidney 55.84
- ovary 65.95
- spermatic cord 63.52
  - with orchiopexy 62.5
- testis 63.52
  - with orchiopexy 62.5
- volvulus 46.80
  - endoscopic (balloon) 46.85

Detoxification therapy 94.25
- alcohol 94.62
  - with rehabilitation 94.63
    - combined alcohol and drug 94.68
      - with rehabilitation 94.69
- drug 94.65
  - with rehabilitation 94.66
    - combined with alcohol and drug 94.68
      - with rehabilitation 94.69

Devascularization, stomach 44.99

Dewebbing
- esophagus 42.01
- syndactyly (fingers) (toes) 86.85

Dextrorotation — see Reduction, torsion

Dialysis
- hemodiafiltration, hemofiltration (extracorporeal) 39.95
- kidney (extracorporeal) 39.95
- peritoneal 54.98
- renal (extracorporeal) 39.95

Diaphanoscopy
- nasal sinuses 89.35
- skull (newborn) 89.16

Diaphysectomy — see category 77.8

Diathermy 93.34
- choroid — see Diathermy, retina
- nasal turbinates 21.61
- retina
  - for
    - destruction of lesion 14.21
    - reattachment 14.51
    - repair of tear 14.31
  - surgical — see Destruction, lesion, by site
- turbinates (nasal) 21.61

Dickson operation (fascial transplant) 83.82

Dickson-Diveley operation (tendon transfer and arthrodesis to correct claw toe) 77.57

Dieffenbach operation (hip disarticulation) 84.18

Dilation
- achalasia 42.92
- ampulla of Vater 51.81
  - endoscopic 51.84
- anus, anal (sphincter) 96.23
- biliary duct
  - endoscopic 51.84
  - pancreatic duct 52.99
  - endoscopic 52.98
  - percutaneous (endoscopy) 51.98
  - sphincter
    - of Oddi 51.81
      - endoscopic 51.84
    - pancreatic 51.82
      - endoscopic 51.85
- bladder 96.25
  - neck 57.92
- bronchus 33.91
- cervix (canal) 67.0
  - obstetrical 73.1
  - to assist delivery 73.1
- choanae (nasopharynx) 29.91
- colon (endoscopic) (balloon) 46.85
  - colostomy stoma 96.24
- duodenum (endoscopic) (balloon) 46.85
- endoscopic — see Dilation, by site
- enterostomy stoma 96.24
- esophagus (by bougie) (by sound) 42.92
- fallopian tube 66.96
- foreskin (newborn) 99.95
- frontonasal duct 96.21
- gastrojejunostomy site, endoscopic 44.22
- heart valve — see Valvulotomy, heart
- ileostomy stoma 96.24
- ileum (endoscopic) (balloon) 46.85
- intestinal stoma (artificial) 96.24
- intestine (endoscopic) (balloon) 46.85
- jejunum (endoscopic) (balloon) 46.85
- lacrimal
  - duct 09.42
  - punctum 09.41
- larynx 31.98
- lymphatic structure(s) (peripheral) 40.9
- nares 21.99
- nasolacrimal duct (retrograde) 09.43
  - with insertion of tube or stent 09.44
- nasopharynx 29.91
- pancreatic duct 52.99
  - endoscopic 52.98
- pharynx 29.91
- prostatic urethra (transurethral) (balloon) 60.95
- punctum, lacrimal papilla 09.41
- pylorus
  - by incision 44.21
  - endoscopic 44.22
- rectum 96.22
- salivary duct 26.91
- sphenoid ostia 22.52
- sphincter
  - anal 96.23
  - cardiac 42.92
  - of Oddi 51.81
    - endoscopic 51.84
  - pancreatic 51.82
    - endoscopic 51.85
- pylorus, endoscopic 44.22
  - by incision 44.21
- Stenson's duct 26.91
- trachea 31.99
- ureter 59.8
  - meatus 56.91
- ureterovesical orifice 59.8
- urethra 58.6
- urethrovesical junction 58.6
- vagina (instrumental) (manual) NEC 96.16
- vesical neck 57.92
- Wharton's duct 26.91
- Wirsung's duct 62.99
  - endoscopic 52.98

Dilation and curettage, uterus (diagnostic) 69.09
- after
  - abortion 69.02
  - delivery 69.02
- to terminate pregnancy 69.01

Diminution, ciliary body 12.74

Disarticulation 84.91
- ankle 84.13
- elbow 84.06
- finger, except thumb 84.01
  - thumb 84.02
- hip 84.18
- knee 84.16
- shoulder 84.08
- thumb 84.02
- toe 84.11
- wrist 84.04

Discission
- capsular membrane 13.64
- cataract (Wheeler knife) (Ziegler knife) 13.2
  - congenital 13.69
  - secondary membranous 13.64
- iris 12.12
- lens (capsule) (Wheeler knife) (Ziegler knife) (with capsulotomy) 13.2
- orbitomaxillary, radical 16.51
- pupillary 13.2
- secondary membrane (after cataract) 13.64
- vitreous strands (posterior approach) 14.74
  - anterior approach 14.73

Discogram, diskogram 87.21

Discolysis (by injection) 80.52

Diskectomy, intervertebral 80.51
- herniated (nucleus pulposus) 80.51
- percutaneous 80.59

Dispensing (with fitting)
- contact lens 95.32
- low vision aids NEC 95.33
- spectacles 95.31

Dissection — see also Excision
- aneurysm 38.60
- artery-vein-nerve bundle 39.91
- branchial cleft fistula or sinus 29.52
- bronchus 32.1
- femoral hernia 53.29
- groin, radical 40.54
- larynx block (en bloc) 30.3
- mediastinum with pneumonectomy 32.5
- neck, radical 40.40
  - with laryngectomy 30.4
  - bilateral 40.42
  - unilateral 40.41
- orbital fibrous bands 16.92
- pterygium (with reposition) 11.31
- radical neck — see Dissection, neck, radical
- retroperitoneal NEC 59.00
- thoracic structures (block) (en bloc) (radical) (brachialplexus, bronchus, lobe of lung, ribs, and sympathetic nerves) 32.6
- vascular bundle 39.91

Distention, bladder (therapeutic) (intermittent) 96.25

Diversion, urinary
- cutaneous 56.61
- ileal conduit 56.51
- internal NEC 56.71
- ureter to
  - intestine 56.71

skin 56.61
uretero-ileostomy 56.61
Diversional therapy 93.81
Diverticulectomy
   bladder (suprapubic) 57.59
      transurethral approach 57.49
   duodenum 45.31
      endoscopic 45.30
   esophagus 42.31
      endoscopic 42.33
   esophagomyotomy 42.7
   hypopharyngeal (by cricopharyngeal
      myotomy) 29.32
   intestine
      large 45.41
         endoscopic 45.43
      small 45.33
   kidney 55.39
   Meckel's 45.33
   pharyngeal (by cricopharyngeal myotomy)
      29.32
   pharyngoesophageal (by cricopharyngeal
      myotomy) 29.32
   stomach 43.42
      endoscopic 43.41
   urethra 58.39
      endoscopic 58.31
Division
   Achilles tendon 83.11
   adductor tendon (hip) 83.12
   adhesions — see Lysis, adhesions
   angle of mandible (open) 76.62
      closed 76.61
   anterior synechiae 12.32
   aponeurosis 83.13
   arcuate ligament (spine) — omit code
   arteriovenous fistula (with ligation) 39.53
   artery (with ligation) 38.80
      abdominal 38.86
      aorta (arch) (ascending) (descending)
         38.84
      head and neck NEC 38.82
      intracranial NEC 38.81
      lower limb 38.88
      thoracic NEC 38.85
      upper limb 38.83
   bladder neck 57.91
   blepharorrhaphy 08.02
   blood vessels, cornea 10.1
   bone (see also Osteotomy) 77.30
   brain tissue 01.32
      cortical adhesions 02.91
   canaliculus 09.52
   canthorrhaphy 08.02
   cartilage 80.40
      ankle 80.47
      elbow 80.42
      foot and toe 80.48
      hand and finger 80.44
      hip 80.45
      knee 80.46
      shoulder 80.41
      specified site NEC 80.49
      spine 80.49
      wrist 80.43
   cerebral tracts 01.32
   chordae tendineae 35.32
   common wall between posterior left atrium
      and coronary sinus(with roofing of
      resultantdefect with patch graft)
      35.82
   congenital web
      larynx 31.98

      pharynx 29.54
   endometrial synechiae 68.21
   fallopian tube — see Ligation, fallopian tube
   fascia 83.14
      hand 82.12
   frenulum, frenum
      labial 27.91
      lingual 25.91
      tongue 25.91
   ganglion, sympathetic 05.0
   glossopharyngeal nerve 29.92
   goniosynechiae 12.31
   hypophyseal stalk (see also
      Hypophysectomy, partial) 07.63
   iliotibial band 83.14
   isthmus
      horseshoe kidney 55.85
      thyroid 06.91
   joint capsule 80.40
      ankle 80.47
      elbow 80.42
      foot and toe 80.48
      hand and finger 80.44
      hip 80.45
      knee 80.46
      shoulder 80.41
      specified site NEC 80.49
      wrist 80.43
   labial frenum 27.91
   lacrimal ductules 09.0
   laryngeal nerve (external) (recurrent)
      (superior) 31.91
   ligament 80.40
      ankle 80.47
      arcuate (spine) — omit code
      canthal 08.36
      elbow 80.42
      foot and toe 80.48
      hand and finger 80.44
      hip 80.45
      knee 80.46
      palpebrae 08.36
      shoulder 80.41
      specified site NEC 80.49
      spine 80.49
         arcuate — omit code
         flavum — omit code
      uterosacral 69.3
      wrist 80.43
   ligamentum flavum (spine) — omit code
   meninges (cerebral) 01.31
   muscle 83.19
      hand 82.19
   nasolacrimal duct stricture (with drainage)
      09.59
   nerve (cranial) (peripheral) NEC 04.03
      acoustic 04.01
      auditory 04.01
      adrenal gland 07.42
      glossopharyngeal 29.92
      lacrimal branch 05.0
      laryngeal (external) (recurrent)
         (superior) 31.91
      phrenic 04.03
         for collapse of lung 33.31
      root, spinal or intraspinal 03.1
      sympathetic 05.0
      tracts
         cerebral 01.32
         spinal cord 03.29
            percutaneous 03.21
      trigeminal 04.02
      vagus (see also Vagotomy) 44.00
      vestibular 04.01

   otosclerotic process or material, middle ear
      19.0
   papillary muscle (heart) 35.31
   patent ductus arteriosus 38.85
   penile adhesions 64.93
   posterior synechiae 12.33
   pylorus (with wedge resection) 43.3
   rectum (stricture) 48.91
   scalenus anticus muscle 83.19
   Skene's gland 71.3
   soft tissue NEC 83.19
      hand 82.19
   sphincter
      anal (external) (internal) 49.59
         left lateral 49.51
         posterior 49.52
      cardiac 42.7
      of Oddi 51.82
         endoscopic 51.85
      pancreatic 51.82
         endoscopic 51.85
   spinal
      cord tracts 03.29
         percutaneous 03.21
      nerve root 03.1
   symblepharon (with insertion of conformer)
      10.5
   synechiae
      endometrial 68.21
      iris (posterior) 12.33
         anterior 12.32
   tarsorrhaphy 08.02
   tendon 83.13
      Achilles 83.11
      adductor (hip) 83.12
      hand 82.11
   trabeculae carneae cordis (heart) 35.35
   tympanum 20.23
   uterosacral ligaments 69.3
   vaginal septum 70.14
   vas deferens 63.71
   vein (with ligation) 38.80
      abdominal 38.87
      head and neck NEC 38.82
      intracranial NEC 38.81
      lower limb 38.89
         varicose 38.59
      thoracic NEC 38.85
      upper limb 38.83
      varicose 38.50
         abdominal 38.57
         head and neck NEC 38.52
         intracranial NEC 38.51
         lower limb 38.59
         thoracic NEC 38.55
         upper limb 38.53
   vitreous, cicatricial bands (posterior
      approach) 14.74
      anterior approach 14.73
Doleris operation (shortening of round
   ligaments) 69.22
D'Ombrain operation (excision of
   pterygium with corneal graft)11.32
Domestic tasks therapy 93.83
Dopplergram, Doppler flow mapping —
   see also Ultrasonography
   aortic arch 88.73
   head and neck 88.71
   heart 88.72
   thorax NEC 88.73
Dorrance operation (push-back operation
   for cleft palate)27.62
Dotter operation (transluminal angioplasty)
   39.59

Douche, vagina 96.44
Douglas operation (suture of tongue to lip for micrognathia) 25.59
Doyle operation (paracervical uterine denervation) 69.3
Drainage
  by
    anastomosis — *see* Anastomosis
    aspiration — *see* Aspiration
    incision — *see* Incision
  abdomen 54.19
    percutaneous 54.91
  abscess — *see also* Drainage, by site and Incision, by site
    appendix 47.2
      with appendectomy 47.0
    parapharyngeal (oral) (transcervical) 28.0
    peritonsillar (oral) (transcervical) 28.0
    retropharyngeal (oral) (transcervical) 28.0
    thyroid (field) (gland) 06.09
      percutaneous (needle) 06.01
      postoperative 06.02
    tonsil, tonsillar (oral) (transcervical) 28.0
  antecubital fossa 86.04
  appendix 47.91
    with appendectomy 47.0
    abscess 47.2
      with appendectomy 47.0
  axilla 86.04
  bladder (without incision) 57.0
    by indwelling catheter 57.94
      percutaneous suprapubic (closed) 57.17
      suprapubic NEC 57.18
  buccal space 27.0
  bursa 83.03
    by aspiration 83.94
      hand 82.92
    hand 82.03
      by aspiration 82.92
    radial 82.03
    ulnar 82.03
  cerebrum, cerebral (meninges) (ventricle) (incision) (trephination) 01.39
    by
      anastomosis — *see* Shunt, ventricular
      aspiration 01.09
        through previously implanted catheter 01.02
  chest (closed) 34.04
    open (by incision) 34.09
  cranial sinus (incision) (trephination) 01.21
    by aspiration 01.09
  cul-de-sac 70.12
    by aspiration 70.0
  cyst — *see also* Drainage, by site and Incision, by site
    pancreas (by catheter) 52.01
      by marsupialization 52.3
      internal (anastomosis) 52.4
    pilonidal 86.03
    spleen, splenic (by marsupialization) 41.41
  duodenum (tube) 46.39
    by incision 45.01
  ear
    external 18.09
    inner 20.79
    middle (by myringotomy) 20.09
      with intubation 20.01
  epidural space, cerebral (incision) (trephination) 01.24
    by aspiration 01.09
  extradural space, cerebral (incision) (trephination) 01.24
    by aspiration 01.09
  extraperitoneal 54.0
  facial region 27.0
  fascial compartments, head and neck 27.0
  fetal hydrocephalic head (needling) (trocar) 73.8
  gallbladder 51.04
    by
      anastomosis 51.35
      aspiration 51.01
      incision 51.04
  groin region (abdominal wall) (inguinal) 54.0
    skin 86.04
    subcutaneous tissue 86.04
  hematoma — *see* Drainage, by site and Incision, by site
  hydrocephalic head (needling) (trocar) 73.8
  hypochondrium 54.0
    intra-abdominal 54.19
  iliac fossa 54.0
  infratemporal fossa 27.0
  intracranial space (epidural) (extradural) (incision) (trephination) 01.24
    by aspiration 01.09
    subarachnoid or subdural (incision) (trephination) 01.31
      by aspiration 01.09
  intraperitoneal 54.19
  kidney (by incision) 55.01
    by
      anastomosis 55.86
      catheter 59.8
    pelvis (by incision) 55.11
  liver 50.0
    by aspiration 50.91
  Ludwig's angina 27.0
  lung (by incision) 33.1
    by punch (needle) (trocar) 33.93
  midpalmar space 82.04
  mouth floor 27.0
  mucocele, nasal sinus 22.00
    by puncture 22.01
    through natural ostium 22.02
  omentum 54.19
    percutaneous 54.91
  ovary (aspiration) 65.91
    by incision 65.0
  palmar space (middle) 82.04
  pancreas (by catheter) 52.01
    by anastomosis 52.96
  parapharyngeal 28.0
  paronychia 86.04
  parotid space 27.0
  pelvic peritoneum (female) 70.12
    male 54.19
  pericardium 37.0
  perigastric 54.19
    percutaneous 54.91
  perineum
    female 71.09
    male 86.04
  perisplenic tissue 54.19
    percutaneous 54.91
  peritoneum 54.19
    pelvic (female) 70.12
    percutaneous 54.91
  peritonsillar 28.0
  pharyngeal space, lateral 27.0
  pilonidal cyst or sinus 86.03
  pleura (closed) 34.04
    open (by incision) 34.09
  popliteal space 86.04
  postural 93.99
  postzygomatic space 27.0
  pseudocyst, pancreas 52.3
    by anastomosis 52.4
  pterygopalatine fossa 27.0
  retropharyngeal 28.0
  scrotum 61.0
  skin 86.04
  spinal (canal) (cord) 03.09
    by anastomosis — *see* Shunt, spinal
    diagnostic 03.31
  spleen 41.2
    cyst (by marsupialization) 41.41
  subarachnoid space, cerebral (incision) (trephination) 01.31
    by aspiration 01.09
  subcutaneous tissue 86.04
  subdiaphragmatic 54.19
    percutaneous 54.91
  subdural space, cerebral (incision) (trephination) 01.31
    by aspiration 01.09
  subhepatic space 54.19
    percutaneous 54.91
  sublingual space 27.0
  submental space 27.0
  subphrenic space 54.19
    percutaneous 54.91
  supraclavicular fossa 86.04
  temporal pouches 27.0
  tendon (sheath) 83.01
    hand 82.01
  thenar space 82.04
  thorax (closed) 34.04
    open (by incision) 34.09
  thyroglossal tract (by incision) 06.09
    by aspiration 06.01
  thyroid (field) (gland) (by incision) 06.09
    by aspiration 06.01
    postoperative 06.02
  tonsil 28.0
  tunica vaginalis 61.0
  ureter (by catheter) 59.8
    by
      anastomosis NEC (*see also* Anastomosis, ureter) 56.79
      incision 56.2
  ventricle (cerebral) (incision) NEC 02.39
    by
      anastomosis — *see* Shunt, ventricular
      aspiration 01.09
        through previously implanted catheter 01.02
  vertebral column 03.09
Drawing test 94.08
Dressing
  burn 93.57
  ulcer 93.56
  wound 93.57
Drilling, bone (*see also* Incision, bone) 77.10
Ductogram, mammary 87.35
Duhamel operation (abdominoperineal pull-through) 48.65
Duhrssen's
  incisions (cervix, to assist delivery) 73.93
  operation (vaginofixation of uterus) 69.22
Dunn operation (triple arthrodesis) 81.12
Duodenectomy 45.62

with
    gastrectomy — *see* Gastrectomy
    pancreatectomy — *see* Pancreatectomy
Duodenocholedochotomy 51.51
Duodenoduodenostomy 45.91
  proximal to distal segment 45.62
Duodenoileostomy 45.91
Duodenojejunostomy 45.91
Duodenorrhaphy 46.71
Duodenoscopy 45.13

  through stoma (artificial) 45.12
  transabdominal (operative) 45.11
Duodenostomy 46.39
Duodenotomy 45.01
Dupuytren operation
  fasciectomy 82.35
  fasciotomy 82.12
    with excision 82.35
  shoulder disarticulation 84.08
Duraplasty 02.12

Durham (-Caldwell) operation (transfer of biceps femoristendon) 83.75
DuToit and Roux operation (staple capsulorrhaphy of shoulder)81.82
DuVries operation (tenoplasty) 83.88
Dwyer operation
  fasciotomy 83.14
  soft tissue release NEC 83.84
  wedge osteotomy, calcaneus 77.28

E

Eagleton operation (extrapetrosal drainage) 20.22
ECG — *see* Electrocardiogram
Echocardiography 88.72
    transesophageal 88.72 [42.23]
        monitoring (Doppler) (ultrasound) 89.68
Echoencephalography 88.71
Echography — *see* Ultrasonography
Echogynography 88.79
Echoplacentogram 88.78
ECMO (extracorporeal membrane oxygenation) 39.65
Eden-Hybinette operation (glenoid bond block) 78.01
Educational therapy (bed-bound children) (handicapped) 93.82
EEG (electroencephalogram) 89.14
    monitoring (radiographic) (video) 89.19
Effler operation (heart) 36.2
Effleurage 93.39
EGD (esophagogastroduodenoscopy) 45.13
    with closed biopsy 45.16
Eggers operation
    tendon release (patellar retinacula) 83.13
    tendon transfer (biceps femoris tendon) (hamstring tendon) 83.75
EKG (*see also* Electrocardiogram) 89.52
Elastic hosiery 93.59
Electrocardiogram (with 12 or more leads) 89.52
    with vectorcardiogram 89.53
    fetal (scalp), intrauterine 75.32
    rhythm (with one to three leads) 89.51
Electrocautery — *see also* Cauterization
    cervix 67.32
    corneal lesion (ulcer) 11.42
    esophagus 42.39
        endoscopic 42.33
Electrocoagulation — *see also* Destruction, lesion, by site
    aneurysm (cerebral) (peripheral vessels) 39.52
    cervix 67.32
    cystoscopic 57.49
    ear
        external 18.29
        inner 20.79
        middle 20.51
    fallopian tube (lesion) 66.61
        for tubal ligation — *see* Ligation, fallopian tube
    gasserian ganglion 04.02
    nasal turbinates 21.61
    nose, for epistaxis (with packing) 21.03
    ovary 65.29
    prostatic bed 60.94
    rectum (polyp) 48.32
        radical 48.31
    retina (for)
        destruction of lesion 14.21
        reattachment 14.51
        repair of tear 14.31
    round ligament 69.19
    semicircular canals 20.79
    urethrovesical junction, transurethral 57.49
    uterine ligament 69.19
    uterosacral ligament 69.19
    uterus 68.29
    vagina 70.33
    vulva 71.3
Electrocochleography 20.31
Electroconization, cervix 67.32
Electroconvulsive therapy (ECT) 94.27
Electroencephalogram (EEG) 89.14
    monitoring (radiographic) (video) 89.19
Electrogastrogram 44.19
Electrokeratotomy 11.49
Electrolysis
    ciliary body 12.71
    hair follicle 86.92
    retina (for)
        destruction of lesion 14.21
    reattachment 14.51
    repair of tear 14.31
    skin 86.92
        subcutaneous tissue 86.92
Electromyogram, electromyography (EMG) (muscle) 93.08
    eye 95.25
    urethral sphincter 89.23
Electronarcosis 94.29
Electronic gaiter 93.59
Electronystagmogram (ENG) 95.24
Electro-oculogram (EOG) 95.22
Electroresection — *see also* Destruction, lesion, by site
    bladder neck (transurethral) 57.49
    esophagus 42.39
        endoscopic 42.33
    prostate (transurethral) 60.2
    stomach 43.49
        endoscopic 43.41
Electroretinogram (ERG) 95.21
Electroshock therapy (EST) 94.27
    subconvulsive 94.26
Elevation
    bone fragments (fractured)
        orbit 76.79
        sinus (nasal)
            frontal 22.79
            maxillary 22.79
        skull (with debridement) 02.02
        spinal 03.53
    pedicle graft 86.71
Elliot operation (scleral trephination with iridectomy) 12.61
Ellis Jones operation (repair of peroneal tendon) 83.88
Ellison operation (reinforcement of collateral ligament) 81.44
Elmslie-Cholmeley operation (tarsal wedge osteotomy) 77.28
Eloesser operation (thoracoplasty) 33.34
Elongation — *see* Lengthening
Embolectomy 38.00
    with endarterectomy — *See* Endarterectomy
    abdominal
        artery 38.06
        vein 38.07
    aorta (arch) (ascending) (descending) 38.04
    head and neck NEC 38.02
    intracranial NEC 38.01
    lower limb
        artery 38.08
        vein 38.09
    thoracic NEC 38.05
    upper limb (artery) (vein) 38.03
Embolization (transcatheter)
    arteriovenous fistula 39.53
    artery (selective) 38.80
        abdominal NEC 38.86
            duodenal (transcatheter) 44.44
            gastric (transcatheter) 44.44
            renal (transcatheter) 38.86
        aorta (arch) (ascending) (descending) 38.84
        duodenal (transcatheter) 44.44
        gastric (transcatheter) 44.44
        head and neck NEC 38.82
        intracranial NEC 38.81
        lower limb 38.88
        renal (transcatheter) 38.86
        thoracic NEC 38.85
        upper limb 38.83
    carotid cavernous fistula 39.53
    vein (selective) 38.80
        abdominal NEC 38.87
            duodenal (transcatheter) 44.44
            gastric (transcatheter) 44.44
        duodenal (transcatheter) 44.44
        gastric (transcatheter) 44.44
Embryotomy 73.8
EMG — *see* Electromyogram
Emmet operation (cervix) 67.61
Encephalocentesis (*see also* Puncture) 01.09
    fetal head, transabdominal 73.8
Encephalography (cisternal puncture) (fractional) (lumbar) (pneumoencephalogram) 87.01
Encephalopuncture 01.09
Encircling procedure — *see also* Cerclage
    sclera, for buckling 14.49
        with implant 14.41
Endarterectomy (gas) (with patch graft) 38.10
    abdominal 38.16
    aorta (arch) (ascending) (descending) 38.14
    coronary artery - *see* category 36.0
        open chest approach 36.03
    head and neck NEC 38.12
    intracranial NEC 38.11
    lower limb 38.18
    thoracic NEC 38.15
    upper limb 38.13
Endoaneurysmorrhaphy (*see also* Aneurysmorrhaphy) 39.52
Endolymphatic (-subarachnoid) shunt 20.71
Endometrectomy (uterine) (internal) 68.29
    bladder 57.59
    cul-de-sac 70.32
Endoprosthesis
    bile duct 51.87
    femoral head (bipolar) 81.52
Endoscopy
    with biopsy — *see* Biopsy, by site, closed
    anus 49.21
    biliary tract (operative) 51.11
        by retrograde cholangiography (ERC) 51.11
        by retrograde cholangiopancreatography (ERCP) 51.10

    intraoperative 51.11
    percutaneous (via T-tube of other tract) 51.98
        with removal of common duct stones 51.96
  bladder 57.32
    through stoma (artificial) 57.31
  bronchus NEC 33.23
    with biopsy 33.24
    fiberoptic 33.22
    through stoma (artificial) 33.21
  colon 45.23
    through stoma (artificial) 45.22
    transabdominal (operative) 45.21
  cul-de-sac 70.22
  ear 18.11
  esophagus NEC 42.23
    through stoma (artificial) 42.22
    transabdominal (operative) 42.21
  ileum 45.13
    through stoma (artificial) 45.12
    transabdominal (operative) 45.11
  intestine NEC 45.24
    large 45.24
      fiberoptic (flexible) 45.23
      through stoma (artificial) 45.22
      transabdominal (intraoperative) 45.21
    small 45.13
      esophagogastroduodenoscopy (EGD) 45.13
        with closed biopsy 45.16
      through stoma (artificial) 45.12
      transabdominal (operative) 45.11
  jejunum 45.13
    through stoma (artificial) 45.12
    transabdominal (operative) 45.11
  kidney 55.21
  larynx 31.42
    through stoma (artificial) 31.41
  lung — see Bronchoscopy
  mediastinum (transpleural) 34.22
  nasal sinus 22.19
  nose 21.21
  pancreatic duct 52.13
  pelvis 55.22
  peritoneum 54.21
  pharynx 29.11
  rectum 48.23
    through stoma (artificial) 48.22
    transabdominal (operative) 48.21
  sinus, nasal 22.19
  stomach NEC 44.13
    through stoma (artificial) 44.12
    transabdominal (operative) 44.11
  thorax (transpleural) 34.21
  trachea NEC 31.42
    through stoma (artificial) 31.41
  transpleural
    mediastinum 34.22
    thorax 34.21
  ureter 56.31
  urethra 58.22
  uterus 68.12
  vagina 70.21
Enema (transanal) NEC 96.39
  for removal of impacted feces 96.38
ENG (electronystagmogram) 95.24
Enlargement
  aortic lumen, thoracic 38.14
  atrial septal defect (pre-existing) 35.41
    in repair of total anomalous pulmonary venous connection 35.82
  eye socket 16.64
  foramen ovale (pre-existing) 35.41
    in repair of total anomalous pulmonary venous connection 35.82
  intestinal stoma 46.40
    large intestine 46.43
    small intestine 46.41
  introitus 96.16
  orbit (eye) 16.64
  palpebral fissure 08.51
  punctum 09.41
  sinus tract 86.89
Enterectomy NEC 45.63
Enteroanastomosis
  large-to-large intestine 45.94
  small-to-large intestine 45.93
  small-to-small intestine 45.91
Enterocelectomy 53.9
▸ female 70.92
▸ vaginal 70.92
Enterocentesis 45.00
  duodenum 45.01
  large intestine 45.03
  small intestine 45.02
Enterocholecystostomy 51.32
Enteroclysis (small bowel) 96.43
Enterocolectomy NEC 45.79
Enterocolostomy 45.93
Enteroentectropy 46.99
Enteroenterostomy 45.90
  small-to-large intestine 45.93
  small-to-small intestine 45.91
Enterogastrostomy 44.39
Enterolithotomy 45.00
Enterolysis 54.5
Enteropancreatostomy 52.96
Enterorrhaphy 46.79
  large intestine 46.75
  small intestine 46.73
Enterostomy NEC 46.39
  cecum (see also Colostomy) 46.10
  colon (transverse) (see also Colostomy) 46.10
    loop 46.03
  delayed opening 46.31
  duodenum 46.39
    loop 46.01
  feeding NEC 46.39
    percutaneous (endoscopic) 46.32
  ileum (Brooke) (Dragstedt) 46.20
    loop 46.01
  jejunum (feeding) 46.39
    loop 46.01
    percutaneous (endoscopic) 46.32
  sigmoid colon (see also Colostomy) 46.10
    loop 46.03
  transverse colon (see also Colostomy) 46.10
    loop 46.03
Enterotomy 45.00
  large intestine 45.03
  small intestine 45.02
Enucleation - see also Excision, lesion, by site
  cyst
    broad ligament 69.19
    dental 24.4
    liver 50.29
    ovarian 65.29
    parotid gland 26.29
    salivary gland 26.29
    skin 86.3
    subcutaneous tissue 86.3
  eyeball 16.49
    with implant (into Tenon's capsule) 16.42
      with attachment of muscles 16.41
EOG (electro-oculogram) 95.22
Epicardiectomy 36.3
Epididymectomy 63.4
  with orchidectomy (unilateral) 62.3
    bilateral 62.41
Epididymogram 87.93
Epididymoplasty 63.59
Epididymorrhaphy 63.81
Epididymotomy 63.92
Epididymovasostomy 63.83
Epiglottidectomy 30.21
Epikeratophakia 11.76
Epilation
  eyebrow (forceps) 08.93
    cryosurgical 08.92
    electrosurgical 08.91
  eyelid (forceps) NEC 08.93
    cryosurgical 08.92
    electrosurgical 08.91
  skin 86.92
Epiphysiodesis (see also Arrest, bone growth) - see category 78.2
Epiphysiolysis (see also Arrest, bone growth) - see category 78.2
Epiploectomy 54.4
Epiplopexy 54.74
Epiplorrhaphy 54.74
Episioperineoplasty 71.79
Episioperineorrhaphy 71.71
  obstetrical 75.69
Episioplasty 71.79
Episioproctotomy 73.6
Episiorrhaphy 71.71
  following routine episiotomy — see Episiotomy
  for obstetrical laceration 75.69
Episiotomy (with subsequent episiorrhaphy) 73.6
  high forceps 72.31
  low forceps 72.1
  mid forceps 72.21
  nonobstetrical 71.09
  outlet forceps 72.1
EPS (electrophysiologic stimulation) 37.26
Equalization, leg
  lengthening - see category 78.3
  shortening - see category 78.2
Equilibration (occlusal) 24.8
Equiloudness balance 95.43
ERC (endoscopic retrograde cholangiography) 51.11
ERCP (endoscopic retrograde cholangiopancreatography) 51.10
  cannulation of pancreatic duct 52.93
ERG (electroretinogram) 95.21
ERP (endoscopic retrograde pancreatography) 52.13
Eruption, tooth, surgical 24.6
Erythrocytapheresis, therapeutic 99.73
Escharectomy 86.22
Escharotomy 86.22
Esophageal voice training (post-laryngectomy) 93.73
Esophagectomy 42.40
  abdominothoracocervical (combined) (synchronous) 42.42

partial or subtotal 42.41
total 42.42
Esophagocologastrostomy (intrathoracic) 42.55
　antesternal or antethoracic 42.65
Esophagocolostomy (intrathoracic) NEC 42.56
　with interposition of colon 42.55
　antesternal or antethoracic NEC 42.66
　　with interposition of colon 42.65
Esophagoduodenostomy (intrathoracic) NEC 42.54
　with
　　complete gastrectomy 43.99
　　interposition of small bowel 42.53
Esophagoenterostomy (intrathoracic) NEC (*see also* Anastomosis, esophagus, tointestinal segment) 42.54
　antesternal or antethoracic (*see also* Anastomosis, esophagus, antesternal, to intestinalsegment) 42.64
Esophagoesophagostomy (intrathoracic) 42.51
　antesternal or antethoracic 42.61
Esophagogastrectomy 43.99
Esophagogastroduodenoscopy (EGD) 45.13
　with closed biopsy 45.16
　through stoma (artificial) 45.12
　transabdominal (operative) 45.11
Esophagogastromyotomy 42.7
Esophagogastroplaxy 44.65
Esophagogastroscopy NEC 44.13
　through stoma (artificial) 44.12
　transabdominal (operative) 44.11
Esophagogastrostomy (intrathoracic) 42.52
　with partial gastrectomy 43.5
　antesternal or antethoracic 42.62
Esophagoileostomy (intrathoracic) NEC 42.54
　with interposition of small bowel 42.53
　antesternal or antethoracic NEC 42.64
　　with interposition of small bowel 42.63
Esophagojejunostomy (intrathoracic) NEC 42.54
　with
　　complete gastrectomy 43.99
　　interposition of small bowel 42.53
　antesternal or antethoracic NEC 42.64
　　with interposition of small bowel 42.63
Esophagomyotomy 42.7
Esophagoplasty NEC 42.89
Esophagorrhaphy 42.82
Esophagoscopy NEC 42.23
　by incision (operative) 42.21
　with closed biopsy 42.24
　through stoma (artificial) 42.22
　transabdominal (operative) 42.21
Esophagostomy 42.10
　cervical 42.11
　thoracic 42.19
Esophagotomy NEC 42.09
Estes operation (ovary) 65.72
Estlander operation (thoracoplasty) 33.34
ESWL (extracorporeal shockwave lithotripsy) NEC 98.59
　bile duct 98.52
　bladder 98.51
　gallbladder 98.52

kidney 98.51
renal pelvis 98.51
specified site NEC 98.59
ureter 98.51
Ethmoidectomy 22.63
Ethmoidotomy 22.51
Evacuation
　abscess — Drainage, by site
　anterior chamber (eye) (aqueous) (hyphema) 12.91
　cyst — *see also* Excision, lesion, by site
　　breast 85.91
　　kidney 55.01
　　liver 50.29
　hematoma — *see also* Incision, hematoma
　　obstetrical 75.92
　　　incisional 75.91
　hemorrhoids (thrombosed) 49.47
　pelvic blood clot (by incision) 54.19
　　by
　　　culdocentesis 70.0
　　　culdoscopy 70.22
　retained placenta
　　with curettage 69.02
　　manual 75.4
　streptothrix from lacrimal duct 09.42
Evaluation (of)
　audiological 95.43
　criminal responsibility, psychiatric 94.11
　functional (physical therapy) 93.01
　hearing NEC 95.49
　orthotic (for brace fitting) 93.02
　prosthetic (for artificial limb fitting) 93.03
　psychiatric NEC 94.19
　　commitment 94.13
　psychologic NEC 94.08
　testamentary capacity, psychiatric 94.11
Evans operation (release of clubfoot) 83.84
Evisceration
　eyeball 16.39
　　with implant (into scleral shell) 16.31
　ocular contents 16.39
　　with implant (into scleral shell) 16.31
　orbit (*see also* Exenteration, orbit) 16.59
　pelvic (anterior) (posterior) (partial) (total) (female) 68.8
　　male 57.71
Evulsion
　nail (bed) (fold) 86.23
　skin 86.3
　　subcutaneous tissue 86.3
Examination (for)
　breast
　　manual 89.36
　　radiographic NEC 87.37
　　thermographic 88.85
　　ultrasonic 88.73
　cervical rib (by x-ray) 87.43
　colostomy stoma (digital) 89.33
　dental (oral mucosa) (peridontal) 89.31
　　radiographic NEC 87.12
　enterostomy stoma (digital) 89.33
　eye 95.09
　　color vision 95.06
　　comprehensive 95.02
　　dark adaptation 95.07
　　limited (with prescription of spectacles) 95.01
　　under anesthesia 95.04
　fetus, intrauterine 75.35
　general physical 89.7
　glaucoma 95.03

gynecological 89.26
hearing 95.47
microscopic (specimen) (of) 91.9
　adenoid 90.3
　adrenal gland 90.1
　amnion 91.4
　anus 90.9
　appendix 90.9
　bile ducts 91.0
　bladder 91.3
　blood 90.5
　bone 91.5
　　marrow 90.6
　brain 90.0
　breast 91.6
　bronchus 90.4
　bursa 91.5
　cartilage 91.5
　cervix 91.4
　chest wall 90.4
　chorion 91.4
　colon 90.9
　cul-de-sac 91.1
　dental 90.8
　diaphragm 90.4
　duodenum 90.8
　ear 90.3
　endocrine gland NEC 90.1
　esophagus 90.8
　eye 90.2
　fallopian tube 91.4
　fascia 91.5
　female genital tract 91.4
　fetus 91.4
　gallbladder 91.0
　hair 91.6
　ileum 90.9
　jejunum 90.9
　joint fluid 91.5
　kidney 91.2
　large intestine 90.9
　larynx 90.3
　ligament 91.5
　liver 91.0
　lung 90.4
　lymph (node) 90.7
　meninges 90.0
　mesentery 91.1
　mouth 90.8
　muscle 91.5
　musculoskeletal system 91.5
　nails 91.6
　nerve 90.0
　nervous system 90.0
　nose 90.3
　omentum 91.1
　operative wound 91.7
　ovary 91.4
　pancreas 91.0
　parathyroid gland 90.1
　penis 91.3
　perirenal tissue 91.2
　peritoneum (fluid) 91.1
　periureteral tissue 91.2
　perivesical (tissue) 91.3
　pharynx 90.3
　pineal gland 90.1
　pituitary gland 90.1
　placenta 91.4
　pleura (fluid) 90.4
　prostate 91.3
　rectum 90.9
　retroperitoneum 91.1
　semen 91.3
　seminal vesicle 91.3
　sigmoid 90.9

skin 91.6
small intestine 90.9
specified site NEC 91.8
spinal fluid 90.0
spleen 90.6
sputum 90.4
stomach 90.8
stool 90.9
synovial membrane 91.5
tendon 91.5
thorax NEC 90.4
throat 90.3
thymus 90.1
thyroid gland 90.1
tonsil 90.3
trachea 90.4
ureter 91.2
urethra 91.3
urine 91.3
uterus 91.4
vagina 91.4
vas deferens 91.3
vomitus 90.8
vulva 91.4
neurologic 89.13
neuro-ophthalmology 95.03
ophthalmoscopic 16.21
panorex, mandible 87.12
pelvic (manual) 89.26
instrumental (by pelvimeter) 88.25
pelvimetric 88.25
physical, general 89.7
postmortem 89.8
rectum (digital) 89.34
endoscopic 48.23
through stoma (artificial) 48.22
transabdominal 48.21
retinal disease 95.03
specified type (manual) NEC 89.39
thyroid field, postoperative 06.02
uterus (digital) 68.11
endoscopic 68.12
vagina 89.26
endoscopic 70.21
visual field 95.05
Exchange transfusion 99.01
intrauterine 75.2
Excision
aberrant tissue — see Excision, lesion, by site of tissue origin
abscess — see Excision, lesion, by site
accessory tissue — see also Excision, lesion, by site of tissue origin
lung 32.29
endoscopic 32.28
spleen 41.93
adenoids (tag) 28.6
with tonsillectomy 28.3
adenoma — see Excision, lesion, by site
adrenal gland (see also Adrenalectomy) 07.22
ampulla of Vater (with reimplantation of common duct) 51.62
anal papilla 49.39
endoscopic 49.31
aneurysm (arteriovenous) (see also Aneurysmectomy) 38.60
coronary artery 36.91
heart 37.32
myocardium 37.32
sinus of Valsalva 35.39
ventricle (heart) 37.32
anus (complete) (partial) 49.6
aortic subvalvular ring 35.35

apocrine gland 86.3
aponeurosis 83.42
hand 82.33
appendiceal stump 47.0
appendices epiploicae 54.4
appendix (see also Appendectomy) 47.0
epididymis 63.3
testis 62.2
arcuate ligament (spine) — omit code
arteriovenous fistula (see also Aneurysmectomy) 38.60
artery (see also Arteriectomy) 38.60
Baker's cyst, knee 83.39
Bartholin's gland 71.24
basal ganglion 01.59
bile duct 51.69
endoscopic 51.64
bladder — see also Cystectomy
bleb (emphysematous), lung 32.29
endoscopic 32.28
blood vessel (see also Angiectomy) 38.60
bond (ends) (partial), except facial — see category 77.8
facial NEC 76.39
total 76.45
with reconstruction 76.44
for graft (autograft) (homograft) — see category 77.7
fragments (chips) (see also Incision, bone) 77.10
joint (see also Arthrotomy) 80.10
necrotic (see also Sequestrectomy, bone) 77.00
heterotopic, from
muscle 83.32
hand 82.22
skin 86.3
tendon 83.31
hand 82.21
mandible 76.31
with arthrodesis — see Arthrodesis
total 76.42
with reconstruction 76.41
spur — see Excision, lesion, bone
total, except facial — see category 77.9
facial NEC 76.45
with reconstruction 76.44
mandible 76.42
with reconstruction 76.41
brain 01.59
hemisphere 01.52
lobe 01.53
branchial cleft cyst or vestige 29.2
breast (see also Mastectomy) 85.41
aberrant tissue 85.24
accessory 85.24
ectopic 85.24
nipple 85.25
accessory 85.24
segmental 85.23
supernumerary 85.24
wedge 85.21
broad ligament 69.19
bronchogenic cyst 32.09
endoscopic 32.01
bronchus (wide sleeve) NEC 32.1
buccal mucosa 27.49
bulbourethral gland 58.92
bulbous tuberosities (mandible) (maxilla) (fibrous) (osseous) 24.31
bunion (see also Bunionectomy) 77.59
bunionette (with osteotomy) 77.54
bursa 83.5
hand 82.31

canal of Nuck 69.19
cardioma 37.33
carotid body (lesion) (partial) (total) 39.8
cartilage (see also Chondrectomy) 80.90
intervertebral 80.5
knee (semilunar) 80.6
larynx 30.29
nasal (submucous) 21.5
caruncle, urethra 58.39
endoscopic 58.31
cataract (see also Extraction, cataract) 13.19
secondary membrane (after cataract) 13.65
cervical
rib 77.91
stump 67.4
cervix (stump) NEC 67.4
cold (knife) 67.2
conization 67.2
cryoconization 67.33
electroconization 67.32
chalazion (multiple) (single) 08.21
cholesteatoma — see Excision, lesion, by site
choroid plexus 02.14
cicatrix (skin) 86.3
cilia base 08.20
ciliary body, prolapsed 12.98
clavicle (head) (partial) 77.81
total (complete) 77.91
clitoris 71.4
coarctation of aorta (end-to-end anastomosis) 38.64
with
graft replacement (interposition)
abdominal 38.44
thoracic 38.45
thoracoabdominal 38.45
[38.44]
common
duct 51.63
wall between posterior and coronary sinus (with roofing of resultant defect with patchgraft) 35.82
condyle — see category 77.8
mandible 76.5
conjunctival ring 10.31
cornea 11.49
epithelium (with chemocauterization) 11.41
for smear or culture 11.21
costal cartilage 80.99
cul-de-sac (Douglas) 70.92
cusp, heart valve 35.10
aortic 35.11
mitral 35.12
tricuspid 35.14
cyst — see also Excision, lesion, by site
apical (tooth) 23.73
with root canal therapy 23.72
Baker's (popliteal) 83.39
breast 85.21
broad ligament 69.19
bronchogenic 32.09
endoscopic 32.01
cervix 67.39
dental 24.4
dentigerous 24.4
epididymis 63.2
fallopian tube 66.61
Gartner's duct 70.33
hand 82.29
labia 71.3
lung 32.29

Excision — INDEX TO PROCEDURES

endoscopic 32.28
mesonephric duct 69.19
Morgagni
    female 66.61
    male 62.2
mullerian duct 60.73
nasolabial 27.49
nasopalatine 27.31
    by wide excision 27.32
ovary 65.29
parovarian 69.19
pericardium 37.31
periodontal (apical) (lateral) 24.4
popliteal (Baker's), knee 83.39
radicular 24.4
spleen 41.42
synovial (membrane) 83.39
thyroglossal (with resection of hyoid bone) 06.7
urachal (bladder) 57.51
    abdominal wall 54.3
vagina (Gartner's duct) 70.33
cystic
    duct remnant 51.61
    hygroma 40.29
dentinoma 24.4
diaphragm 34.81
disc, intervertebral (NOS) 80.50
    herniated (nucleus pulposus) 80.51
        with arthrodesis — see Fusion, spinal
    other specified (diskectomy) 80.51
        with arthrodesis — see Fusion, spinal
diverticulum
    ampulla of Vater 51.62
    anus 49.39
        endoscopic 49.31
    bladder 57.59
        transurethral 57.49
    duodenum 45.31
        endoscopic 45.30
    esophagus (local) 42.31
        endoscopic 42.33
    hypopharyngeal (by cricopharyngeal myotomy) 29.32
    intestine
        large 45.41
            endoscopic 45.43
        small NEC 45.33
    Meckel's 45.33
    pharyngeal (by cricopharyngeal myotomy) 29.32
    pharyngoesophageal (by cricopharyngeal myotomy) 29.32
    stomach 43.42
        endoscopic 43.41
    urethra 58.39
        endoscopic 58.31
    ventricle, heart 37.33
duct
    mullerian 69.19
    paramesonephric 69.19
    thyroglossal (with resection of hyoid bone) 06.7
ear, external (complete) NEC 18.29
    partial 18.29
        radical 18.31
ectopic
    abdominal fetus 74.3
    tissue — see also Excision, lesion, by site of tissue origin
        bone, from muscle 83.32
        breast 85.24
        lung 32.29
            endoscopic 32.28
        spleen 41.93
empyema pocket, lung 34.09
epididymis 63.4
epiglottis 30.21
epithelial downgrowth, anterior chamber (eye) 12.93
epulis (gingiva) 24.31
esophagus (see also Esophagectomy) 42.40
exostosis (see also Excision, lesion, bone) 77.60
    auditory canal, external 18.29
    facial bone 76.2
    first metatarsal (hallux valgus repair) — see Bunionectomy
eye 16.49
    with implant (into Tenon's capsule) 16.42
        with attachment of muscles 16.41
eyelid 08.20
    redundant skin 08.86
falciform ligament 54.4
fallopian tube — see Salpingectomy
fascia 83.44
    for graft 83.43
        hand 82.34
    hand 82.35
        for graft 82.34
fat pad NEC 86.3
    knee (infrapatellar) (prepatellar) 86.3
    scalene 40.21
fibroadenoma, breast 85.21
fissure, anus 49.39
    endoscopic 49.31
fistula — see also Fistulectomy
    anal 49.12
    arteriovenous (see also Aneurysmectomy) 38.60
    ileorectal 46.74
    lacrimal
        gland 09.21
        sac 09.6
    rectal 48.73
    vesicovaginal 57.84
frenulum, frenum
    labial (lip) 27.41
    lingual (tongue) 25.92
ganglion (hand) (tendon sheath) (wrist) 82.21
    gasserian 04.05
    site other than hand or nerve 83.31
    sympathetic nerve 05.29
    trigeminal nerve 04.05
gastrocolic ligament 54.4
gingiva 24.31
glomus jugulare tumor 20.51
goiter — see Thyroidectomy
gum 24.31
hallux valgus — see also Bunionectomy
    with prosthetic implant 77.59
hamartoma, mammary 85.21
hematocele, tunica vaginalis 61.92
hematoma — see Drainage, by site
hemorrhoids (external) (internal) (tag) 49.46
heterotopic bone, from
    muscle 83.32
        hand 82.22
    skin 86.3
    tendon 83.31
        hand 82.21
hydatid of Morgagni
    female 66.61
    male 62.2
hydatid cyst, liver 50.29
hydrocele
    canal of Nuck (female) 69.19
    male 63.1
    round ligament 69.19
    spermatic cord 63.1
    tunica vaginalis 61.2
hygroma, cystic 40.29
hymen (tag) 70.31
hymeno-urethral fusion 70.31
intervertebral disc — see Excision, disc, intervertebral (NOS) 80.50
intestine (see also Resection, intestine) 45.8
    for interposition 45.50
        large 45.52
        small 45.51
    large (total) 45.8
        for interposition 45.52
        local 45.41
            endoscopic 45.43
        segmental 45.79
            multiple 45.71
    small (total) 45.63
        for interposition 45.51
        local 45.33
        partial 45.62
        segmental 45.62
            multiple 45.61
intraductal papilloma 85.21
iris prolapse 12.13
joint (see also Arthrectomy) 80.90
keloid (scar), skin 86.3
labia — see Vulvectomy
lacrimal
    gland 09.20
        partial 09.22
        total 09.23
    passage 09.6
    sac 09.6
lesion (local)
    abdominal wall 54.3
    accessory sinus — see Excision, lesion, nasal sinus
    adenoids 28.92
    adrenal gland(s) 07.21
    alveolus 24.4
    ampulla of Vater 51.62
    anterior chamber (eye) NEC 12.40
    anus 49.39
        endoscopic 49.31
    apocrine gland 86.3
    artery 38.60
        abdominal 38.66
        aorta (arch) (ascending) (descending thoracic) 38.64
            with end-to-end anastomosis 38.45
                abdominal 38.44
                thoracic 38.45
                thoracoabdominal 38.45 [38.44]
            with graft interposition graft replacement 38.45
                abdominal 38.44
                thoracic 38.45
                thoracoabdominal 38.45 [38.44]
        head and neck NEC 38.62
        intracranial NEC 38.61
        lower limb 38.68
        thoracic NEC 38.65
        upper limb 38.63
    atrium 37.33
    auditory canal or meatus, external 18.29
        radical 18.31
    auricle, ear 18.29

Excision — continued

  radical 18.31
biliary ducts 51.69
  endoscopic 51.64
bladder (transurethral) 57.49
  open 57.59
  suprapubic 57.59
blood vessel 38.60
  abdominal
    artery 38.66
    vein 38.67
  aorta (arch) (ascending) (descending) 38.64
  head and neck NEC 38.62
  intracranial NEC 38.61
  lower limb
    artery 38.68
    vein 38.69
  thoracic NEC 38.65
  upper limb (artery) (vein) 38.63
bone 77.60
  carpal, metacarpal 77.64
  clavicle 77.61
  facial 76.2
  femur 77.65
  fibula 77.67
  humerus 77.62
  jaw 76.2
    dental 24.4
  patella 77.66
  pelvic 77.69
  phalanges (foot) (hand) 77.69
  radius 77.63
  scapula 77.61
  skull 01.6
  specified site NEC 77.69
  tarsal, metatarsal 77.68
  thorax (ribs) (sternum) 77.61
  tibia 77.67
  ulna 77.63
  vertebrae 77.69
brain (transtemporal approach) NEC 01.59
breast (segmental) (wedge) 85.21
broad ligament 69.19
bronchus NEC 32.09
  endoscopic 32.01
cerebral (cortex) NEC 01.59
  meninges 01.51
cervix (myoma) 67.39
chest wall 34.4
choroid plexus 02.14
ciliary body 12.44
colon 45.41
  endoscopic NEC 45.43
    polypectomy 45.42
conjunctiva 10.31
cornea 11.49
cranium 01.6
cul-de-sac (Douglas') 70.32
dental (jaw) 24.4
diaphragm 34.81
duodenum (local) 45.31
  endoscopic 45.30
ear, external 18.29
  radical 18.31
endometrium 68.29
epicardium 37.31
epididymis 63.3
epiglottis 30.09
esophagus NEC 42.32
  endoscopic 42.33
eye, eyeball 16.93
  anterior segment NEC 12.40
eyebrow (skin) 08.20
eyelid 08.20
  by
    halving procedure 08.24
    wedge resection 08.24
  major
    full-thickness 08.24
    partial-thickness 08.23
  minor 08.22
fallopian tube 66.61
fascia 83.39
  hand 82.29
groin region (abdominal wall) (inguinal) 54.3
  skin 86.3
  subcutaneous tissue 86.3
gum 24.31
heart 37.33
hepatic duct 51.69
inguinal canal 54.3
intestine
  large 45.41
    endoscopic NEC 45.43
      polypectomy 45.42
  small NEC 45.33
intracranial NEC 01.59
intranasal 21.31
intraspinal 03.4
iris 12.42
jaw 76.2
  dental 24.4
joint 80.80
  ankle 80.87
  elbow 80.82
  foot and toe 80.88
  hand and finger 80.84
  hip 80.85
  knee 80.86
  shoulder 80.81
  specified site NEC 80.89
  spine 80.89
  wrist 80.83
kidney 55.39
  with partial nephrectomy 55.4
labia 71.3
lacrimal
  gland (frontal approach) 09.21
  passage 09.6
  sac 09.6
larynx 30.09
ligament (joint) (see also Excision, lesion, joint) 80.80
  broad 69.19
  round 69.19
  uterosacral 69.19
lip 27.43
  by wide excision 27.42
liver 50.29
lung NEC 32.29
  by wide excision 32.3
  endoscopic 32.28
lymph structure(s) (channel) (vessel) NEC 40.29
  node — see Excision, lymph, node
mammary duct 85.21
mastoid (bone) 20.49
mediastinum 34.3
meninges (cerebral) 01.51
  spinal 03.4
mesentery 54.4
middle ear 20.51
mouth NEC 27.49
muscle 83.32
  hand 82.22
  ocular 15.13
myocardium 37.33
nail 86.23
nasal sinus 22.60
  antrum 22.62
    with Caldwell-Luc approach 22.61
    specified approach NEC 22.62
  ethmoid 22.63
  frontal 22.42
  maxillary 22.62
    with Caldwell-Luc approach 22.61
    specified approach NEC 22.62
  sphenoid 22.64
nasopharynx 29.3
nerve (cranial) (peripheral) 04.07
  sympathetic 05.29
nonodontogenic 24.31
nose 21.30
  intranasal 21.31
  polyp 21.31
  skin 21.32
  specified site NEC 21.32
odontogenic 24.4
omentum 54.4
orbit 16.92
ovary 65.29
  by wedge resection 65.22
palate (bony) 27.31
  by wide excision 27.32
  soft 27.49
pancreas (local) 52.22
  endoscopic 52.21
parathyroid 06.89
parotid gland or duct NEC 26.29
pelvic wall 54.3
pelvirectal tissue 48.82
penis 64.2
pericardium 37.31
perineum (female) 71.3
  male 86.3
periprostatic tissue 60.82
perirectal tissue 48.82
perirenal tissue 59.91
peritoneum 54.4
perivesical tissue 59.91
pharynx 29.39
  diverticulum 29.32
pineal gland 07.53
pinna 18.29
  radical 18.31
pituitary (gland) (see also Hypophysectomy, partial) 07.63
pleura 34.59
pouch of Douglas 70.32
preauricular (ear) 18.21
presacral 54.4
prostate (transurethral) 60.61
pulmonary (fibrosis) 32.29
  endoscopic 32.28
rectovaginal septum 48.82
rectum 48.35
retroperitoneum 54.4
salivary gland or duct NEC 26.29
  en bloc 26.32
sclera 12.84
scrotum 61.3
sinus (nasal) — see Excision, lesion, nasal sinus
Skene's gland 71.3
skin 86.3
  breast 85.21
  nose 21.32
  radical (wide) (involving underlying or adjacent structure) (with flap closure) 86.4
  scrotum 61.3
skull 01.6
soft tissue NEC 83.39
  hand 82.29
spermatic cord 63.3
sphincter of Oddi 51.62

Excision — INDEX TO PROCEDURES — **Excision**

endoscopic 51.64
spinal cord (meninges) 03.4
spleen (cyst) 41.42
stomach NEC 43.42
    endoscopic 43.41
        polyp 43.41
        polyp (endoscopic) 43.41
subcutaneous tissue 86.3
    breast 85.21
subgingival 24.31
sweat gland 86.3
tendon 83.39
    hand 82.29
    ocular 15.13
    sheath 83.31
        hand 82.21
testis 62.2
thorax 34.4
thymus 07.81
thyroid 06.31
    substernal or transsternal route 06.51
tongue 25.1
tonsil 28.92
trachea 31.5
tunica vaginalis 61.92
ureter 56.41
urethra 58.39
    endoscopic 58.31
uterine ligament 69.19
uterosacral ligament 69.19
uterus 68.29
vagina 70.33
vein 38.60
    abdominal 38.67
    head and neck NEC 38.62
    intracranial NEC 38.61
    lower limb 38.69
    thoracic NEC 38.65
    upper limb 38.63
ventricle (heart) 37.33
vocal cords 30.09
vulva 71.3
ligament (*see also* Arthrectomy) 80.90
    broad 69.19
    round 69.19
    uterine 69.19
    uterosacral 69.19
ligamentum flavum (spine) — omit code
lingual tonsil 28.5
lip 27.43
liver (partial) 50.22
loose body
    bone — *see* Sequestrectomy, bone
    joint 80.10
lung (complete) (with mediastinal dissection) 32.5
    accessory or ectopic tissue 32.29
        endoscopic 32.28
    segmental 32.3
    specified type NEC 32.29
        endoscopic 32.28
    wedge 32.29
lymph, lymphatic
    drainage area 40.29
        radical — *see* Excision, lymph, node, radical
        regional (with lymph node, skin, subcutaneous tissue, and fat) 40.3
    node (simple) NEC 40.29
        with
            lymphatic drainage area (including skin, subcutaneous tissue, and fat) 40.3

mastectomy — *see* Mastectomy, radical
muscle and deep facia — *see* Excision, lymph, node, radical
axillary 40.23
    radical 40.51
    regional (extended) 40.3
cervical (deep) (with excision of scalene fat pad) 40.21
    with laryngectomy 30.4
    radical (including muscle and deep fascia) 40.40
        bilateral 40.42
        unilateral 40.41
    regional (extended) 40.3
    superficial 40.29
groin 40.24
    radical 40.53
    regional (extended) 40.3
iliac 40.29
    radical 40.54
    regional (extended) 40.3
inguinal (deep) (superficial) 40.24
    radical 40.54
    regional (extended) 40.3
jugular — *see* Excision, lymph node, cervical
mammary (internal) 40.22
    external 40.29
        radical 40.59
        regional (extended) 40.3
    radical 40.59
        regional (extended) 40.3
paratracheal — *see* Excision, lymph, node, cervical
periaortic 40.29
    radical 40.52
    regional (extended) 40.3
radical 40.50
    with mastectomy — *see* Mastectomy, radical
    specified site NEC 40.59
regional (extended) 40.3
sternal - *see* Excision, lymph, node, mammary
structure(s) (simple) NEC 40.29
    radical 40.59
    regional (extended) 40.3
lymphangioma 40.29
lymphocele 40.29
mastoid (*see also* Mastoidectomy) 20.49
median bar, transurethral approach 60.2
meibomian gland 08.20
meniscus (knee) 80.6
    acromioclavicular 80.91
    jaw 76.5
    sternoclavicular 80.91
    temporomandibular (joint) 76.5
    wrist 80.93
mullerian duct cyst 60.73
muscle 83.45
    for graft 83.43
    hand 82.34
        hand 82.36
        for graft 82.34
myositis ossificans 83.32
    hand 82.22
nail (bed) (fold) 86.23
nasolabial cyst 27.49
nasopalatine cyst 27.31
    by wide excision 27.32
neoplasm — *see* Excision, lesion, by site
nerve (cranial) (peripheral) NEC 04.07
    sympathetic 05.29

neuroma (Morton's) (peripheral nerve) 04.07
    acoustic
        by craniotomy 04.01
        by radiosurgery 04.07
    sympathetic nerve 05.29
nipple 85.25
    accessory 85.24
odontoma 24.4
orbital contents (*see also* Exenteration, orbit) 16.59
osteochondritis dissecans (*see also* Excision, lesion, joint) 80.80
ovary — *see also* Oophorectomy
    partial 65.29
        by wedge resection 65.22
Pancoast tumor (lung) 32.6
pancreas (total) (with synchronous duodenectomy) 52.6
    partial NEC 52.59
        distal (tail) (with part of body) 52.52
        proximal (head) (with part of body) (with synchronous duodenectomy) 52.51
    radical subtotal 52.53
    radical (one-stage) (two-stage) 52.7
    subtotal 52.53
paramesonephric duct 69.19
parathyroid gland (partial)) (subtotal) NEC (*see also* Parathyroidectomy) 06.89
parotid gland (*see also* Excision, salivary gland) 26.30
parovarian cyst 69.19
patella (complete) 77.96
    partial 77.86
pelvirectal tissue 48.82
perianal tissue 49.04
    skin tags 49.03
pericardial adhesions 37.31
periprostatic tissue 60.82
perirectal tissue 48.82
perirenal tissue 59.91
periurethral tissue 58.92
perivesical tissue 59.91
petrous apex cells 20.59
pharyngeal bands 29.54
pharynx (partial) 29.33
pilonidal cyst or sinus (open) (with partial closure) 86.21
pineal gland (complete) (total) 07.54
    partial 07.53
pituitary gland (complete) (total) (*see also* Hypophysectomy) 07.69
pleura NEC 34.59
polyp — *see also* Excision, lesion, by site
    esophagus 42.32
        endoscopic 42.33
    large intestine 45.41
        endoscopic 45.42
    nose 21.31
    stomach (endoscopic) 43.41
preauricular
    appendage (remnant) 18.29
    cyst, fistula, or sinus (congenital) 18.21
    remnant 18.29
prolapsed iris (in wound) 12.13
prostate — *see* Prostatectomy
pterygium (simple) 11.39
    with corneal graft 11.32
radius (head) (partial) 77.83
    total 77.93
ranula, salivary gland NEC 26.29
    rectal mucosa 48.35

rectum — see Resection, rectum
redundant mucosa
    colostomy 45.41
        endoscopic 45.43
    duodenostomy 45.31
        endoscopic 45.30
    ileostomy 45.33
    jejunostomy 45.33
    perineum 71.3
    rectum 48.35
    vulva 71.3
renal vessel, aberrant 38.66
rib (cervical) 77.91
ring of conjunctiva around cornea 10.31
round ligament 69.19
salivary gland 26.30
    complete 26.32
    partial 26.31
    radical 26.32
scalene fat pad 40.21
scar — see also Excision, lesion, by site
    epicardium 37.31
    mastoid 20.92
    pericardium 37.31
    pleura 34.59
    skin 86.3
    thorax 34.4
secondary membrane, lens 13.65
seminal vesicle 60.73
    with radical prostatectomy 60.5
septum — see also Excision, lesion, by site
    uterus (congenital) 68.22
    vagina 70.33
sinus — see also Excision, lesion, by site
    nasal — see Sinusectomy
    pilonidal 86.21
    preauricular (ear) (radical) 18.21
    tarsi 80.88
    thyroglossal (with resection of hyoid bone) 06.7
    urachal (bladder) 57.51
        abdominal wall 54.3
Skene's gland 71.3
skin (local) 86.3
    for graft (with closure of donor site) 86.91
    radical (wide) (involving underlying or adjacent structure) (with flap closure) 86.4
    tags
        perianal 49.03
        periauricular 18.29
soft tissue NEC 83.49
    hand 82.39
spermatocele 63.2
spinous process 77.89
spleen (total) 41.5
    accessory 41.93
    partial 41.43
stomach — see Gastrectomy
sublingual gland (salivary) (see also Excision, salivary gland) 26.30
submaxillary gland (see also Excision, salivary gland) 26.30
supernumerary
    breast 85.24
    digits 86.26
sweat gland 86.3
synechiae — see also Lysis, synechiae
    endometrial 68.21
tarsal plate (eyelid) 08.20
    by wedge resection 08.24
tattoo 86.3
    by dermabrasion 86.25

tendon (sheath) 83.42
    for graft 83.41
    hand 82.32
    hand 82.33
        for graft 82.32
thymus (see also Thymectomy) 07.80
thyroglossal duct or tract (with resection of hyoid bone) 06.7
thyroid NEC (see also Thyroidectomy) 06.39
tongue (complete) (total) 25.3
    partial or subtotal 25.2
    radical 25.4
tonsil 28.2
    with adenoidectomy 28.3
    lingual 28.5
    tag 28.4
tooth NEC (see also Removal, tooth, surgical) 23.19
    from nasal sinus 22.60
torus
    lingual 76.2
    mandible, mandibularis 76.2
    palate, palatinus 27.31
        by wide excision 27.32
trabeculae carneae cordis (heart) 35.35
trochanteric lipomatosis 86.83
tumor — see Excision, lesion, by site
ulcer — see also Excision, lesion, by site
    duodenum 45.31
        endoscopic 45.30
    stomach 43.42
        endoscopic 43.41
umbilicus 54.3
urachus, urachal (cyst) (bladder) 57.51
    abdominal wall 54.3
ureter, ureteral 56.40
    with nephrectomy — see Nephrectomy
    partial 56.41
    stricture 56.41
    total 56.42
ureterocele 56.41
urethra, urethral 58.39
    with complete cystectomy 57.79
    endoscopic 58.31
    septum 58.0
    stricture 58.39
        endoscopic 58.31
    valve (congenital) 58.39
        endoscopic (transurethral) (transvesical) 58.31
urethrovaginal septum 70.33
uterus (corpus) (see also Hysterectomy) 68.9
    cervix 67.4
        lesion 67.39
    lesion 68.29
    septum 68.22
uvula 27.72
vagina (total) 70.4
varicocele, spermatic cord 63.1
vein (see also Phlebectomy) 38.60
    varicose 38.50
        abdominal 38.57
        head and neck NEC 38.52
        intracranial NEC 38.51
        lower limb 38.59
        ovarian 38.67
        thoracic NEC 38.55
        upper limb 38.53
verruca — see also Excision, lesion, by site
    eyelid 08.22
vesicovaginal septum 70.33
vitreous opacity 14.74

    anterior approach 14.73
    vocal cord(s) (submucous) 30.22
    vulva (bilateral) (simple) (see also Vulvectomy) 71.62
    wart — see also Excision, lesion, by site
        eyelid 08.22
    wolffian duct 69.19
    xanthoma (tendon sheath, hand) 82.21
        site other than hand 83.31
Excisional biopsy — see Biopsy
Exclusion, pyloric 44.39
Exenteration
    ethmoid air cells 22.63
    orbit 16.59
        with
            removal of adjacent structures 16.51
            temporalis muscle transplant 16.59
            therapeutic removal of bone 16.52
    pelvic (organs) (female) 68.8
        male 57.71
    petrous pyramid air cells 20.59
Exercise (physical therapy) NEC 93.19
    active musculoskeletal NEC 93.12
    assisting 93.11
        in pool 93.31
    breathing 93.18
    musculoskeletal
        active NEC 93.12
        passive NEC 93.17
    neurologic 89.13
    passive musculoskeletal NEC 93.17
    resistive 93.13
Exfoliation, skin, by chemical 86.24
Exostectomy (see also Excision, lesion, bone) 77.60
    first metatarsal (hallux valgus repair) — see Bunionectomy
    hallux valgus repair (with wedge osteotomy) — see Bunionectomy
Expiratory flow rate 89.38
Exploration — see also Incision
    abdomen 54.11
    abdominal wall 54.0
    adrenal (gland) 07.41
        field 07.00
            bilateral 07.02
            unilateral 07.01
    artery 38.00
        abdominal 38.06
        aorta (arch) (ascending) (descending) 38.04
        head and neck NEC 38.02
        intracranial NEC 38.01
        lower limb 38.08
        thoracic NEC 38.05
        upper limb 38.03
    auditory canal, external 18.02
    axilla 86.09
    bile duct(s) 51.59
        common duct 51.51
            endoscopic 51.11
        for
            relief of obstruction 51.42
                endoscopic 51.84
            removal of calculus 51.41
                endoscopic 51.88
        for relief of obstruction 51.49
            endoscopic 51.84
    bladder (by incision) 57.19
        endoscopic 57.32
            through stoma (artificial) 57.31
    bone (see also Incision, bone) 77.10

brain (tissue) 01.39
breast 85.0
bronchus 33.0
    endoscopic — see Bronchoscopy
bursa 83.03
    hand 82.03
carotid body 39.8
carpal tunnel 04.43
choroid 14.9
ciliary body 12.44
colon 45.03
common bile duct 51.51
    endoscopic 51.11
    for
        relief of obstruction 51.42
            endoscopic 51.84
        removal of calculus 51.41
            endoscopic 51.88
coronary artery 36.99
cranium 01.24
cul-de-sac 70.12
    endoscopic 70.22
disc space 03.09
duodenum 45.01
endoscopic — see Endoscopy, by site
epididymis 63.92
esophagus (by incision) NEC 42.09
    endoscopic — see Esophagoscopy
ethmoid sinus 22.51
eyelid 08.09
fallopian tube 66.01
fascia 83.09
    hand 82.09
flank 54.0
fossa (superficial) NEC 86.09
    pituitary 07.71
frontal sinus 22.41
frontonasal duct 96.21
gallbladder 51.04
groin (region) (abdominal wall) (inguinal) 54.0
    skin and subcutaneous tissue 86.09
heart 37.11
hepatic duct 51.59
hypophysis 07.72
ileum 45.02
inguinal canal (groin) 54.0
intestine (by incision) NEC 45.00
    large 45.03
    small 45.02
intrathoracic 34.02
jejunum 45.02
joint structures (see also Arthrotomy) 80.10
kidney 55.01
    pelvis 55.11
labia 71.09
lacrimal
    gland 09.0
    sac 09.53
laparotomy site 54.12
larynx (by incision) 31.3
    endoscopic 31.42
liver 50.0
lung (by incision) 33.1
lymphatic structure(s) (channel) (node) (vessel) 40.0
mastoid 20.21
maxillary antrum or sinus (Caldwell-Luc approach) 22.39
mediastinum 34.1
    endoscopic 34.22
middle ear (transtympanic) 20.23
muscle 83.02
    hand 82.02
neck (see also Exploration, thyroid) 06.09
nerve (cranial) (peripheral) NEC 04.04
    auditory 04.01
    root (spinal) 03.09
nose 21.1
orbit (see also Orbitotomy) 16.09
pancreas 52.09
    endoscopic 52.13
pancreatic duct 52.09
    endoscopic 52.13
pelvis (by laparotomy) 54.11
    by colpotomy 70.12
penis 64.92
perinephric area 59.09
perineum (female) 71.09
    male 86.09
peripheral vessels
    lower limb
        artery 38.08
        vein 38.09
    upper limb (artery) (vein) 38.03
periprostatic tissue 60.81
perirenal tissue 59.09
perivesical tissue 59.19
petrous pyramid air cells 20.22
pilonidal sinus 86.03
pineal (gland) 07.52
    field 07.51
pituitary (gland) 07.72
    fossa 07.71
pleura 34.09
popliteal space 86.09
prostate 60.0
rectum (see also Proctoscopy) 48.23
    by incision 48.0
retroperitoneum 54.0
retropubic 59.19
salivary gland 26.0
sclera (by incision) 12.89
scrotum 61.0
sinus
    ethmoid 22.51
    frontal 22.41
    maxillary (Caldwell-Luc approach) 22.39
    sphenoid 22.52
    tract, skin and subcutaneous tissue 86.09
skin 86.09
soft tissue NEC 83.09
    hand 82.09
spermatic cord 63.93
sphenoidal sinus 22.52
spinal (canal) (nerve root) 03.09
spleen 41.2
stomach (by incision) 43.0
    endoscopic — see Gastroscopy
subcutaneous tissue 86.09
subdiaphragmatic space 54.11
superficial fossa 86.09
tarsal tunnel 04.44
tendon (sheath) 83.01
    hand 82.01
testes 62.0
thymus (gland) 07.92
    field 07.91
thyroid (field) (gland) (by incision) 06.09
    postoperative 06.02
trachea (by incision) 31.3
    endoscopic — see Tracheoscopy
tunica vaginalis 61.0
tympanum 20.09
transtympanic route 20.23
ureter (by incision) 56.2
    endoscopic 56.31
urethra (by incision) 58.0
    endoscopic 58.22
uterus (corpus) 68.0
    cervix 69.95
    digital 68.11
    postpartal, manual 75.7
vagina (by incision) 70.14
    endoscopic 70.21
vas deferens 63.6
vein 38.00
    abdominal 38.07
    head and neck NEC 38.02
    intracranial NEC 38.01
    lower limb 38.09
    thoracic NEC 38.05
    upper limb 38.03
vulva (by incision) 71.09

Exposure — see also Incision, by site
    tooth (for orthodontic treatment) 24.6
Expression, trachoma follicles 10.33
Exsanguination transfusion 99.01
Extension
    buccolabial sulcus 24.91
    limb, forced 93.25
    lingual sulcus 24.91
    mandibular ridge 76.43
Exteriorization
    esophageal pouch 42.12
    intestine 46.03
        large 46.03
        small 46.01
    maxillary sinus 22.9
    pilonidal cyst or sinus (open excision) (with partial closure) 86.21
Extirpation — see also Excision, by site
    aneurysm — see Aneurysmectomy
    arteriovenous fistula — Aneurysmectomy
    lacrimal sac 09.6
    larynx 30.3
        with radical neck dissection (with synchronous thyroidectomy) (with synchronoustracheostomy) 30.4
    nerve, tooth (see also Therapy, root canal 23.70
    varicose vein (peripheral) (lower limb) 38.59
        upper limb 38.53
Extracorporeal
    circulation (regional), except hepatic 39.61
        hepatic 50.92
        percutaneous 39.66
    hemodialysis 39.95
    membrane oxygenation (ECMO) 39.65
    photopheresis, therapeutic 99.88
    shockwave lithotripsy (ESWL) NEC 98.59
        bile duct 98.52
        bladder 98.51
        gallbladder 98.52
        kidney 98.51
        renal pelvis 98.51
        specified site NEC 98.59
        ureter 98.51
Extracranial-intracranial bypass [EC-IC] 39.28
Extraction
    breech (partial) 72.52
        with forceps to aftercoming head 72.51
        total 72.54

Extraction

with forceps to aftercoming head 72.53
cataract 13.19
  after cataract (by)
    capsulectomy 13.65
    capsulotomy 13.64
    discission 13.64
    excision 13.65
    iridocapsulectomy 13.65
    mechanical fragmentation 13.66
    needling 13.64
    phacofragmentation (mechanical) 13.66
  aspiration (simple) (with irrigation) 13.3
  cryoextraction (intracapsular approach) 13.19
    temporal inferior route (in presence of fistulization bleb) 13.11
  curette evacuation (extracapsular approach) 13.2
  emulsification (and aspiration) 13.41
  erysiphake (intracapsular approach) 13.19
    temporal inferior route (in presence of fistulization bleb) 13.11
  extracapsular approach (with iridectomy) NEC 13.59
    by temporal inferior route (in presence of fistulization bleb) 13.51
    aspiration (simple) (with irrigation) 13.3
    curette evacuation 13.2
    emulsification (and aspiration) 13.41
    linear extraction 13.2
    mechanical fragmentation with aspiration by
      posterior route 13.42
      specified route NEC 13.43
    phacoemulsification (ultrasonic) (with aspiration) 13.41
    phacofragmentation (mechanical) with aspiration by
      posterior route 13.42
      specified route NEC 13.43
    ultrasonic (with aspiration) 13.41
    rotoextraction (mechanical) with aspiration by
      posterior route 13.42
      specified route NEC 13.43
  intracapsular (combined) (simple) (with iridectomy) (with suction) (with zonulolysis) 13.19
    by temporal inferior route (in presence of fistulization bleb) 13.11
  linear extraction (extracapsular approach) 13.2
  phacoemulsification (and aspiration) 13.41
  phacofragmentation (mechanical)
    with aspiration by
      posterior route 13.42
      specified route 13.43
    ultrasonic 13.41
  rotoextraction (mechanical)
    with aspiration by
      posterior route 13.42
      specified route NEC 13.43
  secondary membranous (after cataract) (by)
    capsulectomy 13.65
    capsulotomy 13.64
    discission 13.64
    excision 13.65
    iridocapsulectomy 13.65
    mechanical fragmentation 13.66
    needling 13.64
    phacofragmentation (mechanical) 13.66
common duct stones (percutaneous) (through sinus tract) (with basket) 51.96
foreign body — *see* Removal, foreign body
kidney stone(s), percutaneous 55.03
  with fragmentation procedure 55.04
lens (eye) (*see also* Extraction, cataract) 13.19
Malstrom's 72.79
  with episiotomy 72.71
menstrual, menses 69.6
milk from lactating breast (manual) (pump) 99.98
tooth (by forceps) (multiple) (single) NEC 23.09
  with mucoperiosteal flap elevation 23.19
  deciduous 23.01
  surgical NEC (*see also* Removal, tooth, surgical) 23.19
vacuum, fetus 72.79
  with episiotomy 72.71
vitreous (*see also* Removal, vitreous) 14.72

F

Face lift 86.82
Facetectomy 77.89
Facilitation, intraocular circulation NEC 12.59
Failed (trial) forceps 73.3
Family
    counselling (medical) (social) 94.49
    therapy 94.42
Farabeuf operation (ischiopubiotomy) 77.39
Fasanella-Servatt operation (blepharoptosis repair) 08.35
Fascia sling operation — *see* Operation, sling
Fasciaplasty — *see* Fascioplasty
Fasciectomy 83.44
    for graft 83.43
        hand 82.34
    hand 82.35
        for graft 82.34
    palmar (release of Dupuytren's contracture) 82.35
Fasciodesis 83.89
    hand 82.89
Fascioplasty (*see also* Repair, fascia) 83.89
    hand (*see also* Repair, fascia, hand) 82.89
Fasciorrhaphy — *see* Suture, fascia
Fasciotomy 83.14
    Dupuytren's 82.12
        with excision 82.35
    Dwyer 83.14
    hand 82.12
    Ober-Yount 83.14
    orbital (*see also* Orbitotomy) 16.09
    palmar (release of Dupuytren's contracture) 82.12
        with excision 82.35
Fenestration
    aneurysm (dissecting), thoracic aorta 39.54
    aortic aneurysm 39.54
    cardiac valve 35.10
    chest wall 34.01
    ear
        inner (with graft) 20.61
            revision 20.62
        tympanic 19.55
    labyrinth (with graft) 20.61
    Lempert's (endaural) 19.9
    operation (aorta) 39.54
    oval window, ear canal 19.55
    palate 27.1
    pericardium 37.12
    semicircular canals (with graft) 20.61
    stapes foot plate (with vein graft) 19.19
        with incus replacement 19.11
    tympanic membrane 19.55
    vestibule (with graft) 20.61
Ferguson operation (hernia repair) 53.00
Fetography 87.81
Fetoscopy 75.31
Fiberoscopy — *see* Endoscopy, by site
Fibroidectomy, uterine 68.29
Fick operation (perforation of foot plate) 19.0
Filipuncture (aneurysm) (cerebral) 39.52
Filleting
    hammer toe 77.56
    pancreas 52.3

Filling, tooth (amalgam) (plastic) (silicate) 23.2
    root canal (*see also* Therapy, root canal) 23.70
Fimbriectomy (*see also* Salpingectomy, partial) 66.69
    Uchida (with tubal ligation) 66.32
Finney operation (pyloroplasty) 44.29
Fissurectomy, anal 49.39
    endoscopic 49.31
    skin (subcutaneous tissue) 49.04
Fistulectomy — *see also* Closure, fistula, by site
    abdominothoracic 34.83
    abdominouterine 69.42
    anus 49.12
    appendix 47.92
    bile duct 51.79
    biliary tract NEC 51.79
    bladder (transurethral approach) 57.84
    bone (*see also* Excision, lesion, bone) 77.60
    branchial cleft 29.52
    bronchocutaneous 33.42
    bronchoesophageal 33.42
    bronchomediastinal 34.73
    bronchopleural 34.73
    bronchopleurocutaneous 34.73
    bronchopleuromediastinal 34.73
    bronchovisceral 33.42
    cervicosigmoidal 67.62
    cholecystogastroenteric 51.93
    cornea 11.49
    diaphragm 34.83
    enterouterine 69.42
    esophagopleurocutaneous 34.73
    esophagus NEC 42.84
    fallopian tube 66.73
    gallbladder 51.93
    gastric NEC 44.63
    hepatic duct 51.79
    hepatopleural 34.73
    hepatopulmonary 34.73
    intestine
        large 46.76
        small 46.74
    intestinouterine 69.42
    joint (*see also* Excision, lesion, joint) 80.80
    lacrimal
        gland 09.21
        sac 09.6
    laryngotracheal 31.62
    larynx 31.62
    mediastinocutaneous 34.73
    mouth NEC 27.53
    nasal 21.82
        sinus 22.71
    nasolabial 21.82
    nasopharyngeal 21.82
    oroantral 22.71
    oronasal 21.82
    pancreas 52.95
    perineorectal 71.72
    perineosigmoidal 71.72
    perirectal, not opening into rectum 48.93
    pharyngoesophageal 29.53
    pharynx NEC 29.53
    pleura 34.73
    rectolabial 71.72

    rectourethral 58.43
    rectouterine 69.42
    rectovaginal 70.73
    rectovesical 57.83
    rectovulvar 71.72
    rectum 48.73
    salivary (duct) (gland) 26.42
    scrotum 61.42
    skin 86.3
    stomach NEC 44.63
    subcutaneous tissue 86.3
    thoracoabdominal 34.83
    thoracogastric 34.83
    thoracointestinal 34.83
    thorax NEC 34.73
    trachea NEC 31.73
    tracheoesophageal 31.73
    ureter 56.84
    urethra 58.43
    uteroenteric 69.42
    uterointestinal 69.42
    uterorectal 69.42
    uterovaginal 69.42
    vagina 70.75
    vesicosigmoidovaginal 57.83
    vocal cords 31.62
    vulvorectal 71.72
Fistulization
    appendix 47.91
    arteriovenous 39.27
    cisterna chyli 40.62
    endolymphatic sac (for decompression) 20.79
    esophagus, external 42.10
        cervical 42.11
        specified technique NEC 42.19
    interatrial 35.41
    labyrinth (for decompression) 20.79
    lacrimal sac into nasal cavity 09.81
    larynx 31.29
    lymphatic duct, left (thoracic) 40.62
    orbit 16.09
    peritoneal 54.93
    salivary gland 26.49
    sclera 12.69
        by trephination 12.61
        with iridectomy 12.65
    sinus, nasal NEC 22.9
    subarachnoid space 02.2
    thoracic duct 40.62
    trachea 31.29
    tracheoesophageal 31.95
    urethrovaginal 58.0
    ventricle, cerebral (*see also* Shunt, ventricular) 02.2
Fistulogram
    abdominal wall 88.03
    chest wall 87.38
    retroperitoneum 88.14
Fistulotomy, anal 49.11
Fitting
    arch bars (orthodontic) 24.7
        for immobilization (fracture) 93.55
    artificial limb 84.40
    contact lens 95.32
    denture (total) 99.97
        bridge (fixed) 23.42
            removable 23.43

partial (fixed) 23.42
    removable 23.43
hearing aid 95.48
obturator (orthodontic) 24.7
ocular prosthetics 95.34
orthodontic
  appliance 24.7
  obturator 24.7
  wiring 24.7
orthotic device 93.23
periodontal splint (orthodontic) 24.7
prosthesis, prosthetic device
  above knee 84.45
  arm 84.43
    lower (and hand) 84.42
    upper (and shoulder) 84.41
  below knee 84.46
  hand (and lower arm) 84.42
  leg 84.47
    above knee 84.45
    below knee 84.46
  limb NEC 84.40
  ocular 95.34
  penis (external) 64.94
  shoulder (and upper arm) 84.41
spectacles 95.31

Five-in-one repair, knee 81.42
Fixation
  bone
    external, without reduction 93.59
      with fracture reduction — see
        Reduction, fracture
      cast immobilization NEC 93.53
      splint 93.54
      traction (skeletal) NEC 93.44
        intermittent 93.43
    internal (without fracture reduction)
      78.50
      with fracture reduction — see
        Reduction, fracture
      carpal, metacarpal 78.54
      clavicle 78.51
      femur 78.55
      fibula 78.57
      humerus 78.52
      patella 78.56
      pelvic 78.59
      phalanges (foot) (hand) 78.59
      radius 78.53
      scapula 78.51
      specified site NEC 78.59
      tarsal, metatarsal 78.58
      thorax (ribs) (sternum) 78.51
      tibia 78.57
      ulna 78.53
      vertebrae 78.59
  breast (pendulous) 85.6
  cardinal ligaments 69.22
  duodenum 46.62
    to abdominal wall 46.61
  external (with manipulation for reduction)
    93.59
    with fracture reduction — Reduction,
      fracture
    cast immobilization NEC 93.53
    pressure dressing 93.56
    splint 93.54
    traction (skeletal) NEC 93.44
      intermittent 93.43
  hip 81.40
  ileum 46.62
    to abdominal wall 46.61
  internal
    with fracture reduction — see
      Reduction, fracture

    without fracture reduction — see
      Fixation, bone, internal
  intestine 46.60
    large 46.64
      to abdominal wall 46.63
    small 46.62
      to abdominal wall 46.61
    to abdominal wall 46.60
  iris (bombe) 12.11
  jejunum 46.62
    to abdominal wall 46.61
  joint — see Arthroplasty
  kidney 55.7
  ligament
    cardinal 69.22
    palpebrae 08.36
  omentum 54.74
  parametrial 69.22
  rectum (sling) 48.76
  spine, with fusion (see also Fusion, spinal)
    81.00
  spleen 41.95
  tendon 83.88
    hand 82.85
  testis in scrotum 62.5
  tongue 25.59
  urethrovaginal (to Cooper's ligament) 70.77
  uterus (abdominal) (vaginal)
    (ventrofixation) 69.22
  vagina 70.77
Flooding (psychologic desensitization) 94.33
Flowmetry, Doppler (ultrasonic) — see also
  Ultrasonography
  aortic arch 88.73
  head and neck 88.71
  heart 88.72
  thorax NEC 88.73
Fluoroscopy — see Radiography
Fog therapy (respiratory) 93.94
Folding, eye muscle 15.22
  multiple (two or more muscles) 15.4
Foley operation (pyeloplasty) 55.87
Fontan operation (creation of conduit
  between right atrium and pulmonary
  artery) 35.94
Foraminotomy 03.09
Forced extension, limb 93.25
Forceps delivery — see Delivery, forceps
Formation
  adhesions
    pericardium 36.3
    pleura 34.6
  anus, artificial (see also Colostomy) 46.13
    duodenostomy 46.39
    ileostomy (see also Ileostomy) 46.23
    jejunostomy 46.39
      percutaneous (endoscopic) (PEJ)
        46.32
  arteriovenous fistula (for kidney dialysis)
    (peripheral) (shunt) 39.27
    external cannula 39.93
  bone flap, cranial 02.03
  cardiac pacemaker pocket
    with initial insertion of pacemaker —
      omit code
    new site (skin) (subcutaneous) 37.79
  colostomy (see also Colostomy) 46.13
  conduit
    ileal (urinary) 56.51
    left ventricle and aorta 35.93
    right atrium and pulmonary artery
      35.94

    right ventricle and pulmonary (distal)
      artery 35.92
    in repair of
      pulmonary artery atresia 35.92
      transposition of great vessels
        35.92
      truncus arteriosus 35.83
  endorectal ileal pouch (J-pouch) (H-pouch)
    (S-pouch) (with anastomosis to anus)
    45.95
  fistula
    arteriovenous (for kidney dialysis)
      (peripheral shunt) 39.27
      external cannula 39.93
    bladder to skin NEC 57.18
      with bladder flap 57.21
      percutaneous 57.17
    cutaneoperitoneal 54.93
    gastric 43.19
      percutaneous (endoscopic)
        (transabdominal) 43.11
    mucous (see also Colostomy) 46.13
    rectovaginal 48.99
    tracheoesophageal 31.95
    tubulovalvular (Beck-Jianu) (Frank's)
      (Janeway) (Spivack's)
      (Ssabanejew-Frank) 43.19
    urethrovaginal 58.0
  ileal
    bladder
      closed 57.87 [45.51]]
      open 56.51
    conduit 56.51
  interatrial fistula 35.42
  mucous fistula (see also Colostomy) 46.13
  pericardial
    baffle, interatrial 35.91
    window 37.12
  pleural window (for drainage) 34.09
  pupil 12.39
    by iridectomy 12.14
  rectovaginal fistula 48.99
  reversed gastric tube (intrathoracic)
    (retrosternal) 42.58
    antesternal or antethoracic 42.68
  septal defect, interatrial 35.42
  shunt
    abdominovenous 54.94
    arteriovenous 39.93
    peritoneojugular 54.94
    peritoneo-vascular 54.94
▶   pleuroperitoneal 34.05
▶   transjugular intrahepatic portosystemic
      (TIPS) 39.1
  subcutaneous tunnel for esophageal
    anastomosis 42.86
    with anastomosis — see Anastomosis,
      esophagus, antesternal
  syndactyly (finger) (toe) 86.89
  tracheoesophageal 31.95
  tubulovalvular fistula (Beck-Jianu)
    (Frank's) (Janeway) (Spivack's)
    (Ssabanejew-Frank)43.19
  uretero-ileostomy, cutaneous 56.51
  ureterostomy, cutaneous 56.61
    ileal 56.51
  urethrovaginal fistula 58.0
  window
    pericardial 37.12
    pleural (for drainage) 34.09
Fothergill (-Donald) operation (uterine
  suspension) 69.22
Fowler operation

arthroplasty of metacarpophalangeal joint 81.72
release (mallet finger repair) 82.84
tenodesis (hand) 82.85
thoracoplasty 33.34
Fox operation (entropion repair with wedge resection) 08.43
Fracture, surgical (*see also* Osteoclasis) 78.70
    turbinates (nasal) 21.62
Fragmentation
    lithotriptor — *see* Lithotripsy
    mechanical
        cataract (with aspiration) 13.43
            posterior route 13.42
            secondary membrane 13.66
        secondary membrane (after cataract) 13.66
    ultrasonic
        cataract (with aspiration) 13.41
        stones, urinary 59.95
        urinary stones 59.95
            percutaneous nephrostomy 55.04
Franco operation (suprapubic cystotomy) 57.18
Frank operation 43.19
Frazier (-Spiller) **operation** (subtemporal trigeminal rhizotomy) 04.02
Fredet-Ramstedt operation (pyloromyotomy) (with wedge resection) 43.3
Freeing
    adhesions — *see* Lysis, adhesions
    anterior synechiae (with injection of air or liquid) 12.32
    artery-vein-nerve bundle 39.91
    extraocular muscle, entrapped 15.7
    goniosynechiae (with injection of air or liquid) 12.31
        intestinal segment for interposition 45.50
            large 45.52
            small 45.51
        posterior synechiae 12.33
        synechiae (posterior) 12.33
            anterior (with injection of air or liquid) 12.32
    vascular bundle 39.91
    vessel 39.91
Freezing, gastric 96.32
Frenckner operation (intrapetrosal drainage) 20.22
Frenectomy
    labial 27.41
    lingual 25.92
    lip 27.41
    maxillary 27.41
    tongue 25.92
Frenotomy
    labial 27.91
    lingual 25.91
Frenulumectomy — *see* Frenectomy
Frickman operation (abdominal proctopexy) 48.75
Frommel operation (shortening of uterosacral ligaments) 69.22
Fulguration — *see also* Electrocoagulation and Destruction, lesion, by site
    adenoid fossa 28.7
    anus 49.39
        endoscopic 49.31
    bladder (transurethral) 57.59

    suprapubic 57.59
    choroid 14.21
    duodenum 45.32
        endoscopic 45.30
    esophagus 42.39
        endoscopic 42.33
    large intestine 45.49
        endoscopic 45.43
            polypectomy 45.42
    penis 64.2
    perineum, female 71.3
    prostate, transurethral 60.2
    rectum 48.32
        radical 48.31
    retina 14.21
    scrotum 61.3
    Skene's gland 71.3
    skin 86.3
    small intestine NEC 45.34
        duodenum 45.32
            endoscopic 45.30
    stomach 43.49
        endoscopic 43.41
    subcutaneous tissue 86.3
    tonsillar fossa 28.7
    urethra 58.39
        endoscopic 58.31
    vulva 71.3
Function
    study — *see also* Scan, radioisotope
        gastric 89.39
        muscle 93.08
            ocular 95.25
        nasal 89.12
        pulmonary — (*see* categories 89.37–89.38)
        renal 92.03
        thyroid 92.01
        urethral sphincter 89.23
Fundectomy, uterine 68.3
Fundoplication (esophageal) (Nissen's) 44.66
Fundusectomy, gastric 43.89
Fusion
    atlas-axis (spine) 81.01
        for pseudarthrosis 81.09
    bone (*see also* Osteoplasty) 78.40
    cervical (spine) (C2 level or below) NEC 81.02
        anterior (interbody), anterolateral technique 81.02
        C1-C2 level (anterior interbody) (anterolateral) 81.01
            for pseudarthrosis 81.09
        occiput - C2 81.01
        posterior (interbody), posterolateral technique 81.03
    claw toe 77.57
    craniocervical 81.01
        for pseudarthrosis 81.09
    dorsal, dorsolumbar NEC 81.05
        anterior (interbody), anterolateral technique 81.04
            for pseudarthrosis 81.09
        posterior (interbody) posterolateral technique 81.05
            for pseudarthrosis 81.09
    epiphyseal-diaphyseal (*see also* Arrest, bone growth) 78.20
    epiphysiodesis (*see also* Arrest, bone growth) 78.20
    joint (with bone graft) (*see also* Arthrodesis) 81.20

    ankle 81.11
    claw toe 77.57
    foot NEC 81.17
    hammer toe 77.56
    hip 81.21
    interphalangeal, finger 81.28
    ischiofemoral 81.21
    metatarsophalangeal 81.16
    midtarsal 81.14
    overlapping toe(s) 77.58
    pantalar 81.11
    spinal (*see also* Fusion, spinal) 81.00
    subtalar 81.13
    tarsal joints NEC 81.17
    tarsometatarsal 81.15
    tibiotalar 81.11
    toe NEC 77.58
        claw toe 77.57
        hammer toe 77.56
        overlapping toe(s) 77.58
    lip to tongue 25.59
    lumbar, lumbosacral NEC 81.08
        anterior (interbody), anterolateral technique 81.06
            for pseudarthrosis 81.09
        for pseudarthrosis 81.09
        lateral transverse process technique 81.07
            for pseudarthrosis 81.09
        posterior (interbody), posterolateral technique 81.08
            for pseudarthrosis 81.09
    occiput - C2 (spinal) 81.01
        for pseudarthrosis 81.09
    spinal (with graft) (with internal fixation) (with instrumentation) 81.00
        atlas-axis (anterior transoral) (posterior) 81.01
            for pseudarthrosis 81.09
        cervical (C2 level or below) NEC 81.02
            anterior (interbody), anterolateral technique 81.02
                for pseudarthrosis 81.09
            C1-C2 level (anterior) (posterior) 81.01
                for pseudarthrosis 81.09
            posterior (interbody), posterolateral technique 81.03
                for pseudarthrosis 81.09
        craniocervical (anterior transoral) (posterior) 81.01
            for pseudarthrosis NEC 81.09
        dorsal, dorsolumbar NEC 81.05
            anterior (interbody), anterolateral technique 81.04
                for pseudarthrosis 81.09
            posterior (interbody), posterolateral technique 81.05
                for pseudarthrosis 81.09
        lumbar, lumbosacral NEC 81.08
            anterior (interbody), anterolateral technique 81.06
                for pseudarthrosis 81.09
            for pseudarthrosis 81.09
            lateral transverse process technique 81.07
                for pseudarthrosis 81.09
            posterior (interbody), posterolateral technique 81.08
                for pseudarthrosis 81.09
        occiput - C2 (anterior transoral) (posterior) 81.01
            for pseudarthrosis 81.09
    tongue (to lip) 25.59

G

Gait training 93.22
Galeaplasty 86.89
Galvanoionization 99.27
Games
  competitive 94.39
  organized 93.89
Ganglionectomy
  gasserian 04.05
  lumbar sympathetic 05.23
  nerve (cranial) (peripheral) NEC 04.06
    sympathetic 05.29
  sphenopalatine (Meckel's) 05.21
  tendon sheath (wrist) 82.21
    site other than hand 83.31
  trigeminal 04.05
Ganglionotomy, trigeminal (radiofrequency) 04.02
Gant operation (wedge osteotomy of trochanter) 77.25
Garceau operation (tibial tendon transfer) 83.75
Gardner operation (spinal meningocele repair) 03.51
Gas endarterectomy 38.10
  abdominal 38.16
  aorta (arch) (ascending) (descending) 38.14
  coronary artery 36.09
  head and neck NEC 38.12
  intracranial NEC 38.11
  lower limb 38.18
  thoracic NEC 38.15
  upper limb 38.13
Gastrectomy (partial) (subtotal) NEC 43.89
  with
    anastomosis (to) NEC 43.89
      duodenum 43.6
      esophagus 43.5
      gastrogastric 43.89
      jejunum 43.7
    esophagogastrostomy 43.5
    gastroduodenostomy (bypass) 43.6
    gastroenterostomy (bypass) 43.7
    gastrogastrostomy (bypass) 43.89
    gastrojejunostomy (bypass) 43.7
    jejunal transposition 43.81
  complete NEC 43.99
    with intestinal interposition 43.91
  distal 43.6
  Hofmeister 43.7
  Polya 43.7
  proximal 43.5
  radical NEC 43.99
    with intestinal interposition 43.91
  total NEC 43.99
    with intestinal interposition 43.91
Gastrocamera 44.19
Gastroduodenectomy — Gastrectomy
Gastroduodenoscopy 45.13
  through stoma (artificial) 45.12
  transabdominal (operative) 45.11
Gastroduodenostomy (bypass) (Jaboulay's) 44.39
  with partial gastrectomy 43.6
Gastroenterostomy (bypass) NEC 44.39
  with partial gastrectomy 43.7
Gastrogastrostomy (bypass) 44.39
  with partial gastrectomy 43.89

Gastrojejunostomy (bypass) 44.39
  with partial gastrectomy 43.7
Gastrolysis 54.5
Gastropexy 44.64
Gastroplasty NEC 44.69
Gastroplication 44.69
Gastropylorectomy 43.6
Gastrorrhaphy 44.61
Gastroscopy NEC 44.13
  through stoma (artificial) 44.12
  transabdominal (operative) 44.11
Gastrostomy (Brunschwig's) (decompression) (fine caliber tube) (Kader) (permanent)(Stamm) (Stamm-Kader) (temporary) (tube) (Witzel) 43.19
  Beck-Jianu 43.19
  Frank's 43.19
  Janeway 43.19
  percutaneous (endoscopic) (PEG) 43.11
  Spivack's 43.19
  Ssabanejew-Frank 43.19
Gastrotomy 43.0
  for control of hemorrhage 44.49
Gavage, gastric 96.35
Gelman operation (release of clubfoot) 83.84
Genioplasty (augmentation) (with graft) (with implant) 76.68
  reduction 76.67
Ghormley operation (hip fusion) 81.21
Gifford operation
  destruction of lacrimal sac 09.6
  keratotomy (delimiting) 11.1
    radial (refractive) 11.75
Gill operation
  arthrodesis of shoulder 81.23
  laminectomy 03.09
Gilliam operation (uterine suspension) 69.22
Gill-Stein operation (carporadial arthrodesis) 81.25
Gingivectomy 24.31
Gingivoplasty (with bone graft) (with soft tissue graft) 24.2
Girdlestone operation
  laminectomy with spinal fusion 81.00
  muscle transfer for claw toe repair 77.57
  resection of femoral head and neck 77.85
Girdlestone-Taylor operation (muscle transfer for claw toe repair) 77.57
Glenn operation (anastomosis of superior vena cava to right pulmonary artery 39.21
Glenoplasty, shoulder 81.83
  with
    partial replacement 81.81
    total replacement 81.80
  for recurrent dislocation 81.82
Glomectomy
  carotid 39.8
  jugulare 20.51
Glossectomy (complete) (total) 25.3
  partial or subtotal 25.2
  radical 25.4
Glossopexy 25.59
Glossoplasty NEC 25.59

Glossorrhaphy 25.51
Glossotomy NEC 25.94
  for tongue tie 25.91
Goebel-Frangenheim-Stoeckel operation (urethrovesical suspension) 59.4
Goldner operation (clubfoot release) 80.48
Goldthwaite operation
  ankle stabilization 81.11
  patellar stabilization 81.44
  tendon transfer for stabilization of patella 81.44
Gonadectomy
  ovary 65.3
  testis 62.3
Goniopuncture 12.51
  with goniotomy 12.53
Gonioscopy 12.29
Goniospasis 12.59
Goniotomy (Barkan's) 12.52
  with goniopuncture 12.53
Goodai-Power operation (vagina) 70.8
Gordon-Taylor operation (hindquarter amputation) 84.19
Graber-Duvernay operation (drilling of femoral head) 77.15
Graft, grafting
  aneurysm 39.52
  artery, arterial (patch) 39.58
    with
      excision of resection of vessel — see Arteriectomy, with graft replacement
      synthetic patch (Dacron) (Teflon) 39.57
      tissue patch (vein) (autogenous) (homograft) 39.56
  blood vessel (patch) 39.58
    with
      excision or resection of vessel — see Angiectomy, with graft replacement
      synthetic patch (Dacron) (Teflon) 39.57
      tissue patch (vein) (autogenous) (homograft) 39.56
  bone (autogenous) (bone bank) (dual onlay) (heterogenous) (inlay) (massive only)(multiple) (osteoperiosteal) (peg) (subperiosteal) (with metallic fixation) 78.00
    with
      arthrodesis — see Arthrodesis
      arthroplasty — see Arthroplasty
      gingivoplasty 24.2
      lengthening — see Lengthening, bone
    carpals, metacarpals 78.04
    clavicle 78.01
    facial NEC 76.91
      with total ostectomy 76.44
    femur 78.05
    fibula 78.07
    humerus 78.02
    joint — see Arthroplasty
    mandible 76.91
      with total mandibulectomy 76.41
    marrow — see Transplant, bone, marrow
    nose — see Graft, nose

patella 78.06
pelvic 78.09
pericranial 02.04
phalanges (foot) (hand) 78.09
radius 78.03
scapula 78.01
skull 02.04
specified site NEC 78.09
spine 78.09
    with fusion — *see* Fusion, spinal
tarsal, metatarsal 78.08
thorax (ribs) (sternum) 78.01
thumb (with transfer of skin flap) 82.69
tibia 78.07
ulna 78.03
vertebrae 78.09
    with fusion — *see* Fusion, spinal
breast (*see also* Mammoplasty) 85.89
buccal sulcus 27.99
cartilage (joint) — *see also* Arthroplasty
  nose — *see* Graft, nose
chest wall (mesh) (silastic) 34.79
conjunctiva (free) (mucosa) 10.44
  for symblepharon repair 10.41
cornea (*see also* Keratoplasty) 11.60
dermal-fat 86.69
dura 02.12
ear
  auricle 18.79
  external auditory meatus 18.6
  inner 20.61
  pedicle preparation 86.71
esophagus NEC 42.87
  with interposition (intrathoracic) NEC 42.58
    antesternal or antethoracic NEC 42.68
    colon (intrathoracic) 42.55
      antesternal or antethoracic 42.65
    small bowel (intrathoracic) 42.53
      antesternal or antethoracic 42.63
eyebrow (*see also* Reconstruction, eyelid, with graft) 08.69
eyelid (*see also* Reconstruction, eyelid, with graft) 08.69
  free mucous membrane 08.62
eye socket (skin) (cartilage) (bone) 16.63
fallopian tube 66.79
fascia 83.82
  with hernia repair — *see* Repair, hernia
  eyelid 08.32
  hand 82.72
  tarsal cartilage 08.69
fat pad NEC 86.89
  with skin graft — *see* Graft, skin, full-thickness
flap (advanced) (rotating) (sliding) — *see also* Graft, skin, pedicle
  tarsoconjunctival 08.64
hair-bearing skin 86.64
hand
  fascia 82.72
  free skin 86.62
  muscle 82.72
  pedicle (flap) 86.73
  tendon 82.79
heart, for revascularization 36.3
joint — *see* Arthroplasty
larynx 31.69
lip 27.56
  full-thickness 27.55
lymphatic structure(s) (channel) (node) (vessel) 40.9
mediastinal fat to myocardium 36.3
meninges (cerebral) 02.12
mouth, except palate 27.56
  full-thickness 27.55
muscle 83.82
  hand 82.72
myocardium, for revascularization 36.3
nasolabial flaps 21.86
nerve (cranial) (peripheral) 04.5
nipple 85.86
nose 21.89
  with
    augmentation 21.85
    rhinoplasty — *see* Rhinoplasty
    total reconstruction 21.83
  septum 21.88
  tip 21.86
omentum 54.74
  to myocardium 36.3
orbit (bone) (cartilage) (skin) 16.63
outflow tract (patch) (pulmonary valve) 35.26
  in total repair of tetralogy of Fallot 35.81
ovary 65.92
palate 27.69
  for cleft palate repair 27.62
pedicle — *see* Graft, skin, pedicle
penis (rib) (skin) 64.49
pigskin 86.65
pinch — *see* Graft, skin, free
pocket — *see* Graft, skin, pedicle
porcine 86.65
postauricular (Wolff) 18.79
razor — *see* Graft, skin, free
rope — *see* Graft, skin, pedicle
saphenous vein in aortocoronary bypass — *see* Bypass, aortocoronary
scrotum 61.49
skin (partial-thickness) 86.99
  amnionic membrane 86.66
  auditory meatus (ear) 18.6
  dermal-fat 86.99
    for breast augmentation 85.50
  ear
    auditory meatus 18.6
    postauricular 18.79
  eyelid 08.61
  flap — *see* Graft, skin, pedicle
  free (autogenous) NEC 86.60
    lip 27.56
    thumb 86.62
      for
        pollicization 82.61
        reconstruction 82.69
  full-thickness 86.63
    breast 85.53
    hand 86.61
  hair-bearing 86.64
    eyelid or eyebrow 08.63
  hand 86.62
    full-thickness 86.61
  heterograft 86.65
  homograft 86.66
  island flap 86.70
  mucous membrane 86.69
    eyelid 08.62
  nose — *see* Graft, nose
  pedicle (flap) (tube) 86.70
    advancement 86.72
    attachment to site (advanced) (double) (rotating) (sliding) 86.74
      hand (cross finger) (pocket) 86.73
      lip 27.57
      mouth 27.57
      thumb 86.73
        for
          pollicization 82.61
          reconstruction NEC 82.69
    breast 85.84
    defatting 86.75
    delayed 86.71
    design and raising 86.71
    elevation 86.71
    preparation of (cutting) 86.71
    revision 86.75
    sculpturing 876.71
    transection 86.71
    transfer 86.74
    trimming 86.71
  postauricular 18.79
  rotation flap 86.70
  specified site NEC 86.69
    full-thickness 86.63
tarsal cartilage 08.69
temporalis muscle to orbit 16.63
  with exenteration of orbit 16.59
tendon 83.81
  for joint repair — *see* Arthroplasty
  hand 82.79
testicle 62.69
thumb (for reconstruction) NEC 82.69
tongue (mucosal) (skin) 25.59
trachea 31.79
tubular (tube) — *see* Graft, skin, pedicle
tunnel — *see* Graft, skin, pedicle
tympanum (*see also* Tympanoplasty) 19.4
ureter 56.89
vein (patch) 39.58
  with
    excision or resection of vessel — *see* Phlebectomy, with graft replacement
    synthetic patch (Dacron) (Teflon) 39.57
    tissue patch (vein) (autogenous) (homograft) 39.56
vermilion border (lip) 27.56

Grattage, conjunctiva 10.31
Green operation (scapulopexy) 78.41
Grice operation (subtalar arthrodesis) 81.13
Grip, strength 93.04
Gritti-Stokes operation (knee disarticulation) 84.16
Gross operation (herniorrhaphy) 53.49
Group therapy 94.44
Guttering, bone (*see also* Excision, lesion, bone) 77.60
Guyon operation (amputation of ankle) 84.13

H

Hagner operation (epididymotomy) 63.92
Halsted operation — see Repair, hernia, inguinal
Hampton operation (anastomosis small intestine to rectal stump) 45.92
Hanging hip operation (muscle release) 83.19
Harelip operation 27.54
Harrison-Richardson operation (vaginal suspension) 70.77
Hartmann resection (of intestine) (with pouch) — see Colectomy, by site
Harvesting
   bone marrow 41.91
▸ stem cells 99.79
Hauser operation
   achillotenotomy 83.11
   bunionectomy with adductor tendon transfer 77.53
   stabilization of patella 81.44
Heaney operation (vaginal hysterectomy) 68.5
Hearing aid (with battery replacement) 95.49
Hearing test 95.47
Hegar operation (perineorrhaphy) 71.79
Heine operation (cyclodialysis) 12.55
Heineke-Mikulicz operation (pyloroplasty) 44.29
Heller operation (esophagomyotomy) 42.7
Hellstom operation (transplantation of aberrant renal vessel) 39.55
Hemicolectomy
   left 45.75
   right (extended) 45.73
Hemicystectomy 57.6
Hemigastrectomy — see Gastrectomy
Hemiglossectomy 25.2
Hemilaminectomy (decompression) (exploration) 03.09
Hemilaryngectomy (anterior) (lateral) (vertical) 30.1
Hemimandibulectomy 76.31
Hemimastectomy (radical) 85.23
Hemimaxillectomy (with bone graft) (with prosthesis) 76.39
Heminephrectomy 55.4
Hemipelvectomy 84.19
Hemispherectomy (cerebral) 01.52
Hemithyroidectomy (with removal of isthmus) (with removal of portion of remaining lobe) 06.2
Hemodiafiltration (extracorporeal) 39.95
Hemodialysis (extracorporeal) 39.95
Hemofiltration (extracorporeal) 39.95
Hemorrhage control - see Control, hemorrhage
Hemorrhoidectomy 49.46
   by
      cautery, cauterization 49.43
      crushing 49.45
      cryotherapy, cryosurgery 49.44
      excision 49.46
      injection 49.42
      ligation 49.45
Hemostasis — see Control, hemorrhage
Henley operation (jejunal transposition) 43.81

Hepatectomy (complete) (total) 50.4
   partial or subtotal 50.22
Hepatic assistance, extracorporeal 50.92
Hepaticocholangiojejunostomy 51.37
Hepaticocystoduodenostomy 51.37
Hepaticodochotomy 51.59
Hepaticoduodenostomy 51.37
Hepaticojejunostomy 51.37
Hepaticolithectomy 51.49
   endoscopic 51.88
Hepaticolithotomy 51.49
   endoscopic 51.88
Hepaticostomy 51.59
Hepaticotomy 51.59
Hepatocholangiocystoduodenostomy 51.37
Hepatocholedochostomy 51.43
   endoscopic 51.87
Hepatoduodenostomy 50.69
Hepatogastrostomy 50.69
Hepatojejunostomy 50.69
Hepatolithotomy
   hepatic duct 51.49
   liver 50.0
Hepatopexy 50.69
Hepatorrhaphy 50.61
Hepatostomy (external) (internal) 50.69
Hepatotomy (with packing) 50.0
Herniorrhaphy — see Repair, hernia
Herniotomy — see Repair, hernia
Heterograft — see Graft
Heterotransplant, heterotransplantation — see Transplant
Hey operation (amputation of foot) 84.12
Hey-Groves operation (reconstruction of anterior cruciate ligament) 81.45
Heyman operation (soft tissue release for clubfoot) 83.84
Heyman-Herndon (-Strong) **operation** (correction of metatarsus varus) 80.48
Hibbs operation (lumbar spinal fusion) — see Fusion, lumbar
Higgins operation — see Repair, hernia, femoral
High forceps delivery 72.39
   with episiotomy 72.31
Hill-Allison operation (hiatal hernia repair, transpleural approach) 53.80
Hinging, mitral valve 35.12
His bundle recording 37.29
Hitchcock operation (anchoring tendon of biceps) 83.88
Hofmeister operation (gastrectomy) 43.7
Hoke operation
   midtarsal fusion 81.14
   triple arthrodesis 81.12
Holth operation
   iridencleisis 12.63
   sclerectomy 12.65
Homan operation (correction of lymphedema) 40.9
Homograft — see Graft
Homotransplant, homotransplantation — see Transplant
Hosiery, elastic 93.59

Hutch operation (ureteroneocystostomy) 56.74
Hybinette-Eden operation (glenoid bone block) 78.01
Hydrocelectomy
   canal of Nuck (female) 69.19
      male 63.1
   round ligament 69.19
   spermatic cord 63.1
   tunica vaginalis 61.2
Hydrotherapy 93.33
   assisted exercise in pool 93.31
   whirlpool 93.32
Hymenectomy 70.31
Hymenoplasty 70.76
Hymenorrhaphy 70.76
Hymenotomy 70.11
Hyperalimentation 99.15
Hyperbaric oxygenation 93.95
   wound 93.59
Hyperextension, joint 93.25
Hyperthermia NEC 93.35
   for cancer treatment (interstitial) (radiofrequency) (ultrasound) 99.85
Hypnodrama, psychiatric 94.32
Hypnosis (psychotherapeutic) 94.32
   for anesthesia — omit code
Hypnotherapy 94.32
Hypophysectomy (complete) (total) 07.69
   partial or subtotal 07.63
      transfrontal approach 07.61
      transsphenoidal approach 07.62
   specified approach NEC 07.68
      (complete) (total) 07.64
      partial 07.61
   transsphenoidal approach (complete) (total) 07.65
      partial 07.62
Hypothermia (central) (local) 99.81
   gastric (cooling) 96.31
      freezing 96.32
   systemic (in open heart surgery) 39.62
Hypotympanotomy 20.23
Hysterectomy (abdominal) (complete) (extended) (total) 68.9
   abdominal 68.4
   partial or subtotal (supracervical) (supravaginal) 68.3
   radical (modified) (Wertheim's) 68.6
   vaginal (complete) (partial) (subtotal) (total) 68.5
      radical (Schauta) 68.7
Hysterocolpectomy (radical) (vaginal) 68.7
   abdominal 68.6
Hysterogram NEC 87.85
   percutaneous 87.84
Hysterolysis 54.5
Hysteromyomectomy 68.29
Hysteropexy 69.22
Hysteroplasty 69.49
Hysterorrhaphy 69.41
Hysterosalpingography
   gas (contrast) 87.82
   opaque dye (contrast) 87.83
Hysterosalpingostomy 66.74
Hysteroscopy 68.12
   with biopsy 68.16

Hysterotomy (with removal of foreign body) (with removal of hydatidiform mole) 68.0
   for intrauterine transfusion 75.2
   obstetrical 74.99
      for termination of pregnancy 74.91
Hysterotrachelectomy 67.4
Hysterotracheloplasty 69.49
Hysterotrachelorrhaphy 69.41
Hysterotrachelotomy 69.95

I

ICCE (intracapsular cataract extraction) 13.19
Ileal
  bladder
    closed 57.87 [45.51]
    open (ileoureterostomy) 56.51
  conduit (ileoureterostomy) 56.51
Ileocecostomy 45.93
Ileocolectomy 45.73
Ileocolostomy 45.93
Ileocolotomy 45.00
Ileocystoplasty (isolated segment anastomosis) (open loop) 57.87 [45.51]
Ileoduodenotomy 45.01
Ileoectomy (partial) 45.62
  with cecectomy 45.72
Ileoentectropy 46.99
Ileoesophagostomy 42.54
Ileoileostomy 45.91
  proximal to distal segment 45.62
Ileoloopogram 87.78
Ileopancreatostomy 52.96
Ileopexy 46.61
Ileoproctostomy 45.93
Ileorectostomy 45.93
Ileorrhaphy 46.73
Ileoscopy 45.13
  through stoma (artificial) 45.12
  transabdominal (operative) 45.11
Ileosigmoidostomy 45.93
Ileostomy 46.20
  continent (permanent) 46.22
  delayed opening 46.24
  Hendon (temporary) 46.21
  loop 46.01
  Paul (temporary) 46.21
  permanent 46.23
    continent 46.22
  repair 46.41
  revision 46.41
  tangential (temporary) 46.21
  temporary 46.21
  transplantation to new site 46.23
  tube (temporary) 46.21
  ureteral
    external 56.51
    internal 56.71
Ileotomy 45.02
Ileotransversostomy 45.93
Ileoureterostomy (Bricker's) ileal bladder) 56.51
Imaging (diagnostic)
  diagnostic, not elsewhere classified 88.90
  magnetic resonance (nuclear) (proton) NEC 88.97
    abdomen 88.97
    bladder (urinary) 88.95
    bone marrow blood supply 88.94
    brain (brain stem) 88.91
    chest (hilar) (mediastinal) 88.92
    extremity (upper) (lower) 88.94
    eye orbit 88.97
    face 88.97
    head NEC 88.97
    musculoskeletal 88.94
    myocardium 88.92
    neck 88.97
    orbit of eye 88.97
    prostate 88.95
    specified site NEC 88.97
    spinal canal (cord) (spine) 88.93
Immobilization (by)
  with fracture reduction — *see* Reduction, fracture
  bandage 93.59
  bone 93.53
  cast NEC 93.53
    with reduction of fracture or dislocation — *see* Reduction, fracture, and Reduction, dislocation
  device NEC 93.59
  pressure dressing 93.56
  splint (plaster) (tray) 93.54
    with reduction of fracture or dislocation — *see* Reduction, fracture, and Reduction, dislocation
Immunization — *see also* Vaccination
  allergy 99.12
  autoimmune disease 99.13
  BCG 99.33
  brucellosis 99.55
  cholera 99.31
  diphtheria 99.36
  DPT 99.39
  epidemic parotitis 99.46
  German measles 99.47
  Hemophilus influenzae 99.52
  influenza 99.52
  measles 99.45
  meningococcus 99.55
  mumps 99.46
  pertussis 99.37
  plague 99.34
  poliomyelitis 99.41
  rabies 99.44
  rubella 99.47
  salmonella 99.55
  smallpox 99.42
  staphylococcus 99.55
  TAB 99.32
  tetanus 99.38
  triple vaccine 99.48
  tuberculosis 99.33
  tularemia 99.35
  typhoid-paratyphoid 99.32
  typhus 99.55
  viral NEC 99.55
  whooping cough 99.37
  yellow fever 99.43
Immunotherapy, antineoplastic 99.28
  C-Parvum 99.28
  Interferon 99.28
  Interleukin-2 99.28
  Levamisole 99.28
  Thymosin 99.28
Implant, implantation
  artery
    aortic branches to heart muscle 36.2
    mammary to ventricular wall (Vineberg) 36.2
  baffle, atrial or interatrial 35.91
  biliary fistulous tract into stomach or intestine 51.39
  bipolar endoprosthesis (femoral head) 81.52
  bladder sphincter, artificial (inflatable) 58.93
  blood vessels to myocardium 36.2
  bone growth stimulator (invasive) (percutaneous) (semi-invasive) — *see* category 78.9
  breast (for augmentation) (bilateral) 85.54
    unilateral 85.53
  cardioverter/defibrillator (automatic) 37.94
    leads only (patch electrodes) (sensing) (pacing) 37.95
    pulse generator only 37.96
    total system 37.94
  chest wall (mesh) (silastic) 34.79
  chin (polyethylene) (silastic) 76.68
  cochlear (electrode) 20.96
    prosthetic device (electrode and receiver) 20.96
      channel (single) 20.97
        multiple 20.98
    electrode only 20.99
    internal coil only 20.99
  cornea 11.73
  custodis eye 14.41
  dental (endosseous) (prosthetic) 23.6
  device, vascular access 86.07
  diaphragmatic pacemaker 34.85
  electrode(s)
    brain 02.93
      depth 02.93
      foramen ovale 02.93
      sphenoidal 02.96
    cardiac (initial) (transvenous) 37.70
      atrium (initial) 37.73
        replacement 37.76
      atrium and ventricle (initial) 37.72
        replacement 37.76
      epicardium (sternotomy or thoracotomy approach) 37.74
      temporary transvenous pacemaker system 37.78
        during and immediately following cardiac surgery 39.64
      ventricle (initial) 37.71
        replacement 37.76
    depth 02.93
    foramen ovale 02.93
    heart (*see also* Implant, electrode(s), cardiac) 37.70
    intracranial 02.93
    osteogenic (invasive) for bone growth stimulation - *see* category 78.9
    peripheral nerve 04.92
    sphenoidal 02.96
    spine 03.93
  electroencephalographic receiver
    brain 02.93
    intracranial 02.93
  electronic stimulator
    anus (subcutaneous) 49.92
    bladder 57.96
    bone growth (invasive) (percutaneous) (semi-invasive) 78.9
    brain 02.93
    carotid sinus 39.8
    cochlear 20.96
      channel (single) 20.97
        multiple 20.98
    intracranial 02.93
    peripheral nerve 04.92
    phrenic nerve 34.85
    skeletal muscle 83.92
    spine 03.93
    ureter 56.92

Implant, implantation

electrostimulator — *see* Implant, electronic stimulator, by site
endoprosthesis
    bile duct 51.87
    femoral head (bipolar) 81.52
    pancreatic duct 52.93
endosseous (dental) 23.6
epidural pegs 02.93
epikeratoprosthesis 11.73
estradiol (pellet) 99.23
eye (Iowa type) 16.61
    integrated 16.41
facial bone, synthetic (alloplastic) 76.92
fallopian tube (Mulligan hood) (silastic tube) (stent) 66.93
    into uterus 66.74
half-heart 37.62
hearing device, electromagnetic 20.95
heart
    artificial 37.62
    assist system NEC 37.62
    auxiliary ventricle 37.62
    pacemaker (*see also* Implant, pacemaker, cardiac) 37.80
    valve(s)
        prosthesis or synthetic device (partial) (synthetic) (total) 35.20
            aortic 35.22
            mitral 35.24
            pulmonary 35.26
            tricuspid 35.28
        tissue graft 35.20
            aortic 35.21
            mitral 35.23
            pulmonary 35.25
            tricuspid 35.27
inert material
    breast (for augmentation) (bilateral) 85.54
        unilateral 85.53
    larynx 31.0
    nose 21.85
    orbit (eye socket) 16.69
        reinsertion 16.62
    scleral shell (cup) (with evisceration of eyeball) 16.31
        reinsertion 16.62
    Tenon's capsule (with enucleation of eyeball) 16.42
        with attachment of muscles 16.41
        reinsertion 16.62
    urethra 59.70
    vocal cord(s) 31.0
infusion pump 86.06
joint (prosthesis) (silastic) (Swanson type) NEC 81.96
    ankle (total) 81.56
        revision 81.59
    carpocarpal, carpometacarpal 81.74
    elbow (total) 81.84
        revision 81.97
    extremity (bioelectric) (cineplastic) (kineplastic) 84.40
        lower 84.48
            revision 81.59
        upper 84.44
            revision 81.97
    finger 81.71
    femoral (bipolar endoprosthesis) 81.52
    hand (metacarpophalangeal) (interphalangeal) 81.71
        revision 81.97
    hip (partial) 81.52
        revision 81.53
        total 81.51
            revision 81.53
    interphalangeal 81.71
        revision 81.97
    knee (partial) (total) 81.54
        revision 81.55
    metacarpophalangeal 81.71
        revision 81.97
    shoulder (partial) 81.81
        revision 81.97
        total replacement 81.80
    toe 81.57
        for hallux valgus repair 77.59
        revision 81.59
    wrist (partial) 81.74
        revision 81.97
        total replacement 81.73
kidney, mechanical 55.97
larynx 31.0
leads (cardiac) — *see* Implant, electrode(s), cardiac
mammary artery
    in ventricle (Vineberg) 36.2
    to coronary artery (single vessel) 36.15
        double vessel 36.16
Mulligan hood, fallopian tube 66.93
nerve (peripheral) 04.79
neuropacemaker
    brain 02.93
    intracranial 02.93
    peripheral nerve 04.92
    spine 03.93
neurostimulator
    brain 02.93
    intracranial 02.93
    peripheral nerve 04.92
    spine 03.93
nose 21.85
Ommaya reservoir 02.2
orbit 16.69
    reinsertion 16.62
outflow tract prosthesis (heart) (gusset type)
    in
        pulmonary valvuloplasty 35.26
        total repair of tetralogy of Fallot 35.81
ovary into uterine cavity 65.72
pacemaker
    brain 02.93
    cardiac (device) (initial) (permanent) (replacement) 37.80
        dual-chamber device (initial) 37.83
            replacement 37.87
        single-chamber device (initial) 37.81
            rate responsive 37.82
            replacement 37.85
                rate responsive 37.86
        temporary transvenous pacemaker system 37.78
            during and immediately following cardiac surgery 39.64
    carotid sinus 39.8
    diaphragm 34.85
    intracranial 02.93
    neural
        brain 02.93
        intracranial 02.93
        peripheral nerve 04.92
        spine 03.93
    peripheral nerve 04.92
    spine 03.93
pancreas (duct) 52.96
penis, prosthesis (internal)
    inflatable 64.97
    non-inflatable 64.95
port, vascular access device 86.07
premaxilla 76.68
progesterone (subdermal) 99.23
prosthesis, prosthetic device
    acetabulum (Aufranc-Turner) 81.52
    ankle (total) 81.56
    arm (bioelectric) (cineplastic) (kineplastic) 84.44
    breast (Cronin) (Dow-Corning) (Perras-Pappillon) (bilateral) 85.54
        unilateral 85.53
    cochlear 20.96
        channel (single) 20.97
            multiple 20.98
    extremity (bioelectric) (cineplastic) (kineplastic) 84.40
        lower 84.48
        upper 84.44
    fallopian tube (Mulligan hood) (stent) 66.93
    femoral head (Austin-Moore) (bipolar) (Eicher) (Thompson) 81.52
    joint (Swanson type) NEC 81.96
        ankle (total) 81.56
        carpocarpal, carpometacarpal 81.74
        elbow (total) 81.84
        finer 81.71
        hand (metacarpophalangeal) (interphalangeal) 81.71
        hip (partial) 81.52
            total 81.51
        interphalangeal 81.71
        knee (partial) (total) 81.54
            revision 81.55
        metacarpophalangeal 81.71
        shoulder (partial) 81.81
            total 81.80
        toe 81.57
            for hallux valgus repair 77.59
        wrist (partial) 81.74
            total 81.73
    leg (bioelectric) (cineplastic) (kineplastic) 84.48
    outflow tract (heart) (gusset type)
        in
            pulmonary valvuloplasty 35.26
            total repair of tetralogy of Fallot 35.81
    penis (internal) (non-inflatable) 64.95
        inflatable (internal) 64.97
    testicular (bilateral) (unilateral) 62.7
pulsation balloon (phase-shift) 37.61
pump, infusion 86.06
radioactive isotope 92.27
radium (radon) 92.27
retinal attachment 14.41
    with buckling 14.41
Rickham reservoir 02.2
silicone
    breast (bilateral) 85.54
        unilateral 85.53
    skin (for filling of defect) 86.02
        for augmentation NEC 86.89
stimoceiver
    brain 02.93
    intracranial 02.93
    peripheral nerve 04.92
    spine 03.93
subdural
    grids 02.93
    strips 02.93

Implosion   INDEX TO PROCEDURES   **Incision**

    Swanson prosthesis (joint) (silastic) NEC 81.96
        carpocarpal, carpometacarpal 81.74
        finger 81.71
        hand (metacarpophalangeal) (interphalangeal) 81.71
        interphalangeal 81.71
        knee (partial) (total) 81.54
            revision 81.55
        metacarpophalangeal 81.71
        toe 81.57
            for hallux valgus repair 77.59
        wrist (partial) 81.74
            total 81.72
    systemic arteries into myocardium (Vineberg type operation) 36.2
    testicular prothesis (bilateral) (unilateral) 62.7
    tissue expander (skin) NEC 86.93
        breast 85.95
    tissue mandril (for vascular graft) 39.99
        with
            blood vessel repair 39.56
            vascular bypass or shunt — see Bypass, vascular
    tooth (bud) (germ) 23.5
        prosthetic 23.6
    umbrella, vena cava 38.7
    ureters into
        bladder 56.74
        intestine 56.71
            external diversion 56.51
        skin 56.61
    urethral sphincter, artificial (inflatable) 58.93
    urinary sphincter, artificial (inflatable) 58.93
    vascular access device 86.07
    vitreous (silicone) 14.75
        for retinal reattachment 14.41
            with buckling 14.41
    vocal cord(s) 31.0
Implosion (psychologic desensitization) 94.33
Incision (and drainage)
    with
        exploration — see Exploration
        removal of foreign body — see Removal, foreign body
    abdominal wall 54.0
        as operative approach — omit code
    abscess — see also Incision, by site
        appendix 47.2
            with appendectomy 47.0
        extraperitoneal 54.0
        ischiorectal 49.01
        lip 27.0
        omental 54.19
        perianal 49.01
        perigastric 54.19
        perisplenic 54.19
        peritoneal NEC 54.19
            pelvic (female) 70.12
        retroperitoneal 54.0
        sclera 12.89
        skin 86.04
        subcutaneous tissue 86.04
        subdiaphragmatic 54.19
        subhepatic 54.19
        subphrenic 54.19
        vas deferens 63.6
    adrenal gland 07.41
    alveolus, alveolar bone 24.0
    antecubital fossa 86.09
    anus NEC 49.93
    fistula 49.11
    septum 49.91
    appendix 47.2
    artery 38.00
        abdominal 38.06
            aorta (arch) (ascending) (descending) 38.04
        head and neck NEC 38.02
        intracranial NEC 38.01
        lower limb 38.08
        thoracic NEC 38.05
        upper limb 38.03
    atrium (heart) 37.11
    auditory canal or meatus, external 18.02
    auricle 18.09
    axilla 86.09
    Bartholin's gland or cyst 71.22
    bile duct (with T or Y tube insertion) NEC 51.59
        common (exploratory) 51.51
            for
                relief of obstruction NEC 51.42
                removal of calculus 51.41
        for
            exploration 51.59
            relief of obstruction 51.49
    bladder 57.19
        neck (transurethral) 57.91
        percutaneous suprapubic (closed) 57.17
        suprapubic NEC 57.18
    blood vessel (see also Angiotomy) 38.00
    bone 77.10
        alveolus, alveolar 24.0
        carpals, metacarpals 77.14
        clavicle 77.11
        facial 76.09
        femur 77.15
        fibula 77.17
        humerus 77.12
        patella 77.16
        pelvic 77.19
        phalanges (foot) (hand) 77.19
        radius 77.13
        scapula 77.11
        skull 01.24
        specified site NEC 77.19
        tarsals, metatarsals 77.18
        thorax (ribs) (sternum) 77.11
        tibia 77.17
        ulna 77.13
        vertebrae 77.19
    brain 01.39
        cortical adhesions 02.91
    breast (skin) 85.0
        with removal of tissue expander 85.96
    bronchus 33.0
    buccal space 27.0
    bulbourethral gland 58.91
    bursa 83.03
        hand 82.03
        pharynx 29.0
    carotid body 39.8
    cerebral (meninges) 01.39
        epidural or extradural space 01.24
        subarachnoid or subdural space 01.31
    cerebrum 01.39
    cervix 69.95
        to
            assist delivery 73.93
            replace inverted uterus 75.93
    chalazion 08.09
        with removal of capsule 08.21
    cheek 86.09
    chest wall (for extrapleural drainage) (for removal of foreign body) 34.01
        as operative approach — omit code
    common bile duct (for exploration) 51.51
        for
            relief of obstruction 51.42
            removal of calculus 51.41
    common wall between posterior left atrium and coronary sinus (with roofing of resultantdefect with patch graft) 35.82
    conjunctiva 10.1
    cornea 11.1
        radial (refractive) 11.75
    cranial sinus 01.21
    craniobuccal pouch 07.72
    cul-de-sac 70.12
    cyst
        dentigerous 24.0
        radicular (apical) (periapical) 24.0
    Duhrssen's (cervix, to assist delivery) 73.93
    duodenum 45.01
    ear
        external 18.09
        inner 20.79
        middle 20.23
    endocardium 37.11
    endolymphatic sac 20.79
    epididymis 63.92
    epidural space, cerebral 01.24
    epigastric region 54.0
        intra-abdominal 54.19
    esophagus, esophageal NEC 42.09
        web 42.01
    exploratory — see Exploration
    extradural space (cerebral) 01.24
    extrapleural 34.01
    eyebrow 08.09
    eyelid 08.09
        margin (trichiasis) 08.01
    face 86.09
    fallopian tube 66.01
    fascia 83.09
        with division 83.14
            hand 82.12
        hand 82.09
            with division 82.12
    fascial compartments, head and neck 27.0
    fistula, anal 49.11
    flank 54.0
    furuncle — see Incision, by site
    gallbladder 51.04
    gingiva 24.0
    gluteal 86.09
    groin region (abdominal wall) (inguinal) 54.0
        skin 86.09
        subcutaneous tissue 86.09
    gum 24.0
    hair follicles 86.09
    heart 37.10
        valve — see Valvulotomy
    hematoma — see also Incision, by site
        axilla 86.04
        broad ligament 69.98
        ear 18.09
        episiotomy site 75.91
        fossa (superficial) NEC 86.04
        groin region (abdominal wall) (inguinal) 54.0
            skin 86.04
            subcutaneous tissue 86.04
        laparotomy site 54.12
        mediastinum 34.1

perineum (female) 71.09
    male 86.04
popliteal space 86.04
scrotum 61.0
skin 86.04
space of Retzius 59.19
subcutaneous tissue 86.04
vagina (cuff) 70.14
    episotomy site 75.91
    obstetrical NEC 75.92
hepatic duct 51.59
hordeolum 08.09
hygroma — see also Incision, by site
    cystic 40.0
hymen 70.11
hypochondrium 54.0
    intra-abdominal 54.19
hypophysis 07.72
iliac fossa 54.0
infratemporal fossa 27.0
ingrown nail 86.09
intestine 45.00
    large 45.03
    small 45.02
intracerebral 01.39
intracranial (epidural space) (extradural space) 01.24
    subarachnoid or subdural space 01.31
intraperitoneal 54.19
ischiorectal tissue 49.02
    abscess 49.01
joint structures (see also Arthrotomy) 80.10
kidney 55.01
    pelvis 55.11
labia 71.09
lacrimal
    canaliculus 09.52
    gland 09.0
    passage NEC 09.59
    punctum 09.51
    sac 09.53
larynx NEC 31.3
ligamentum flavum (spine) — omit code
liver 50.0
lung 33.1
lymphangioma 40.0
lymphatic structure (channel) (node) (vessel) 40.0
mastoid 20.21
mediastinum 34.1
meibomian gland 08.09
meninges (cerebral) 01.31
    spinal 03.09
midpalmar space 82.04
mouth NEC 27.92
    floor 27.0
muscle 83.02
    with division 83.19
        hand 82.19
    hand 82.02
        with division 82.19
myocardium 37.11
nailbed or nailfold 86.09
    nasolacrimal duct (stricture) 09.59
neck 86.09
nerve (cranial) (peripheral) NEC 04.04
    root (spinal) 03.1
nose 21.1
omentum 54.19
orbit (see also Orbitotomy) 16.09
ovary 65.0
palate 27.1
palmar space (middle) 82.04
pancreas 52.09

pancreatic sphincter 51.82
    endoscopic 51.85
parapharyngeal (oral) (transcervical) 28.0
paronychia 86.09
parotid
    gland or duct 26.0
    space 27.0
pelvirectal tissue 48.81
penis 64.92
perianal (skin) (tissue) 49.02
    abscess 49.01
perigastric 54.19
perineum (female) 71.09
    male 86.09
peripheral vessels
    lower limb
        artery 38.08
        vein 38.09
    upper limb (artery) (vein) 38.03
periprostatic tissue 60.81
perirectal tissue 48.81
perirenal tissue 59.09
perisplenic 54.19
peritoneum 54.95
    by laparotomy 54.19
    pelvic (female) 70.12
        male 54.19
periureteral tissue 59.09
periurethral tissue 58.91
perivesical tissue 59.19
petrous pyramid (air cells) (apex) (mastoid) 20.22
pharynx, pharyngeal (bursa) 29.0
    space, lateral 27.0
pilonidal sinus (cyst) 86.03
pineal gland 07.52
pituitary (gland) 07.72
pleura NEC 34.09
popliteal space 86.09
postzygomatic space 27.0
pouch of Douglas 70.12
prostate (perineal approach) (transurethral approach) 60.0
pterygopalatine fossa 27.0
pulp canal (tooth) 24.0
Rathke's pouch 07.72
rectovaginal septum 48.81
rectum 48.0
    stricture 48.91
renal pelvis 55.11
retroperitoneum 54.0
retropharyngeal (oral) (transcervical) 28.0
salivary gland or duct 26.0
sclera 12.89
scrotum 61.0
sebaceous cyst 86.04
seminal vesicle 60.72
sinus — see Sinusotomy
Skene's duct or gland 71.09
skin 86.09
    with drainage 86.04
    breast 85.0
    ear 18.09
    nose 21.1
skull (bone) 01.24
soft tissue NEC 83.09
    with division 83.19
        hand 82.19
    hand 82.09
        with division 82.19
space of Retzius 59.19
spermatic cord 63.93
sphincter of Oddi 51.82

    endoscopic 51.85
spinal
    cord 03.09
    nerve root 03.1
spleen 41.2
stomach 43.0
stye 08.09
subarachnoid space, cerebral 01.31
subcutaneous tissue 86.09
    with drainage 86.04
subdiaphragmatic space 54.19
subdural space, cerebral 01.31
sublingual space 27.0
submandibular space 27.0
submaxillary 86.09
    with drainage 86.04
submental space 27.0
subphrenic space 54.19
supraclavicular fossa 86.09
    with drainage 86.04
sweat glands, skin 86.04
temporal pouches 27.0
tendon (sheath) 83.01
    with division 83.13
        hand 82.11
    hand 82.01
        with division 82.11
testis 62.0
thenar space 82.04
thymus 07.92
thyroid (field) (gland) NEC 06.09
    postoperative 06.02
tongue NEC 25.94
    for tongue tie 25.91
tonsil 28.0
trachea NEC 31.3
tunica vaginalis 61.0
umbilicus 54.0
urachal cyst 54.0
ureter 56.2
urethra 58.0
uterus (corpus) 68.0
    cervix 69.95
    for termination of pregnancy 74.91
    septum (congenital) 68.22
uvula 27.71
vagina (cuff) (septum) (stenosis) 70.14
    for
        incisional hematoma (episiotomy) 75.91
        obstetrical hematoma NEC 75.92
        pelvic abscess 70.12
vas deferens 63.6
vein 38.00
    abdominal 38.07
    head and neck NEC 38.02
    intracranial NEC 38.01
    lower limb 38.09
    thoracic NEC 38.05
    upper limb 38.03
vertebral column 03.09
vulva 71.09
    obstetrical 75.92
web, esophageal 42.01
Incudectomy NEC 19.3
    with
        stapedectomy (see also Stapedectomy) 19.19
        tympanoplasty — see Tympanoplasty
Incudopexy 19.19
Incudostapediopexy 19.19
    with incus replacement 19.11

Indentation, sclera, for buckling (see also Buckling, scleral) 14.49
Indicator dilution flow measurement 89.68
Induction
   abortion
      by
         D and C 69.01
         insertion of prostaglandin suppository 96.49
         intra-amniotic injection (prostaglandin) (saline) 75.0
   labor
      medical 73.4
      surgical 73.01
         intra- and extra-amniotic injection 73.1
         stripping of membranes 73.1
Inflation
   belt wrap 93.99
   Eustachian tube 20.8
   fallopian tube 66.8
      with injection of therapeutic agent 66.95
Infolding, sclera, for buckling (see also Buckling, scleral) 14.49
Infraction, turbinates (nasal) 21.62
Infundibulectomy
   hypophyseal (see also Hypophysectomy, partial) 07.63
   ventricle (heart) (right) 35.34
      in total repair of tetralogy of Fallot 35.81
▶ **Infusion** (intra-arterial) (intravenous)
▶   antineoplastic agent (chemotherapeutic) 99.25
▶   biological response modifier [BRM] 99.28
▶   biological response modifier [BRM], antineoplastic agent 99.28
   cancer chemotherapy agent NEC 99.25
   electrolytes 99.18
   hormone substance NEC 99.24
   nutritional substance — see Nutrition
   prophylactic substance NEC 99.29
   therapeutic substance NEC 99.29
   thrombolytic agent (streptokinase) 99.29
      with percutaneous transluminal angioplasty
         coronary (single vessel) 36.02
            multiple vessels 36.05
         specified site NEC 39.59
      direct intracoronary artery 36.04
Injection (into) (hypodermically) (intramuscularly) (intravenously) (acting locally or systemically)
   Actinomycin D, for cancer chemotherapy 99.25
   alcohol
      nerve — see Injection, nerve
      spinal 03.8
   anterior chamber, eye (air) (liquid) (medication) 12.92
   antibiotic 99.21
   anticoagulant 99.19
   anti-D (Rhesus) globulin 99.11
   antidote NEC 99.16
   anti-infective NEC 99.22
▶   antineoplastic agent (chemotherapeutic) NEC 99.25
▶   biological response modifier [BRM] 99.28
   antivenin 99.16
   BCG
      for chemotherapy 99.25
      vaccine 99.33
▶   biological response modifier [BRM], antineoplastic agent 99.28
   bone marrow 41.92
      transplant — see Transplant, bone, marrow
   breast (therapeutic agent) 85.92
      inert material (silicone) (bilateral) 85.52
         unilateral 85.51
   bursa (therapeutic agent) 83.96
      hand 82.94
   cancer chemotherapeutic agent 99.25
   caudal — see Injection, spinal
   cortisone 99.23
   costochondral junction 81.92
   dinoprost-tromethine, intra-amniotic 75.0
   ear, with alcohol 20.72
   electrolytes 99.18
   epidural, spinal — see Injection, spinal
   esophageal varices or blood vessel (endoscopic) (sclerosing agent) 42.33
   Eustachian tube (inert material) 20.8
   eye (orbit) (retrobulbar) 16.91
      anterior chamber 12.92
      subconjunctival 10.91
   fascia 83.98
      hand 82.96
   gamma globulin 99.14
   ganglion, sympathetic 05.39
      ciliary 12.79
      paravertebral stellate 05.39
   globulin
      anti-D (Rhesus) 99.11
      gamma 99.14
      Rh immune 99.11
   heart 37.92
   heavy metal antagonist 99.16
   hemorrhoids (sclerosing agent) 49.42
   hormone NEC 99.24
   immune sera 99.14
   inert material — see Implant, inert material
   inner ear, for destruction 20.72
   insulin 99.17
   intervertebral space for herniated disc 80.52
   intra-amniotic
      for induction of
         abortion 75.0
         labor 73.1
   intrathecal — see Injection, spinal
   joint (therapeutic agent) 81.92
      temporomandibular 76.96
   kidney (cyst) (therapeutic substance) NEC 55.96
   larynx 31.0
   ligament (joint) (therapeutic substance) 81.92
   liver 50.94
   lung, for surgical collapse 33.32
   Methotrexate, for cancer chemotherapy 99.25
   nerve (cranial) (peripheral) 04.80
      agent NEC 04.89
         alcohol 04.2
         anesthetic for analgesia 04.81
            for operative anesthesia — omit code
         neurolytic 04.2
         phenol 04.2
      laryngeal (external) (recurrent) (superior) 31.91
      optic 16.91
      sympathetic 05.39
         alcohol 05.32
         anesthetic for analgesia 05.31
         neurolytic agent 05.32
         phenol 05.32
   orbit 16.91
   pericardium 37.93
   peritoneal cavity
      air 54.96
      locally-acting therapeutic substance 54.97
   prophylactic substances NEC 99.29
   prostate 60.92
   radioisotopes (intracavitary) (intravenous) 92.28
   renal pelvis (cyst) 55.96
   retrobulbar (therapeutic substance) 16.91
      for anesthesia — omit code
   Rh immune globulin 99.11
   RhoGAM 99.11
   sclerosing agent NEC 99.29
      esophageal varices (endoscopic) 42.33
      hemorrhoids 49.42
      pleura 34.92
         treatment of malignancy (cytotoxic agent) 34.92 [99.25]
         with tetracycline 34.92 [99.21]
      varicose vein 39.92
      vein NEC 39.92
   semicircular canals, for destruction 20.72
   silicone — see Implant, inert material
   skin (sclerosing agent) (filling material) 86.02
   soft tissue 83.98
      hand 82.96
   spinal (canal) NEC 03.92
      alcohol 03.8
      anesthetic for analgesia 03.91
         for operative anesthesia — omit code
      contrast material (for myelogram) 87.21
      destructive agent NEC 03.8
      neurolytic agent NEC 03.8
      phenol 03.8
      proteolytic enzyme (chemopapain) (chemodiactin) 80.52
      saline (hypothermic) 03.92
      steroid 03.92
   spinal nerve root (intrathecal — see Injection, spinal
   steroid NEC 99.23
   subarachnoid, spinal — see Injection, spinal
   subconjunctival 10.91
   tendon 83.97
      hand 82.95
   testis 62.92
   therapeutic agent NEC 99.29
   thoracic cavity 34.92
   thrombolytic agent (streptokinase)
      direct intracoronary artery 36.04
   trachea 31.94
   tranquilizer 99.26
   tunica vaginalis (with aspiration) 61.91
   tympanum 20.94
   urethra (inert material) (Polytef) 59.79
   varices, esophagus (endoscopic) (sclerosing agent) 42.33
   varicose vein (sclerosing agent) 39.92
      esophagus (endoscopic) 42.33
   vestibule, for destruction 20.72

vitreous substitute (silicone) 14.75
   for reattachment of retina 14.59
vocal cords 31.0

Inlay, tooth 23.3

Inoculation
  antitoxins — see Administration, antitoxins
  toxoids — see Administration, toxoids
  vaccine — see Administration, vaccine

Insemination, artificial 69.92

Insertion
  airway
    esophageal obturator 96.03
    nasopharynx 96.01
    oropharynx 96.02
  Allen-Brown cannula 39.93
  arch bars (orthodontic) 24.7
    for immobilization (fracture) 93.55
  atrial septal umbrella 35.52
  Austin-Moore prosthesis 81.52
  baffle, heart (atrial) (interatrial) (intra-atrial) 35.91
  bag, cervix (nonobstetrical) 67.0
    after delivery or abortion 75.8
    to assist delivery or induce labor 73.1
  Baker's (tube) (for stenting) 46.85
  balloon
    gastric 44.93
    heart (pulsation-type) (Kantrowitz) 37.61
    intestine (for decompression) (for dilation) 46.85
  Barton's tongs (skull) (with synchronous skeletal traction) 02.94
  bipolar endoprosthesis (femoral head) 81.52
  Blakemore-Sengstaken tube 96.06
  bone growth stimulator (invasive) (percutaneous) (semi-invasive) — see category 78.9
  bougie, cervix, nonobstetrical 67.0
    to assist delivery or induce labor 73.1
  breast implant (for augmentation) (bilateral) 85.54
    unilateral 85.53
  bridge (dental) (fixed) 23.42
    removable 23.43
  bubble (balloon), stomach 44.93
  caliper tongs (skull) (with synchronous skeletal traction) 02.94
  cannula
    Allen-Brown 39.93
    for extracorporeal membrane oxygenation (ECMO) — omit code
    nasal sinus (by puncture) 22.01
      through natural ostium 22.02
    pancreatic duct 52.92
      endoscopic 52.93
    vessel to vessel 39.93
  catheter
    abdomen of fetus, for intrauterine transfusion 75.2
    anterior chamber (eye), for permanent drainage (glaucoma) 12.79
    artery 38.91
    bile duct(s) 51.59
      common 51.51
        endoscopic 51.87
      endoscopic 51.87
    bladder, indwelling 57.94
      suprapubic 57.18
        percutaneous (closed) 57.17
    bronchus 96.05
      with lavage 96.56
    central venous NEC 38.93
      for
        hemodialysis 38.95
        pressure monitoring 89.62
    chest 34.04
    esophagus (nonoperative) 96.06
      permanent tube 42.81
    intercostal (with water seal), for drainage 34.04
    spinal canal space (epidural) (subarachnoid) subdural) for infusion of therapeutic orpalliative substances 03.90
    Swan-Ganz (pulmonary) 89.64
    transtracheal for oxygenation 31.99
    vein NEC 38.93
      for renal dialysis 38.95
  chest tube 34.04
  choledochohepatic tube (for decompression) 51.43
    endoscopic 51.87
  cochlear prosthetic device — see Implant, cochlear prosthetic device
  contraceptive device (intrauterine) 69.7
  cordis cannula 54.98
  Crosby-Cooney button 54.98
  Crutchfield tongs (skull) (with synchronous skeletal traction) 02.94
  Davidson button 54.98
  denture (total) 99.97
  device, vascular access 86.07
  diaphragm, vagina 96.17
  drainage tube
    kidney 55.02
      pelvis 55.12
    renal pelvis 55.12
  elbow prosthesis (total) 81.84
    revision 81.97
  electrode(s)
    bone growth stimulator (invasive) (percutaneous) (semi-invasive) — see category 78.9
    brain 02.93
      depth 02.93
      foramen ovale 02.93
      sphenoidal 02.96
    depth 02.93
    foramen ovale 02.93
    heart (initial) (transvenous) 37.70
      atrium (initial) 37.73
        replacement 37.76
      atrium and ventricle (initial) 37.72
        replacement 37.76
      epicardium (sternotomy or thoracotomy approach) 37.74
      temporary transvenous pacemaker system 37.78
        during and immediately following cardiac surgery 39.64
      ventricle (initial) 37.71
        replacement 37.76
    intracranial 02.93
    osteogenic (for bone growth stimulation) - see category 78.9
    peripheral nerve 04.92
    sphenoidal 02.96
    spine 03.93
  electroencephalographic receiver — see Implant, electroencephalographic receiver, by site
  electronic stimulator — see Implant, electronic stimulator, by site
  electrostimulator — see Implant, electronic stimulator, by site
  endoprosthesis
    bile duct 51.87
    femoral head (bipolar) 81.52
    pancreatic duct 52.93
  epidural pegs 02.93
  external fixation device (bone) — see category 78.1
  facial bone implant (alloplastic) (synthetic) 76.92
  filling material, skin (filling of defect) 86.02
  filter
    vena cava (inferior) (superior) (transvenous) 38.7
  fixator, mini device (bone) - see category 78.1
  Gardner Wells tongs (skull) (with synchronous skeletal traction) 02.94
  gastric bubble (balloon) 44.93
  globe, into eye socket 16.69
  Greenfield filter 38.7
  halo device (skull) (with synchronous skeletal traction) 02.94
  Harrington rod — see also Fusion, spinal, by level
    with dorsal, dorsolumbar fusion 81.05
  Harris pin 79.15
  heart
    pacemaker — see Insertion, pacemaker, cardiac
    pump (Kantrowitz) 37.62
    valve — see Replacement, heart, valve
  hip prosthesis (partial) 81.52
    revision 81.53
    total 81.51
      revision 81.53
  Holter valve 02.2
  Hufnagel valve — see Replacement, heart valve
  implant — see Insertion, prosthesis
  infusion pump 86.06
  intercostal catheter (with water seal) for drainage 34.04
  intrauterine
    contraceptive device 69.7
    radium (intracavitary) 69.91
    tamponade (nonobstetric) 69.91
  Kantrowitz
    heart pump 37.62
    pulsation balloon (phase-shift) 37.61
  keratoprosthesis 11.73
  King-Mills umbrella device (heart) 35.52
  Kirschner wire 93.44
    with reduction of fracture or dislocation — see Reduction, fracture and Reduction,dislocation
  laminaria, cervix 69.93
  larynx, valved tube 31.75
  leads (cardiac) — see Insertion, electrode(s), heart
  lens, prosthetic (intraocular) 13.70
    with cataract extraction, one-stage 13.71
    secondary (subsequent to cataract extraction) 13.72
  metal staples into epiphyseal plate (see also Stapling, epiphyseal plate) 78.20
  minifixator device (bone) — see category 78.14
  Mobitz-Uddin umbrella, vena cava 38.7
  mold, vagina 96.15
  Moore (cup) 81.52
  myringotomy device (button) (tube) 20.01
    with intubation 20.01

Insertion — INDEX TO PROCEDURES — Insertion

nasobiliary drainage tube (endoscopic) 51.86
nasolacrimal tube or stent 09.44
nasopancreatic drainage tube (endoscopic) 52.97
neuropacemaker — *see* Implant, neuropacemaker, by site
neurostimulator — *see* Implant, neurostimulator, by site
non-invasive (transcutaneous) (surface) stimulator 99.86
obturator (orthodontic) 24.7
ocular implant
  with synchronous
    enucleation 16.42
      with muscle attachment to implant 16.41
    evisceration 16.31
  following or secondary to
    enucleation 16.61
    evisceration 16.61
Ommaya reservoir 02.2
orbital implant (stent) (outside muscle cone) 16.69
  with orbitotomy 16.02
orthodontic appliance (obturator) (wiring) 24.7
outflow tract prosthesis (gusset type) (heart)
  in
    pulmonary valvuloplasty 35.26
    total repair of tetralogy of Fallot 35.81
pacemaker
  brain 02.93
  cardiac (device) (initial) (permanent) (replacement) 37.80
    dual-chamber device (initial) 37.83
      replacement 37.87
    during and immediately following cardiac surgery 39.64
    single-chamber device (initial) 37.81
      rate responsive 37.82
      replacement 37.85
        rate responsive 37.86
    temporary transvenous pacemaker system 37.78
      during and immediately following cardiac surgery 39.64
  carotid 39.8
  heart — *see* Insertion, pacemaker, cardiac
  intracranial 02.93
  neural
    brain 02.93
      intracranial 02.93
    peripheral nerve 04.92
    spine 03.93
  peripheral nerve 04.92
  spine
pacing catheter — *see* Insertion, pacemaker, cardiac
pack
  auditory canal, external 96.11
  cervix (nonobstetrical) 67.0
    after delivery or abortion 75.8
    to assist delivery or induce labor 73.1
  rectum 96.19
  sella turcica 07.79
  vagina (nonobstetrical) 96.14
    after delivery or abortion 75.8

penile prosthesis (non-inflatable) (internal) 64.95
  inflatable (internal) 64.97
peridontal splint (orthodontic) 24.7
pessary
  cervix 96.18
    to assist delivery or induce labor 73.1
  vagina 96.18
pharyngeal valve, artificial 31.75
port, vascular access 86.07
prostaglandin suppository (for abortion) 96.49
prosthesis, prosthetic device
  acetabulum (partial) 81.52
    hip 81.52
    revision 81.53
  ankle (total) 81.56
  arm (bioelectric) (cineplastic) (kineplastic) 84.44
  biliary tract 51.99
  breast (bilateral) 85.54
    unilateral 85.53
  chin (polyethylene) (silastic) 76.68
  elbow (total) 81.84
    revision 81.97
  extremity (bioelectric) (cineplastic) (kineplastic) 84.40
    lower 84.48
    upper 84.44
  fallopian tube 66.93
  femoral head (Austin-Moore) (bipolar) (Eicher) (Thompson) 81.52
  hip (partial) 81.52
    revision 81.53
    total 81.51
      revision 81.53
  joint — *see* Arthroplasty
  knee (partial) (total) 81.54
    revision 81.55
  leg (bioelectric) (cineplastic) (kineplastic) 84.48
  ocular (secondary) 16.61
    with orbital exenteration 16.42
  outflow tract (gusset type) (heart)
    in
      pulmonary valvuloplasty 35.26
      total repair of tetralogy of Fallot 35.81
  penis (internal) (non-inflatable) 64.95
    with
      construction 64.43
      reconstruction 64.64
    inflatable (internal) 64.97
  Rosen (for urinary incontinence) 56.79
  shoulder
    partial 81.81
    revision 81.97
    total 81.80
  testicular (bilateral) (unilateral) 62.7
  toe 81.57
    for hallux valgus repair 77.59
pseudophakos (*see also* Insertion, lens) 13.70
pump, infusion 86.06
radioactive isotope 92.27
radium 92.27
radon seeds 92.27
Reuter bobbin (with intubation) 20.01
Rickham reservoir 02.2
Rosen prosthesis (for urinary incontinence) 59.79
Scribner shunt 39.93
Sengstaken-Blakemore tube 96.06
sieve, vena cava 38.7

skeletal muscle stimulator 83.92
skull
  plate 02.05
  tongs (Barton) (caliper) (Garder Wells) (Vinke) (with synchronous skeletal traction) 02.94
sphenoidal electrodes 02.96
Spitz-Holter valve 02.2
Steinmann pin 93.44
  with reduction of fracture or dislocation — *see* Reduction, fracture, and Reduction, dislocation
stent
  bile duct 51.43
    endoscopic 51.87
  pancreatic duct 52.92
    endoscopic 52.93
stimoceiver — *see* Implant, stimoceiver, by site
stimulator for bone growth — *see* category 78.9
subdural
  grids 02.93
  strips 02.93
suppository
  prostaglandin (for abortion) 96.49
  vagina 96.49
Swan-Ganz catheter (pulmonary) 89.64
tampon
  esophagus 96.06
  uterus 69.91
  vagina 96.14
    after delivery or abortion 75.8
testicular prosthesis (bilateral) (unilateral) 62.7
tissue expander (skin) NEC 86.93
  breast 85.95
tissue mandril (peripheral vessel) (Dacron) (Spark's type) 39.99
  with
    blood vessel repair 39.56
    vascular bypass or shunt — *see* Bypass, vascular
tongs, skull (with synchronous skeletal traction) 02.94
totally implanted device for bone growth (invasive) - *see* category 78.9
tube — *see also* Catheterization and Intubation
  bile duct 51.43
    endoscopic 51.87
  endotracheal 96.04
  esophagus (nonoperative) (Sengstaken) 96.06
    permanent (silicone) (Souttar) 42.81
  feeding
    esophageal 42.81
    gastric 96.6
    nasogastric 96.6
  gastric
    by gastrostomy — *see* categories 43.1
    for
      decompression, intestinal 96.07
      feeding 96.6
  Miller-Abbott (for intestinal decompression) 96.08
  nasobiliary (drainage) 51.86
  nasogastric (for intestinal decompression) NEC 96.07
  nasopancreatic drainage (endoscopic) 52.97
  pancreatic duct 52.92
    endoscopic 52.93

rectum 96.09
stomach (nasogastric) (for intestinal decompression) NEC 96.07
for feeding 96.6
umbrella device
atrial septum (King-Mills) 35.52
vena cava (Mobitz-Uddin) 38.7
ureteral stent (transurethral) 59.8
with ureterotomy 59.8 [56.2]
urinary sphincter, artificial (AUS) (inflatable) 58.93
vaginal mold 96.15
valve
Holter 02.2
Hufnagel — see Replacement, heart valve
pharyngeal (artificial) 31.75
Spitz-Holter 02.2
vas deferens 63.95
vascular access device 86.07
vena cava sieve or umbrella 38.7
Vinke tongs (skull) (with synchronous skeletal traction) 02.94
Instillation
bladder 96.49
digestive tract, except gastric gavage 96.43
genitourinary NEC 96.49
radioisotope (intracavitary) (intravenous) 92.28
Insufflation
Eustachian tube 20.8
fallopian tube (air) (dye) (gas) (saline) 66.8
for radiography — see Hysterosalpingography
therapeutic substance 66.95
lumbar retroperitoneal, bilateral 88.15
Intercricothyroidotomy (for assistance in breathing) 31.1
Intermittent positive pressure breathing (IPPB) 93.91
Interposition operation
antesternal or antethoracic NEC (see also Anastomosis, esophagus, antesternal, with, interposition) 42.68
esophageal reconstruction (intrathoracic) (retrosternal) NEC (see also Anastomosis, esophagus, with, interposition 42.58
uterine suspension 69.21
Interruption
vena cava (inferior) (superior) 38.7
Interview (evaluation) (diagnostic)
medical, except psychiatric 89.05
brief (abbreviated history) 89.01
comprehensive (history and evaluation of new problem) 89.03
limited (interval history) 89.02
specified type NEC 89.04
psychiatric NEC 94.19
follow-up 94.19
initial 94.19
pre-commitment 94.13
Intimectomy 38.10
abdominal 38.16
aorta (arch) (ascending) (descending) 38.14
head and neck NEC 38.12
intracranial NEC 38.11
lower limb 38.18
thoracic NEC 38.15
upper limb 38.13

Introduction
orthodontic appliance 24.7
therapeutic substance (acting locally or systemically) NEC 99.29
bursa 83.96
hand 82.94
fascia 83.98
hand 82.96
heart 37.92
joint 81.92
temporomandibular 76.96
ligament (joint) 81.92
pericardium 37.93
soft tissue NEC 83.98
hand 82.96
tendon 83.97
hand 82.95
vein 39.92
Intubation — see also Catheterization and Insertion
bile duct(s) 51.59
common 51.51
endoscopic 51.87
endoscopic 51.87
esophagus (nonoperative) (Sengstaken) 96.06
permanent tube (silicone) (Souttar) 42.81
Eustachian tube 20.8
intestine (for decompression) 96.08
lacrimal for
dilation 09.42
tear drainage, intranasal 09.81
larynx 96.05
nasobiliary (drainage) 51.86
nasogastric
for
decompression, intestinal 96.07
feeding 96.6
nasolacrimal (duct) (with irrigation) 09.44
nasopancreatic drainage (endoscopic) 52.97
respiratory tract NEC 96.05
small intestine (Miller-Abbott) 96.08
stomach (nasogastric) (for intestinal decompression) NEC 96.07
for feeding 96.6
trachea 96.04
ventriculocisternal 02.2
Invagination, diverticulum
gastric 44.69
pharynx 29.59
stomach 44.69
Inversion
appendix 47.99
diverticulum
gastric 44.69
intestine
large 45.49
endoscopic 45.43
small 45.24
stomach 44.69
tunica vaginalis 61.49
Ionization, medical 99.27
Iontherapy 99.27
Iontophoresis 99.27
Iridectomy (basal) (buttonhole) (optical) (peripheral) (total) 12.14
with
capsulectomy 13.65
cataract extraction — see Extraction, cataract

filtering operation (for glaucoma) NEC 12.65
scleral
fistulization 12.65
thermocauterization 12.62
trephination 12.61
Iridencleisis 12.63
Iridesis 12.63
Irido-capsulectomy 13.65
Iridocyclectomy 12.44
Iridocystectomy 12.42
Iridodesis 12.63
Iridoplasty NEC 12.39
Iridosclerectomy 12.65
Iridosclerotomy 12.69
Iridotasis 12.63
Iridotomy 12.12
by photocoagulation 12.12
with transfixion 12.11
for iris bombe 12.11
specified type NEC 12.12
Iron lung 93.99
Irrigation
anterior chamber (eye) 12.91
bronchus NEC 96.56
canaliculus 09.42
catheter
ureter 96.46
urinary, indwelling NEC 96.48
vascular 96.57
ventricular 02.41
wound 96.58
cholecystostomy 96.41
cornea 96.51
with removal of foreign body 98.21
corpus cavernosum 64.98
cystostomy 96.47
ear (removal of cerumen) 96.52
enterostomy 96.36
eye 96.51
with removal of foreign body 98.21
gastrostomy 96.36
lacrimal
canaliculi 09.42
punctum 09.41
muscle 83.02
hand 82.02
nasal
passages 96.53
sinus 22.00
nasolacrimal duct 09.43
with insertion of tube or stent 09.44
nephrostomy 96.45
peritoneal 54.25
pyelostomy 96.45
rectal 96.39
stomach 96.33
tendon (sheath) 83.01
hand 82.01
trachea NEC 96.56
traumatic cataract 13.3
tube
biliary NEC 96.41
nasogastric NEC 96.34
pancreatic 96.42
ureterostomy 96.46
ventricular shunt 02.41
wound (cleaning) NEC 96.59
Irving operation (tubal ligation) 66.32
Irwin operation (see also Osteotomy) 77.30
Ischiectomy (partial) 77.89
total 77.99

Ischiopubiotomy 77.39
Isolation
    after contact with infectious disease 99.84

ileal loop 45.51
intestinal segment or pedicle flap
    large 45.52

    small 45.51
Isthmectomy, thyroid (see also
    Thyroidectomy, partial) 06.39

J

Jaboulay operation (gastroduodenostomy) 44.39
Janeway operation (permanent gastrostomy) 43.19
Jatene operation (arterial switch) 35.84
Jejunectomy 45.62
Jejunocecostomy 45.93
Jejunocholecystostomy 51.32
Jejunocolostomy 45.93
Jejunoileostomy 45.91
Jejunojejunostomy 45.91

Jejunopexy 46.61
Jejunorrhaphy 46.73
Jejunostomy (feeding) 46.39
   delayed opening 46.31
   loop 46.01
   percutaneous (endoscopic) (PEJ) 46.32
   revision 46.41
Jejunotomy 45.02
Johanson operation (urethral reconstruction) 58.46
Jones operation
   claw toe (transfer of extensor hallucis longus tendon) 77.57
     modified (with arthrodesis) 77.57
   dacryocystorhinostomy 09.81
   hammer toe (interphalangeal fusion) 77.56
     modified (tendon transfer with arthrodesis) 77.57
   repair of peroneal tendon 83.88
Joplin operation (exostectomy with tendon transfer) 77.53

K

Kader operation (temporary gastrostomy) 43.19
Kaufman operation (for urinary stress incontinence) 59.79
Kazanjiian operation (buccal vestibular sulcus extension) 24.91
Kehr operation (hepatopexy) 50.69
Keller operation (bunionectomy) 77.59
Kelly (-Kennedy) **operation** (urethrovesical plication) 59.3
Kelly-Stoeckel operation (urethrovesical plication) 59.3
Kelotomy 53.9
Keratectomy (complete) (partial) (superficial) 11.49
   for pterygium 11.39
      with corneal graft 11.32
Keratocentesis (for hyphema) 12.91
Keratomeieusis 11.71
Keratophakia 11.72

Keratoplasty (tectonic) (with autograft) (with homograft) 11.60
   lamellar (nonpenetrating) (with homograft) 11.62
      with autograft 11.61
   penetrating (full-thickness) (with homograft) 11.64
      with autograft 11.63
   perforating — *see* Keratoplasty, penetrating
   refractive 11.71
   specified type NEC 11.69
Keratoprosthesis 11.73
Keratotomy (delimiting) (posterior) 11.1
   radial (refractive) 11.75
Kerr operation (low cervical cesarean section) 74.1
Kessler operation (arthroplasty, carpometacarpal joint) 81.74
Kidner operation (excision of accessory navicular bone) (with tendon transfer) 77.98

Killian operation (frontal sinusotomy) 22.41
Kineplasty — *see* Cineplasty
King-Steelquist operation (hindquarter amputation) 84.19
Kirk operation (amputation through thigh) 84.17
Kondoleon operation (correction of lymphedema) 40.9
Krause operation (sympathetic denervation) 05.29
Kroener operation (partial salpingectomy) 66.69
Kroenlein operation (lateral orbitotomy) 16.01
Kronig operation (low cervical cesarean section) 74.1
Krukenberg operation (reconstruction of below-elbow amputation) 82.89
Kuhnt-Szymanowski operation (ectropion repair with lid reconstruction) 08.44

L

Labbe operation (gastrotomy) 43.0
Labiectomy (bilateral) 71.62
   unilateral 71.61
Labyrinthectomy (transtympanic) 20.79
Labyrinthotomy (transtympanic) 20.79
Ladd operation (mobilization of intestine) 54.95
Lagrange operation (iridosclerectomy) 12.65
Lambrinudi operation (triple arthrodesis) 81.12
Laminectomy (decompression) (for exploration) 03.09
   as operative approach — omit code
   with
      excision of herniated intervertebral disc (nucleus pulposus) 80.51
      excision of other intraspinal lesion (tumor) 03.4
   reopening of site 03.02
Laminography — see Radiography
Laminotomy (decompression) (for exploration) 03.09
   as operative approach — omit code
   reopening of site 03.02
Langenbeck operation (cleft palate repair) 27.62
Laparoamnioscopy 75.31
Laparorrhaphy 54.63
Laparoscopy 54.21
   with
      biopsy (intra-abdominal) 54.24
         uterine ligaments 68.15
         uterus 68.16
      destruction of fallopian tubes — see Destruction, fallopian tube
Laparotomy NEC 54.19
   as operative approach — omit code
   exploratory (pelvic) 54.11
   reopening of recent operative site (for control of hemorrhage) (for exploration) (for incision of hematoma) 54.12
Laparotracheiotomy 74.1
Lapidus operation (bunionectomy with metatarsal osteotomy) 77.51
Larry operation (shoulder disarticulation) 84.08
Laryngectomy
   with radical neck dissection (with synchronous thyroidectomy) (with synchronoustracheostomy) 30.4
   complete (with partial laryngectomy) (with synchronous tracheostomy) 30.3
      with radical neck dissection (with synchronous thyroidectomy) (with synchronoustracheostomy) 30.4
   frontolateral partial (extended) 30.29
   glottosupraglottic partial 30.29
   lateral partial 30.29
   partial (frontolateral) (glottosupraglottic) (lateral) (submucous) (supraglottic) (vertical) 30.29
   radial (with synchronous thyroidectomy) (with synchronous tracheostomy) 30.4
   submucous (partial) 30.29
   supraglottic partial 30.29
   total (with partial pharyngectomy) (with synchronous tracheostomy) 30.3
      with radical neck dissection (with synchronous thyroidectomy) (with synchronoustracheostomy) 30.4
   vertical partial 30.29
   wide field 30.3
Laryngocentesis 31.3
Laryngoesophagectomy 30.4
Laryngofissure 30.29
Laryngogram 87.09
   contrast 87.07
Laryngopharyngectomy (with synchronous tracheostomy) 30.3
   radical (with synchronous thyroidectomy) 30.4
Laryngopharyngoesophagectomy (with synchronous tracheostomy) 30.3
   with radical neck dissection (with synchronous thyroidectomy) 30.4
Laryngoplasty 31.69
Laryngorrhaphy 31.61
Laryngoscopy (suspension) (through artificial stoma) 31.42
Laryngostomy (permanent) 31.29
   revision 31.63
   temporary (emergency) 31.1
Laryngotomy 31.3
Laryngotracheobronchoscopy 33.23
   with biopsy 33.24
Laryngotracheoscopy 31.42
Laryngotracheostomy (permanent) 31.29
   temporary (emergency) 31.1
Laryngotracheotomy (temporary) 31.1
   permanent 31.29
Laser — see also Coagulation, Destruction, and Photocoagulation by site
   angioplasty, percutaneous transluminal 39.59
      coronary — see Angioplasty, coronary
Lash operation (internal cervical os repair) 67.5
Latzko operation
   cesarean section 74.2
   colpocleisis 70.4
Lavage
   antral 22.00
   bronchus NEC 96.56
   endotracheal 96.56
   gastric 96.33
   nasal sinus(es) 22.00
      by puncture 22.01
      through natural ostium 22.02
   peritoneal (diagnostic) 54.25
   trachea NEC 96.56
Leadbetter operation (urethral reconstruction) 58.46
Leadbetter-Politano operation (ureteroneocystostomy) 56.74
▶**LeFort operation** (colpocleisis) 70.8
LeMesurier operation (cleft lip repair) 27.54
Lengthening
   bone (with bone graft) 78.30
      femur 78.35
      for reconstruction of thumb 82.69
      specified site NEC (see also category 78.3) 78.39
      tibia 78.37
      ulna 78.33
   extraocular muscle NEC 15.21
      multiple (two or more muscles) 15.4
   fascia 83.89
      hand 82.89
   hamstring NEC 83.85
   heel cord 83.85
   leg
      femur 78.35
      tibia 78.37
   levator palpebrae muscle 08.38
   muscle 83.85
      extraocular 15.21
         multiple (two or more muscles) 15.4
      hand 82.55
   palate 27.62
      secondary or subsequent 27.63
   tendon 83.85
      for claw toe repair 77.57
      hand 82.55
Leriche operation (periarterial sympathectomy) 39.7
Leucotomy, leukotomy 01.32
Leukopheresis, therapeutic 99.72
Lid suture operation (blepharoptosis) 08.31
Ligation
   adrenal vessel (artery) (vein) 07.43
   aneurysm 39.52
   appendages, dermal 86.26
   arteriovenous fistula 39.53
      coronary artery 36.99
   artery 38.80
      abdominal 38.86
      adrenal 07.43
      aorta (arch) (ascending) (descending) 38.84
      coronary (anomalous) 36.99
      ethmoidal 21.04
      external carotid 21.06
      for control of epistaxis — see Control, epistaxis
      head and neck NEC 38.82
      intracranial NEC 38.81
      lower limb 38.88
      maxillary (transantral) 21.05
      middle meningeal 02.13
      thoracic NEC 38.85
      thyroid 06.92
      upper limb 38.83
   atrium, heart 37.99
   auricle, heart 37.99
   bleeding vessel — see Control, hemorrhage
   blood vessel 38.80
      abdominal
         artery 38.86
         vein 38.87
      adrenal 07.43
      aorta (arch) (ascending) (descending) 38.84
      esophagus 42.91
         endoscopic 42.33
      head and neck NEC 38.82
      intracranial NEC 38.81
      lower limb
         artery 38.88

vein 38.89
    meningeal (artery) (longitudinal sinus) 02.13
    thoracic NEC 38.85
    thyroid 06.92
    upper limb (artery) (vein) 38.83
bronchus 33.92
cisterna chyli 40.64
coronary
    artery (anomalous) 36.99
    sinus 36.3
dermal appendage 86.26
ductus arteriosus, patent 38.85
esophageal vessel 42.91
    endoscopic 42.33
ethmoidal artery 21.04
external carotid artery 21.06
fallopian tube (bilateral) (remaining) (solitary) 66.39
    by endoscopy (culdoscopy) (hysteroscopy) (laparoscopy) (peritoneoscopy) 66.29
    with
        crushing 66.31
            by endoscopy (laparoscopy) 66.21
        division 66.32
            by endoscopy (culdoscopy) (laparoscopy) (peritoneoscopy) 66.22
        Falope ring 66.39
            by endoscopy (laparoscopy) 66.29
    unilateral 66.92
fistula, arteriovenous 39.53
    coronary artery 36.99
gastric
    artery 38.86
    varices 44.91
        endoscopic 43.41
hemorrhoids 49.45
longitudinal sinus (superior) 02.13
lymphatic (channel) (peripheral) 40.9
    thoracic duct 40.64
maxillary artery 21.05
meningeal vessel 02.13
spermatic
    cord 63.72
        varicocele 63.1
    vein (high) 63.1
splenic vessels 38.86
subclavian artery 38.85
superior longitudinal sinus 02.13
supernumerary digit 86.26
thoracic duct 40.64
thyroid vessel (artery) (vein) 06.92
toes (supernumerary) 86.26
tooth 93.55
    impacted 24.6
ulcer (peptic) (base) (bed) (bleeding vessel) 44.40
    duodenal 44.42
    gastric 44.41
ureter 56.95
varices
    esophageal 42.91
        endoscopic 42.33
    gastric 44.91
        endoscopic 43.41
    peripheral vein (lower limb) 38.59
    upper limb 38.53
varicocele 63.1
vas deferens 63.71
vein
    abdominal 38.87
    adrenal 07.43
    head and neck NEC 38.82
    intracranial NEC 38.81
    lower limb 38.89
    spermatic, high 63.1
    thoracic NEC 38.85
    thyroid 06.92
    upper limb 38.83
    varicose 38.50
        abdominal 38.57
        esophagus 42.91
            endoscopic 42.33
        gastric 44.91
            endoscopic 43.41
        head and neck NEC 38.52
        intracranial NEC 38.51
        lower limb 38.59
        stomach 44.91
        thoracic NEC 38.55
        upper limb 38.53
vena cava, inferior 38.7
venous connection between anomalous vein to
    left innominate vein 35.82
    superior vena cava 35.82
wrist 86.26
Light coagulation — *Photocoagulation*
Lindholm operation (repair of ruptured tendon) 83.88
Lingulectomy, lung 32.3
Linton operation (varicose vein) 38.59
Lip reading training 95.49
Lip shave 27.43
Lipectomy (subcutaneous tissue) (abdominal) (submental) 86.83
Lisfranc operation
    foot amputation 84.12
    shoulder disarticulation 84.08
Litholapaxy, bladder 57.0
    by incision 57.19
Lithotomy
    bile passage 51.49
    bladder (urinary) 57.19
    common duct 51.41
        percutaneous 51.96
    gallbladder 51.04
    hepatic duct 51.49
    kidney 55.01
        percutaneous 55.03
    ureter 56.2
Lithotripsy
    bile duct NEC 51.49
        extracorporeal shockwave (ESWL) 98.52
    bladder 57.0
        with ultrasonic fragmentation 57.0 [59.95]
        extracorporeal shockwave (ESWL) 98.51
    extracorporeal shockwave (ESWL) NEC 98.59
        bile duct 98.52
        bladder (urinary) 98.51
        gallbladder 98.52
        kidney 98.51
        renal pelvis 98.51
        specified site NEC 98.59
        ureter 98.51
    gallbladder NEC 51.04
        endoscopic 51.88
        extracorporeal shockwave (ESWL) 98.52
    kidney 56.0
        extracorporeal shockwave (ESWL) 98.51
        percutaneous nephrostomy with fragmentation (laser) (ultrasound) 55.04
    renal pelvis 56.0
        extracorporeal shockwave (ESWL) 98.51
        percutaneous nephrostomy with fragmentation (laser) (ultrasound) 55.04
    ureter 56.0
        extracorporeal shockwave (ESWL) 98.51
Littlewood operation (forequarter amputation) 84.09
Lloyd-Davies operation (abdominoperineal resection) 48.5
Lobectomy
    brain 01.53
        partial 01.59
    liver (with partial excision of adjacent lobes) 50.3
    lung (complete) 32.4
        partial 32.3
        segmental (with resection of adjacent lobes) 32.4
    thyroid (total) (unilateral) (with removal of isthmus) (with removal of portion of remaininglobe) 06.2
        partial (*see also* Thyroidectomy, partial) 06.39
        substernal 06.51
        subtotal (*see also* Thyroidectomy, partial) 06.39
Lobotomy, brain 01.32
Localization, placenta 88.78
    by RISA injection 92.17
Longmire operation (bile duct anastomosis) 51.39
Loop ileal stoma (*see also* Ileostomy) 46.01
Loopogram 87.78
Looposcopy (ileal conduit) 56.35
Lord operation
    dilation of anal canal for hemorrhoids 49.49
    hemorrhoidectomy 49.49
    orchidopexy 62.5
Lower GI series (x-ray) 87.64
Lucas and Murray operation (knee arthrodesis with plate) 81.22
Lumpectomy
    breast 85.21
    specified site — *see* Excision, lesion, by site
Lymphadenectomy (simple) (*see also* Excision, lymph, node) 40.29
Lymphadenotomy 40.0
Lymphangiectomy (radical) (*see also* Excision, lymph, node, by site, radical) 40.50
Lymphangiogram
    abdominal 88.04
    cervical 87.08
    intrathoracic 87.34
    lower limb 88.36
    pelvic 88.04
    upper limb 88.34
Lymphangioplasty 40.9
Lymphangiorrhaphy 40.9
Lymphangiotomy 40.0
Lymphaticostomy 40.9

Lysis
  adhesions
    abdominal 54.5
    appendiceal 54.5
    artery-vein-nerve bundle 39.91
    biliary tract 54.5
    bladder (neck) (intraluminal) 57.12
      external 59.11
      transurethral 57.41
    blood vessels 39.91
    bone — *see* category 78.4
    bursa 83.91
      by stretching or manipulation 93.28
      hand 82.91
    cartilage of joint 93.26
    chest wall 33.99
    choanae (nasopharynx) 29.54
    conjunctiva 10.5
    corneovitreal 12.34
    cortical (brain) 02.91
    ear, middle 20.23
    Eustachean tube 20.8
    extraocular muscle 15.7
    extrauterine 54.5
    eyelid 08.09
      and conjunctiva 10.5
    eye muscle 15.7
    fallopian tube 65.8
    fascia 83.91
      hand 82.91
        by stretching or manipulation 93.26
    gallbladder 54.5
    ganglion (peripheral) NEC 04.49
      cranial NEC 04.42
    hand 82.91
      by stretching or manipulation 93.26
    heart 37.10
    intestine 54.5
    iris (posterior) 12.33
      anterior 12.32
    joint (capsule) (structure) (*see* also Division, joint capsule) 80.40
    kidney 59.02
    labia (vulva) 71.01
    larynx 31.92
    liver 54.5
    lung (for collapse of lung) 33.39
    mediastinum 34.99
    meninges (spinal) 03.6
      cortical 02.91
    middle ear 20.23
    muscle 83.91
      by stretching or manipulation 93.27
      extraocular 15.7
      hand 82.91
        by stretching or manipulation 93.26
    nasopharynx 29.54
    nerve (peripheral) NEC 04.49
      cranial NEC 04.42
      roots, spinal 03.6
      trigeminal 04.41
    nose, nasal 21.91
    ocular muscle 15.7
    ovary 65.8
    pelvic 54.5
    penile 64.93
    pericardium 37.12
    perineal (female) 71.01
    peripheral vessels 39.91
    perirectal 48.81
    perirenal 59.02
    peritoneum (pelvic) 54.5
    periureteral 59.02
    perivesical 59.11
    pharynx 29.54
    pleura (for collapse of lung) 33.39
    spermatic cord 63.94
    spinal (cord) (meninges) (nerve roots) 03.6
    spleen 54.5
    tendon 83.91
      by stretching or manipulation 93.27
      hand 82.91
        by stretching or manipulation 93.26
    thorax 34.99
    tongue 25.93
    trachea 31.92
    tubo-ovarian 65.8
    ureter 59.02
      with freeing or repositioning of ureter 59.01
      intraluminal 56.81
    urethra (intraluminal) 58.5
    uterus 54.5
      intraluminal 68.21
      peritoneal 54.5
    vagina (intraluminal) 70.13
    vitreous (posterior approach) 14.74
      anterior approach 14.73
    vulva 71.01
  goniosynechiae (with injection of air or liquid) 12.31
  synechiae (posterior) 12.33
    anterior (with injection of air or liquid) 12.32

thoracic duct 40.62

M

Madlener operation (tubal ligation) 66.31
Magnet extraction
  foreign body
    anterior chamber, eye 12.01
    choroid 14.01
    ciliary body 12.01
    conjunctiva 98.22
    cornea 11.0
    eye, eyeball NEC 98.21
      anterior segment 12.01
      posterior segment 14.01
    intraocular (anterior segment) 12.01
    iris 12.01
    lens 13.01
    orbit 98.21
    retina 14.01
    sclera 12.01
    vitreous 14.01
Magnetic resonance imaging (nuclear) — see Imaging, magnetic resonance
Magnuson (-Stack) operation (arthroplasty for recurrent shoulder dislocation) 81.82
Malleostapediopexy 19.19
  with incus replacement 19.11
Malstrom's vacuum extraction 72.79
  with episiotomy 72.71
Mammaplasty — see Mammoplasty
Mammectomy — see also Mastectomy
  subcutaneous (unilateral) 85.34
    with synchronous implant 85.33
    bilateral 85.36
      with synchronous implant 85.35
Mammilliplasty 85.87
Mammography NEC 87.37
Mammoplasty 85.89
  with
    full-thickness graft 85.83
    muscle flap 85.85
    pedicle flap 85.84
    split-thickness 85.82
  amputative (reduction) (bilateral) 85.32
    unilateral 85.31
  augmentation 85.50
    with
      breast implant (bilateral) 85.54
        unilateral 85.53
      injection into breast (bilateral) 85.52
        unilateral 85.51
  reduction (bilateral) 85.32
    unilateral 85.31
  revision 85.89
  size reduction (gynecomastial) (bilateral) 85.32
    unilateral 85.31
Mammotomy 85.0
Manchester (-Donald) (-Fothergill) operation (uterine suspension) 69.22
Mandibulectomy (partial) 76.31
  total 76.42
    with reconstruction 76.41
Maneuver (method)
  Bracht 72.52
  Crede 73.59
  De Lee (key-in-lock) 72.4
  Kristeller 72.54
  Lovset's (extraction of arms in breech birth) 72.52
  Mauriceau (-Smellie-Veit) 72.52
  Pinard (total breech extraction) 72.54
  Prague 72.52
  Ritgen 73.59
  Scanzoni (rotation) 72.4
  Van Hoorn 72.52
  Wigand-Martin 72.52
Manipulation
  with reduction of fracture or dislocation — see Reduction, fracture and Reduction, dislocation
  enterostomy stoma (with dilation) 96.24
  intestine (intra-abdominal) 46.80
    large 46.82
    small 46.81
  joint
    adhesions 93.26
      temporomandibular 76.95
    dislocation — see Reduction, dislocation
  lacrimal passage (tract) NEC 09.49
  muscle structures 93.27
  musculoskeletal (physical therapy) NEC 93.29
  nasal septum, displaced 21.88
  osteopathic NEC 93.67
    for general mobilization (general articulation) 93.61
    high-velocity, low-amplitude forces (thrusting) 93.62
    indirect forces 93.65
    isotonic, isometric force 93.64
    low-velocity, high amplitude forces (springing) 93.63
    to move tissue fluids 93.66
  rectum 96.22
  salivary duct 26.91
  stomach, intraoperative 44.92
  temporomandibular joint NEC 76.95
  ureteral calculus by catheter 56.0
  uterus NEC 69.98
    gravid 75.99
    inverted
      manual replacement (following delivery) 75.94
      surgical — see Repair, inverted uterus
Manometry
  esophageal 89.32
  spinal fluid 89.15
  urinary 89.21
Manual arts therapy 93.81
Mapping
  cardiac (electrophysiologic) 37.27
    doppler (flow) 88.72
  electrocardiogram only 89.52
Marckwald operation (cervical os repair) 67.5
Marshall-Marchetti (-Krantz) operation (retropubic urethral suspension) 59.5
Marsupialization — see also Destruction, lesion, by site
  cyst
    Bartholin's 71.23
    brain 01.59
    cervical (nabothian) 67.31
    dental 24.4
    dentigerous 24.4
    kidney 55.31
    larynx 30.01
    liver 50.21
    ovary 65.21
    pancreas 52.3
    pilonidal (open excision) (with partial closure) 86.21
    salivary gland 26.21
    spinal (intraspinal) (meninges) 03.4
    spleen, splenic 41.41
  lesion
    brain 01.59
    cerebral 01.59
    liver 50.21
  pilonidal cyst or sinus (open excision) (with partial closure) 86.21
  pseudocyst, pancreas 52.3
  ranula, salivary gland 26.21
Massage
  cardiac (external) (manual) (closed) 99.63
    open 37.91
  prostatic 99.94
  rectal (for levator spasm) 99.93
MAST (military anti-shock trousers) 93.58
Mastectomy (complete) (prophylactic) (simple) (unilateral) 85.41
  with
    excision of regional lymph nodes 85.43
      bilateral 85.44
    preservation of skin and nipple 85.34
      with synchronous implant 85.33
      bilateral 85.36
        with synchronous implant 85.35
  bilateral 85.42
  extended
    radical (Urban) (unilateral) 85.47
      bilateral 85.48
    simple (with regional lymphadenectomy) (unilateral) 85.43
      bilateral 85.44
  modified radical (unilateral) 85.43
    bilateral 85.44
  partial 85.23
  radical (Halsted) (Meyer) (unilateral) 85.45
    bilateral 85.46
    extended (Urban) (unilateral) 85.47
      bilateral 85.48
    modified (unilateral) 85.43
      bilateral 85.44
  subcutaneous 85.34
    with synchronous implant 85.33
    bilateral 85.36
      with synchronous implant 85.35
  subtotal 85.23
Masters' stress test (two-step) 89.42
Mastoidectomy (cortical) (conservative) 20.49
  complete (simple) 20.41
  modified radical 20.49
  radical 20.42
    modified 20.49
  simple (complete) 20.41
Mastoidotomy 20.21
Mastoidotympanectomy 20.42
Mastopexy 85.6
Mastoplasty — see Mammoplasty
Mastorrhaphy 85.81
Mastotomy 85.0
Matas operation (aneurysmorrhaphy) 39.52
Mayo operation
  bunionectomy 77.59

herniorrhaphy 53.49
vaginal hysterectomy 68.5
Mazet operation (knee disarticulation) 84.16
McBride operation (bunionectomy with soft tissue correction) 77.53
McBurney operation — *see* Repair, hernia, inguinal
▶**McCall operation** (enterocele repair) 70.92
McCauley operation (release of clubfoot) 83.84
McDonald operation (encirclement suture, cervix) 67.5
McIndoe operation (vaginal construction) 70.61
McKeever operation (fusion of first metatarsophalangeal joint for hallux valgus repair) 77.52
McKissock operation (breast reduction) 85.33
McReynolds operation (transposition of pterygium) 11.31
McVay operation
    femoral hernia — *see* Repair, hernia, femoral
    inguinal hernia — *see* Repair, hernia, inguinal
Measurement
    airway resistance 89.38
    anatomic NEC 89.39
    arterial blood gases 89.65
    basal metabolic rate (BMR) 89.39
    blood gases
        arterial 89.65
        venous 89.66
    body 93.07
    cardiac output (by)
        Fick method 89.67
        indicator dilution technique 89.68
        oxygen consumption technique 89.67
        thermodilution indicator 89.68
    cardiovascular NEC 89.59
    central venous pressure 89.62
    coronary blood flow 89.69
    gastric function NEC 89.39
    girth 93.07
    intelligence 94.01
    intracranial pressure 01.18
    intraocular tension or pressure 89.11
        as part of extended ophthalmologic work-up 95.03
    intrauterine pressure 89.62
    limb length 93.06
    lung volume 89.37
    mixed venous blood gases 89.66
    physiologic NEC 89.39
    portovenous pressure 89.62
    range of motion 93.05
    renal clearance 89.29
    respiratory NEC 89.38
    skin fold thickness 93.07
    skull circumference 93.07
    sphincter of Oddi pressure 51.15
    systemic arterial
        blood gases 89.65
        pressure 89.61
    urine (bioassay) (chemistry) 89.29
    vascular 89.59
    venous blood gases 89.66
    vital capacity (pulmonary) 89.37
Meatoplasty
    ear 18.6

urethra 58.47
Meatotomy
    ureter 56.1
    urethra 58.1
        internal 58.5
▶**Mechanical ventilation** — *see* Ventilation
Mediastinectomy 34.3
Mediastinoscopy (transpleural) 34.22
Mediastinotomy 34.1
    with pneumonectomy 32.5
Meloplasty, facial 86.82
Meningeorrhaphy (cerebral) 02.12
    spinal 03.59
        for
            meningocele 03.51
            myelomeningocele 03.52
Meniscectomy (knee) NEC 80.6
    acromioclavicular 80.91
    sternoclavicular 80.91
    temporomandibular (joint) 76.5
    wrist 80.93
Menstrual extraction or regulation 69.6
Mentoplasty (augmentation) (with graft) (with implant) 76.68
    reduction 76.67
Mesenterectomy 54.4
Mesenteriopexy 54.75
Mesenteriplication 54.75
Mesocoloplication 54.75
Mesopexy 54.75
Metatarsectomy 77.98
Metroplasty 69.49
Mid forceps delivery 72.29
Mikulicz operation (exteriorization of intestine) (first stage) 46.03
    second stage 46.04
Miles operation (proctectomy) 48.5
Military anti-shock trousers (MAST) 93.58
Millard operation (cheiloplasty) 27.54
Miller operation
    midtarsal arthrodesis 81.14
    urethrovesical suspension 59.4
Millin-Read operation (urethrovesical suspension) 59.4
Mist therapy 93.94
Mitchell operation (hallux valgus repair) 77.51
Mobilization
    joint NEC 93.16
    mandible 76.95
    neostrophingic (mitral valve) 35.12
    spine 93.15
    stapes (transcrural) 19.0
    testis in scrotum 62.5
Mohs operation (chemosurgical excision of skin) 86.24
Molegraphy 87.81
Monitoring
    cardiac output (by)
        ambulatory (ACM) 89.50
        electrographic 89.54
            during surgery — omit code
        Fick method 89.67
        Holter-type device 89.50
        indicator dilution technique 89.68
        oxygen consumption technique 89.67
        specified technique NEC 89.68
        telemetry (cardiac) 89.54
        thermodilution indicator 89.68

        transesophageal (Doppler) (ultrasound) 89.68
    central venous pressure 89.62
    circulatory NEC 89.69
    coronary blood flow (coincidence counting technique) 89.69
    electroencephalographic 89.19
        radio-telemetered 89.19
        video 89.19
    fetus (fetal heart)
        antepartum
            nonstress (fetal activity acceleration determinations) 75.35
            oxytocin challenge (contraction stress test) 75.35
            ultrasonography (early pregnancy) (Doppler) 88.78
        intrapartum (during labor)
            (extrauterine) (external) 75.34
            auscultatory (stethoscopy) — omit code
            internal (with contraction measurements) (ECG) 75.32
            intrauterine (direct) (ECG) 75.32
            phonocardiographic (extrauterine) 75.34
            pulsed ultrasound (Doppler) 88.78
    Holter (cardiac) 89.54
    intracranial pressure 01.18
    pulmonary artery
        pressure 89.63
        wedge 89.64
    sleep (recording) — (*see* categories 89.17–89.18)
    systemic arterial pressure 89.61
    transesophageal cardiac output (Doppler) 89.68
    ventricular pressure (cardiac) 89.62
Moore operation (arthroplasty) 81.52
Moschowitz
▶   enterocele repair 70.92
    herniorrhaphy — *see* Repair, hernia, femoral
    sigmoidopexy 46.63
Mountain resort sanitarium 93.98
Mouth-to-mouth resuscitation 93.93
Moxibustion 93.35
MRI — *see* Imaging, magnetic resonance
Muller operation (banding of pulmonary artery) 38.85
Multiple sleep latency test (MSLT) 89.18
Mumford operation (partial claviculectomy) 77.81
Musculoplasty (*see also* Repair, muscle) 83.87
    hand (*see also* Repair, muscle, hand) 82.89
Music therapy 93.84
Mustard operation (interatrial transposition of venous return) 35.91
Myectomy 83.45
    anorectal 48.92
    eye muscle 15.13
        multiple 15.3
    for graft 83.43
        hand 82.34
    hand 82.36
        for graft 82.34
    levator palpebrae 08.33
    rectal 48.92
Myelogram, myelography (air) (gas) 87.21
    posterior fossa 87.02
Myelotomy

spine, spinal (cord) (tract) (one-stage) (two-stage) 03.29
    percutaneous 03.21
Myocardiectomy (infarcted area) 37.33
Myocardiotomy 37.11
Myoclasis 83.99
  hand 82.99
Myomectomy (uterine) 68.29
  broad ligament 69.19
Myoplasty (see also Repair, muscle) 83.87
  hand (see also Repair, muscle, hand) 82.89
  mastoid 19.9
Myorrhaphy 83.65
  hand 82.46
Myosuture 83.65
  hand 82.46
Myotasis 93.27

Myotenontoplasty (see also Repair, tendon) 83.88
Myotenoplasty (see also Repair, tendon) 83.88
  hand 82.86
Myotenotomy 83.13
  hand 82.11
Myotomy 83.02
  with division 83.19
    hand 82.19
  colon NEC 46.92
    sigmoid 46.91
  cricopharyngeal 29.31
    that for pharyngeal (pharyngoesophageal) diverticulectomy 29.32
  esophagus 42.7
  eye (oblique) (rectus) 15.21

  multiple (two or more muscles) 15.4
  hand 82.02
    with division 82.19
  levator palpebrae 08.38
  sigmoid (colon) 46.91
Myringectomy 20.59
Myringodectomy 20.59
Myringomalleolabyrinthopexy 19.52
Myringoplasty (epitympanic, type I) (by cauterization) (by graft) 19.4
  revision 19.6
Myringostapediopexy 19.53
Myringostomy 20.01
Myringotomy (with aspiration) (with drainage) 20.29
  with insertion of tube or drainage device (button) (grommet) 20.01

N

Nailing, intramedullary 79.30
    femur 79.35
    fibula 79.36
    humerus 79.31
    radius 79.32
    tibia 79.36
    ulna 79.32
Narcoanalysis 94.21
Narcosynthesis 94.21
Narrowing, palpebral fissure 08.51
Nasopharyngogram 87.09
    contrast 87.06
Necropsy 89.8
Needleoscopy (fetus) 75.31
Needling
    Bartholin's gland (cyst) 71.21
    cataract (secondary) 13.64
    fallopian tube 66.91
    hydrocephalic head 73.8
    lens (capsule) 13.2
    pupillary membrane (iris) 12.35
Nephrectomy (complete) (total) (unilateral) 55.51
    bilateral 55.54
    partial (wedge) 55.4
    remaining or solitary kidney 55.52
    removal transplanted kidney 55.53
Nephrocolopexy 55.7
Nephrocystanastomosis NEC 56.73
Nephrolithotomy 55.01
Nephrolysis 59.02
Nephropexy 55.7
Nephroplasty 55.89
Nephropyeloplasty 55.87
Nephropyeloureterostomy 55.86

Nephrorrhaphy 55.81
Nephroscopy 55.21
Nephrostolithotomy, percutaneous 55.03
Nephrostomy (with drainage tube) 55.02
    closure 55.82
    percutaneous 55.03
        with fragmentation (ultrasound) 55.04
Nephrotomogram, nephrotomography NEC 87.72
Nephrotomy 55.01
Nephroureterectomy (with bladder cuff) 55.51
Nephroureterocystectomy 55.51 [57.79]
Nerve block (cranial) (peripheral) NEC (*see also* Block, by site) 04.81
Neurectasis (cranial) (peripheral) 04.91
Neurectomy (cranial) (infraorbital) (occipital) (peripheral) (spinal) NEC 04.07
    gastric (vagus) (*see also* Vagotomy) 44.00
    opticociliary 12.79
    paracervical 05.22
    presacral 05.24
    retrogasserian 04.07
    sympathetic — *see* Sympathectomy
    trigeminal 04.07
    tympanic 20.91
Neurexeresis NEC 04.07
Neuroanastomosis (cranial) (peripheral) NEC 04.74
    accessory-facial 04.72
    accessory-hypoglossal 04.73
    hypoglossal-facial 04.71
Neurolysis (peripheral nerve) NEC 04.49
    carpal tunnel 04.43

    cranial nerve NEC 04.42
    spinal (cord) (nerve roots) 03.6
    tarsal tunnel 04.44
    trigeminal nerve 04.41
Neuroplasty (cranial) (peripheral) NEC 04.79
    of old injury (delayed repair) 04.76
    revision 04.75
Neurorrhaphy (cranial) (peripheral) 04.3
Neurotomy (cranial) (peripheral) (spinal) NEC 04.04
    acoustic 04.01
    glossopharyngeal 29.92
    lacrimal branch 05.0
    retrogasserian 04.02
    sympathetic 05.0
    vestibular 04.01
Neurotripsy (peripheral) NEC 04.03
    trigeminal 04.02
Nicola operation (tenodesis for recurrent dislocation of shoulder) 81.82
Nissen operation (fundoplication of stomach) 44.66
Noble operation (plication of small intestine) 46.62
Norman Miller operation (vaginopexy) 70.77
Norton operation (extraperitoneal cesarean section) 74.2
Nuclear magnetic resonance imaging — *see* Imaging, magnetic resonance
Nutrition, concentrated substances
    enteral infusion (of) 96.6
        parenteral, total 99.15
        peripheral parenteral 99.15

O

Ober (-Yount) operation (glutealiliotibial fasciotomy) 83.14
Obliteration
   bone cavity (*see also* Osteoplasty) 78.40
   calyceal diverticulum 55.39
   canaliculi 09.6
   cerebrospinal fistula 02.12
   cul-de-sac 70.92
   frontal sinus (with fat) 22.42
   lacrimal punctum 09.91
   lumbar pseudomeningocele 03.51
   lymphatic structure(s) (peripheral) 40.9
   maxillary sinus 22.31
   meningocele (sacral) 03.51
   pleural cavity 34.6
   sacral meningocele 03.51
   Skene's gland 71.3
   tympanomastoid cavity 19.9
   vagina, vaginal (partial) (total) 70.4
      vault 70.8
Occlusal molds (dental) 89.31
Occlusion
   artery — *see* Ligation, artery
   fallopian tube — *see* Ligation, fallopian tube
   vein — *see* Ligation, vein
   vena cava (surgical) 38.7
Occupational therapy 93.83
O'Donoghue operation (triad knee repair) 81.43
Odontectomy NEC (*see also* Removal, tooth, surgical) 23.19
Oleothorax 33.39
Olshausen operation (uterine suspension) 69.22
Omentectomy 54.4
Omentofixation 54.74
Omentopexy 54.74
Omentoplasty 54.74
Omentorrhaphy 54.74
Omentotomy 54.19
Omphalectomy 54.3
Onychectomy 86.23
Onychoplasty 86.86
Onychotomy 86.09
   with drainage 86.04
Oophorectomy (unilateral) 65.3
   with salpingectomy 65.4
   bilateral (same operative episode) 65.51
      with salpingectomy 65.61
   partial 65.29
      wedge 65.22
   remaining ovary 65.52
      with tube 65.62
Oophorocystectomy 65.29
Oophoropexy 65.79
Oophoroplasty 65.79
Oophororrhaphy 65.71
Oophorostomy 65.0
Oophorotomy 65.0
Opening
   bony labyrinth (ear) 20.79
   cranial suture 02.01
   heart valve
      closed heart technique — *see* Valvulotomy, by site
      open heart technique — *see* Valvuloplasty, by site
   spinal dura 03.09

Operation
   Abbe
      construction of vagina 70.61
      intestinal anastomosis — *see* Anastomosis, intestine
   abdominal (region) NEC 54.99
   abdominoperineal NEC 48.5
   Aburel (intra-amniotic injection for abortion) 75.0
   Adams
      advancement of round ligament 69.22
      crushing of nasal septum 21.88
      excision of palmar fascia 82.35
   adenoids NEC 28.99
   adrenal (gland) (nerve) (vessel) NEC 07.49
   Albee
      bone peg, femoral neck 78.05
      graft for slipping patella 78.06
      sliding inlay graft, tibia 78.07
   Albert (arthrodesis, knee) 81.22
   Aldridge (—Studdiford) (urethral sling) 59.5
   Alexander
      prostatectomy
         perineal 60.62
         suprapubic 60.3
      shortening of round ligaments of uterus 69.22
   Alexander-Adams (shortening of round ligaments of uterus) 69.22
   Almoor (extrapetrosal drainage) 20.22
   Altemeier (perineal rectal pull-through) 48.49
   Ammon (dacryocystotomy) 09.53
   Anderson (tibial lengthening) 78.37
   Anel (dilation of lacrimal duct) 09.42
   anterior chamber (eye) NEC 12.99
   anti-incontinence NEC 59.79
   antrum window (nasal sinus) 22.2
      with Caldwell-Luc approach 22.39
   anus NEC 49.99
   aortic body NEC 39.8
   aorticopulmonary window 39.59
   appendix NEC 47.99
   Arslan (fenestration of inner ear) 20.61
   artery NEC 39.99
   Asai (larynx) 31.75
   Baffes (interatrial transposition of venous return) 35.91
   Baldy-Webster (uterine suspension) 69.22
   Ball
      herniorrhaphy — *see* Repair, hernia, inguinal
      undercutting 49.02
   Bankhart (capsular repair into glenoid, for shoulder dislocation) 81.82
   Bardenheuer (ligation of innominate artery) 38.85
   Barkan (goniotomy) 12.52
      with goniopuncture 12.53
   Barr (transfer of tibialis posterior tendon) 83.75
   Barsky (closure of cleft hand) 82.82
   Bassett (vulvectomy with inguinal lymph node dissection) 71.5 [40.3]
   Bassini (herniorrhaphy) — *see* Repair, hernia, inguinal
   Batch-Spittler-McFaddin (knee disarticulation) 84.16
   Beck I (epicardial poudrage) 36.3

   Beck II (aorta-coronary sinus shunt) 36.3
   Beck-Jianu (permanent gastrostomy) 43.19
   Bell-Beuttner (subtotal abdominal hysterectomy) 68.3
   Belsey (esophagogastric sphincter) 44.65
   Benenenti (rotation of bulbous urethra) 58.49
   Berke (levator resection eyelid) 08.33
   Biesenberger (size reduction of breast, bilateral) 85.32
      unilateral 85.31
   Bigelow (litholapaxy) 57.0
   biliary (duct) (tract) NEC 51.99
   Billroth I (partial gastrectomy with gastroduodenostomy) 43.6
   Billroth II (partial gastrectomy with gastrojejunostomy) 43.7
   Binnie (hepatopexy) 50.69
   Bischoff (ureteroneocystostomy) 56.74
   bisection hysterectomy 68.3
   Bishoff (spinal myelotomy) 03.29
   bladder NEC 57.99
      flap 56.74
   Blalock (systemic-pulmonary anastomosis) 39.0
   Blalock-Hanlon (creation of atrial septal defect) 35.42
   Blalock-Taussig (subclavian-pulmonary anastomosis) 39.0
   Blascovic (resection and advancement of levator palpebrae superioris) 08.33
   blood vessel NEC 39.99
   Blount
      femoral shortening (with blade plate) 78.25
      by epiphyseal stapling 78.25
   Boari (bladder flap) 56.74
   Bobb (cholelithotomy) 51.04
   bone NEC — *see* category 78.4
      facial 76.99
      injury NEC — *see* category 79.9
      marrow NEC 41.98
      skull NEC 02.99
   Bonney (abdominal hysterectomy) 68.4
   Borthen (iridotasis) 12.63
   Bost
      plantar dissection 80.48
      radiocarpal fusion 81.26
   Bosworth
      arthroplasty for acromioclavicular separation 81.83
      fusion of posterior lumbar spine 81.08
         for pseudarthrosis 81.09
      resection of radial head ligaments (for tennis elbow) 80.92
      shelf procedure, hip 81.40
   bottle (repair if hydrocele of tunica vaginalis) 61.2
   Boyd (hip disarticulation) 84.18
   brain NEC 02.99
   Brauer (cardiolysis) 37.10
   breast NEC 85.99
   Bricker (ileoureterostomy) 56.51
   Bristow (repair of shoulder dislocation) 81.82
   Brock (pulmonary valvulotomy) 35.03
   Brockman (soft tissue release for clubfoot) 83.84
   bronchus NEC 33.98

Browne (-Denis) (hypospadias repair) 58.45
Brunschwig (temporary gastrostomy) 43.19
buccal cavity NEC 27.99
Bunnell (tendon transfer) 82.56
Burgess (amputation of ankle) 84.14
bursa NEC 83.99
    hand 82.99
bypass — see Bypass
Caldwell (sulcus extension) 24.91
Caldwell-Luc (maxillary sinusotomy) 22.39
    with removal of membrane lining 22.31
Callander (knee disarticulation) 84.16
Campbell
    bone block, ankle 81.11
    fasciotomy (iliac crest) 83.14
    reconstruction of anterior cruciate ligaments 81.45
canthus NEC 08.99
cardiac NEC 37.99
    septum NEC 35.98
    valve NEC 35.99
carotid body or gland NEC 39.8
Carroll and Taber (arthroplasty proximal interphalangeal joint) 81.72
Cattell (herniorrhaphy) 53.51
Cecil (urethral reconstruction) 58.46
cecum NEC 46.99
cerebral (meninges) NEC 02.99
cervix NEC 69.99
Chandler (hip fusion) 81.21
Charles (correction of lymphedema) 40.9
Charnley (compression arthrodesis)
    ankle 81.11
    hip 81.21
    knee 81.22
Cheatle-Henry — see Repair, hernia, femoral
chest cavity NEC 34.99
Chevalier-Jackson (partial laryngectomy) 30.29
Child (radical subtotal pancreatectomy) 52.53
Chopart (midtarsal amputation) 84.12
chordae tendineae NEC 35.32
choroid NEC 14.9
ciliary body NEC 12.98
cisterna chyli NEC 40.69
Clagett (closure of chest wall following open flap drainage) 34.72
Clayton (resection of metatarsal heads and bases of phalanges) 77.88
clitoris NEC 71.4
cocked hat (metacarpal lengthening and transfer of local flap) 82.69
Cockett (varicose vein)
    lower limb 38.59
    supper limb 38.53
Cody tack (perforation of footplate) 19.0
Coffey (uterine suspension) (Meigs' modification) 69.22
Cole (anterior tarsal wedge osteotomy) 77.28
Collis-Nissen (hiatal hernia repair) 53.80
colon NEC 46.99
Colonna
    adductor tenotomy (first stage) 83.12
    hip arthroplasty (second stage) 81.40
    reconstruction of hip (second stage) 81.40
commando (radical glossectomy) 25.4
conjunctiva NEC 10.99
    destructive NEC 10.33

cornea NEC 11.99
Coventry (tibial wedge osteotomy) 77.27
Crawford (tarso-frontalis sling of eyelid) 08.32
cul-de-sac NEC 70.92
Culp-Deweerd (spiral flap pyeloplasty) 55.87
Culp-Scardino (ureteral flap pyeloplasty) 55.87
Curtis (interphalangeal joint arthroplasty) 81.72
cystocele NEC 70.51
Dahlman (excision of esophageal diverticulum) 42.31
Dana (posterior rhizotomy) 03.1
Danforth (fetal) 73.8
Darrach (ulnar resection) 77.83
Davis (intubated ureterotomy) 56.2
de Grandmont (tarsectomy) 08.35
Delorme
    pericardiectomy 37.31
    proctopexy 48.76
    repair of prolapsed rectum 48.76
    thoracoplasty 33.34
Denker (radical maxillary antrotomy) 22.31
Dennis-Varco (herniorrhaphy) — see Repair, hernia, femoral
Denonvillier (limited rhinoplasty) 21.86
dental NEC 24.99
    orthodontic NEC 24.8
Derlacki (tympanoplasty) 19.4
diaphragm NEC 34.89
Dickson (fascial transplant) 83.82
Dickson-Diveley (tendon transfer and arthrodesis to correct claw toe) 77.57
Dieffenbach (hip disarticulation) 84.18
digestive tract NEC 46.99
Doleris (shortening of round ligaments) 69.22
D'Ombrain (excision of pterygium with corneal graft) 11.32
Dorrance (push-back operation for cleft palate) 27.62
Dotter (transluminal angioplasty) 39.59
Douglas (suture of tongue to lip for micrognathia) 25.59
Doyle (paracervical uterine denervation) 69.3
Duhamel (abdominoperineal pull-through) 48.65
Duhrssen (vaginofixation of uterus) 69.22
Dunn (triple arthrodesis) 81.12
duodenum NEC 46.99
Dupuytren
    fasciectomy 82.35
    fasciotomy 82.12
        with excision 82.35
    shoulder disarticulation 84.08
Durham (-Caldwell) (transfer of biceps femoris tendon) 83.75
DuToit and Roux (staple capsulorrhaphy of shoulder) 81.82
DuVries (tenoplasty) 83.88
Dwyer
    fasciotomy 83.14
    soft tissue release NEC 83.84
    wedge osteotomy, calcaneus 77.28
Eagleton (extrapetrosal drainage) 20.22
ear (external) NEC 18.9
    middle or inner NEC 20.99
Eden-Hybinette (glenoid bone block) 78.01
Effler (heart) 36.2

Eggers
    tendon release (patellar retinacula) 83.13
    tendon transfer (biceps femoris tendon) (hamstring tendon) 83.75
Elliot (scleral trephination with iridectomy) 12.61
Ellis Jones (repair of peroneal tendon) 83.88
Ellison (reinforcement of collateral ligament) 81.44
Elmslie-Cholmeley (tarsal wedge osteotomy) 77.28
Eloesser (thoracoplasty) 33.34
Emmet (cervix) 67.61
endorectal pull-through 48.41
epididymis NEC 63.99
esophagus NEC 42.99
Estes (ovary) 65.72
Estlander (thoracoplasty) 33.34
Evans (release of clubfoot) 83.84
extraocular muscle NEC 15.9
    multiple (two or more muscles) 15.4
        with temporary detachment from globe 15.3
    revision 15.6
    single 15.29
        with temporary detachment from globe 15.19
eyeball NEC 16.99
eyelid(s) NEC 08.99
face NEC 27.99
facial bone or joint NEC 76.99
fallopian tube NEC 66.99
Farabeuf (ischiopubiotomy) 77.39
Fasanella-Servatt (blepharoptosis repair) 08.35
fascia NEC 83.99
    hand 82.99
female (genital organs) NEC 71.9
    hysterectomy NEC 68.9
fenestration (aorta) 39.54
Ferguson (hernia repair) 53.00
Fick (perforation of footplate) 19.0
filtering (for glaucoma) 12.79
    with iridectomy 12.65
Finney (pyloroplasty) 44.2
fistulizing, sclera NEC 12.69
Foley (pyeloplasty) 55.87
Fontan (creation of conduit between right atrium and pulmonary artery) 35.94
Fothergill (-Donald) (uterine suspension) 69.22
Fowler
    arthroplasty of metacarpophalangeal joint 81.72
    release (mallet finger repair) 82.84
    tenodesis (hand) 82.85
    thoracoplasty 33.34
Fox (entropion repair with wedge resection) 08.43
Franco (suprapubic cystotomy) 57.19
Frank (permanent gastrostomy) 43.19
Frazier (-Spiller) (subtemporal trigeminal rhizotomy) 04.02
Fredet-Ramstedt (pyloromyotomy) (with wedge resection) 43.3
Frenckner (intrapetrosal drainage) 20.22
Frickman (abdominal proctopexy) 48.75
Frommel (shortening of uterosacral ligaments) 69.22
Gabriel (abdominoperineal resection of rectum) 48.5

gallbladder NEC 51.99
ganglia NEC 04.99
    sympathetic 04.89
Gant (wedge osteotomy of trochanter) 77.25
Garceau (tibial tendon transfer) 83.75
Gardner (spinal meningocele repair) 03.51
gastric NEC 44.99
Gelman (release of clubfoot) 83.84
genital organ NEC
    female 71.9
    male 64.99
Ghormley (hip fusion) 81.21
Gifford
    destruction of lacrimal sac 09.6
    keratotomy (delimiting) 11.1
Gill
    arthrodesis of shoulder 81.23
    laminectomy 03.09
Gill-Stein (carporadial arthrodesis) 81.25
Gilliam (uterine suspension) 69.22
Girdlestone
    laminectomy with spinal fusion 81.00
    muscle transfer for claw toe 77.57
    resection of femoral head and neck 77.85
Girdlestone-Taylor (muscle transfer for claw toe repair) 77.57
glaucoma NEC 12.79
Glenn (anastomosis of superior vena cava to right pulmonary artery) 39.21
globus pallidus NEC 01.42
Goebel-Frangenheim-Stoeckel (urethrovesical suspension) 59.4
Goldner (clubfoot release) 80.48
Goldthwait
    ankle stabilization 81.11
    patella stabilization 81.44
    tendon transfer for patella dislocation 81.44
Goodall-Power (vagina) 70.4
Gordon-Taylor (hindquarter amputation) 84.19
Graber-Duvernay (drilling femoral head) 77.15
Green (scapulopexy) 78.41
Grice (subtalar arthrodesis) 81.13
Gritti-Stokes (knee disarticulation) 84.16
Gross (herniorrhaphy) 53.49
gum NEC 24.39
Guyon (amputation of ankle) 84.13
Hagner (epididymotomy) 63.92
Halsted — see Repair, hernia, inguinal
Hampton (anastomosis small intestine to rectal stump) 45.92
hanging hip (muscle release) 83.19
harelip 27.54
Harrison-Richardson (vaginal suspension) 70.77
Hartmann — see Colectomy, by site
Hauser
    achillotenotomy 83.11
    bunionectomy with adductor tendon transfer 77.53
    stabilization of patella 81.44
Heaney (vaginal hysterectomy) 68.5
heart NEC 37.99
    valve NEC 35.99
        adjacent structure NEC 35.39
Hegar (perineorrhaphy) 71.79
Heine (cyclodialysis) 12.55
Heineke-Mikulicz (pyloroplasty) 44.2
Heller (esophagomyotomy) 42.7

Hellstrom (transplantation of aberrant renal vessel) 39.55
hemorrhoids NEC 49.49
Henley (jejunal transposition) 43.81
hepatic NEC 50.99
hernia — see Repair, hernia
Hey (amputation of foot) 84.12
Hey-Groves (reconstruction of anterior cruciate ligament) 81.45
Heyman (soft tissue release for clubfoot) 83.84
Heyman-Herndon (-Strong) (correction of metatarsus varus) 80.48
Hibbs (lumbar spinal fusion) — see Fusion, lumbar
Higgins — see Repair, hernia, femoral
Hill-Allison (hiatal hernia repair, transpleural approach) 53.80
Hitchcock (anchoring tendon of biceps) 83.88
Hofmeister (gastrectomy) 43.7
Hoke
    midtarsal fusion 81.14
    triple arthrodesis 81.12
Holth
    iridencleisis 12.63
    sclerectomy 12.65
Homan (correction of lymphedema) 40.9
Hutch (ureteroneocystostomy) 56.74
Hybinette-eden (glenoid bone block) 78.01
hymen NEC 70.91
hypopharynx NEC 29.99
hypophysis NEC 07.79
ileal loop 56.51
ileum NEC 46.99
intestine NEC 46.99
iris NEC 12.97
    inclusion 12.63
Irving (tubal ligation) 66.32
Irwin (see also Osteotomy) 77.30
Jaboulay (gastroduodenostomy) 44.39
Janeway (permanent gastrostomy) 43.19
Jatene (arterial switch) 35.84
jejunum NEC 46.99
Johanson (urethral reconstruction) 58.46
joint (capsule) (ligament) (structure) NEC 81.99
    facial NEC 76.99
Jones
    claw toe (transfer of extensor hallucis longus tendon) 77.57
        modified (with arthrodesis) 77.57
    dacryocystorhinostomy 09.81
    hammer toe (interphalangeal fusion) 77.56
        modified (tendon transfer with arthrodesis) 77.57
    repair of peroneal tendon 83.88
Joplin (exostectomy with tendon transfer) 77.53
Kader (temporary gastrostomy) 43.19
Kaufman (for urinary stress incontinence) 59.79
Kazanjiian (buccal vestibular sulcus extension) 24.91
Kehr (hepatopexy) 50.69
Keller (bunionectomy) 77.59
Kelly (-Kennedy) (urethrovesical plication) 59.3
Kelly-Stoeckel (urethrovesical plication) 59.3
Kerr (cesarean section) 74.1

Kessler (arthroplasty, carpometacarpal joint) 81.74
Kidner (excision of accessory navicular bone) (with tendon transfer) 77.98
kidney NEC 55.99
Killian (frontal sinusotomy) 22.41
King-Steelquist (hindquarter amputation) 84.19
Kirk (amputation through thigh) 84.17
Kondoleon (correction of lymphedema) 40.9
Krause (sympathetic denervation) 05.29
Kroener (partial salpingectomy) 66.69
Kroenlein (lateral orbitotomy) 16.01
Kronig (low cervical cesarean section) 74.1
Krukenberg (reconstruction of below-elbow amputation) 82.89
Kuhnt-Szymanowski (ectropion repair with lid reconstruction) 08.44
Labbe (gastrotomy) 43.0
labia NEC 71.8
lacrimal
    gland 09.3
    system NEC 09.99
Ladd (mobilization of intestine) 54.95
Lagrange (iridosclerectomy) 12.65
Lambrinudi (triple arthrodesis) 81.12
Langenbeck (cleft palate repair) 27.62
Lapidus (bunionectomy with metatarsal osteotomy) 77.51
Larry (shoulder disarticulation) 84.08
larynx NEC 31.98
Lash (internal cervical os repair) 67.5
Latzko
    cesarean section, extraperitoneal 74.2
    colpocleisis 70.8
Leadbetter (urethral reconstruction) 58.46
Leadbetter-Politano (ureteroneocystostomy) 56.74
Le Fort (colpocleisis) 70.8
LeMesurier (cleft lip repair) 27.54
lens NEC 13.9
Leriche (periarterial sympathectomy) 39.7
levator muscle sling
    eyelid ptosis repair 08.33
    urethrovesical suspension 59.71
    urinary stress incontinence 59.71
lid suture (blepharoptosis) 08.31
ligament NEC 81.99
    broad NEC 69.98
    round NEC 69.98
    uterine NEC 69.98
Lindholm (repair of ruptured tendon) 83.88
Linton (varicose vein) 38.59
lip NEC 27.99
Lisfranc
    foot amputation 84.12
    shoulder disarticulation 84.08
Littlewood (forequarter amputation) 84.09
liver NEC 50.99
Lloyd-Davies (abdominoperineal resection) 48.5
Longmire (bile duct anastomosis) 51.39
Lord
    dilation of anal canal for hemorrhoids 49.49
    hemorrhoidectomy 49.49
    orchidopexy 62.5
Lucas and Murray (knee arthrodesis with plate) 81.22
lung NEC 33.99
lymphatic structure(s) NEC 40.9
    duct, left (thoracic) NEC 40.69

Madlener (tubal ligation) 66.31
Magnuson (-Stack) (arthroplasty for
    recurrent shoulder dislocation) 81.82
male genital organs NEC 64.99
Manchester (-Donald) (-Fothergill),
    (uterine suspension) 69.22
mandible NEC 76.99
    orthognathic 76.64
Marckwald (cervical os repair) 67.5
Marshall-Marchetti (-Krantz) (retropubic
    urethral suspension) 59.5
Matas (aneurysmorrhaphy) 39.52
Mayo
    bunionectomy 77.59
    herniorrhaphy 53.49
    vaginal hysterectomy 68.5
Mazet (knee disarticulation) 84.16
McBride (bunionectomy with soft tissue
    correction) 77.53
McBurney — see Repair, hernia, inguinal
McCall (enterocele repair) 70.92
McCauley (release of clubfoot) 83.84
McDonald (encirclement suture, cervix)
    67.5
McIndoe (vaginal construction) 70.61
McKeever (fusion of first
    metatarsophalangeal joint for hallux
    valgus repair) 77.52
McKissock (breast reduction) 85.33
McReynolds (transposition of pterygium)
    11.31
McVay
    femoral hernia — see Repair, hernia,
        femoral
    inguinal hernia — see Repair, hernia,
        inguinal
meninges (spinal) NEC 03.99
    cerebral NEC 02.99
mesentery NEC 54.99
Mikulicz (exteriorization of intestine) (first
    stage) 46.03
    second stage 46.04
Miles (complete proctectomy) 48.5
Millard (cheiloplasty) 27.54
Miller
    midtarsal arthrodesis 81.14
    urethrovesical suspension 59.4
Millin-Read (urethrovesical suspension)
    59.4
Mitchell (hallux valgus repair) 77.51
Mohs (chemosurgical excision of skin)
    86.24
Moore (arthroplasty) 81.52
Moschowitz
    enterocele repair 70.92
    herniorrhaphy — see Repair, hernia,
        femoral
    sigmoidopexy 46.63
mouth NEC 27.09
Muller (banding of pulmonary artery)
    38.85
Mumford (partial claviculectomy) 77.81
muscle NEC 83.99
    extraocular — see Operation,
        extraocular
    hand NEC 82.99
    papillary heart NEC 35.31
musculoskeletal system NEC 84.99
Mustard (interatrial transposition of venous
    return) 35.91
nail (finger) (toe) NEC 86.99
nasal sinus NEC 22.9
nasopharynx NEC 29.99

nerve (cranial) (peripheral) NEC 04.99
    adrenal NEC 07.49
    sympathetic NEC 05.89
nervous system NEC 05.9
Nicola (tenodesis for recurrent dislocation
    of shoulder) 81.82
nipple NEC 85.99
Nissen (fundoplication of stomach) 44.66
Noble (plication of small intestine) 46.62
node (lymph) NEC 40.9
Norman Miller (vaginopexy) 70.77
Norton (extraperitoneal cesarean
    operation) 74.2
nose, nasal NEC 21.99
    sinus NEC 22.9
Ober (-Yount) (gluteal-iliotibial fasciotomy)
    83.14
obstetric NEC 75.99
ocular NEC 16.99
    muscle — see Operation, extraocular
        muscle
O'Donoghue (triad knee repair) 81.43
Olshausen (uterine suspension) 69.22
omentum NEC 54.99
ophthalmologic NEC 16.99
oral cavity NEC 27.99
orbicularis muscle sling 08.36
orbit NEC 16.98
oropharynx NEC 29.99
orthodontic NEC 24.8
orthognathic NEC 76.69
Oscar Miller (midtarsal arthrodesis) 81.14
Osmond-Clark (soft tissue release with
    peroneus brevis tendon transfer)
    83.75
ovary NEC 65.99
Oxford (for urinary incontinence) 59.4
palate NEC 27.99
palpebral ligament sling 08.36
Panas (linear proctotomy) 48.0
Pancoast (division of trigeminal nerve at
    foramen ovale) 04.02
pancreas NEC 52.99
pantaloon (revision of gastric anastomosis)
    44.5
papillary muscle (heart) NEC 35.31
Paquin (ureteroneocystostomy) 56.74
parathyroid gland(s) NEC 06.99
parotid gland or duct NEC 26.99
Partsch (marsupialization of dental cyst)
    24.4
Pattee (auditory canal) 18.6
Peet (splanchnic resection) 05.29
Pemberton
    osteotomy of ilium 77.39
    rectum (mobilization and fixation for
        prolapse repair) 48.76
penis NEC 64.98
Pereyra (paraurethral suspension) 59.6
pericardium NEC 37.99
perineum (female) NEC 71.8
    male NEC 86.99
perirectal tissue NEC 48.99
perirenal tissue NEC 59.92
peritoneum NEC 54.99
periurethral tissue NEC 58.99
perivesical tissue NEC 59.92
pharyngeal flap (cleft palate repair) 27.62
    secondary or subsequent 27.63
pharynx, pharyngeal (pouch) NEC 29.99
pineal gland NEC 07.59

Pinsker (obliteration of nasoseptal
    telangiectasia) 21.07
Piper (forceps) 72.6
Pirogoff (ankle amputation through
    malleoli of tibia and fibula) 84.14
pituitary gland NEC 07.79
plastic — see Repair, by site
pleural cavity NEC 34.99
Politano-Leadbetter (ureteroneocystostomy)
    56.74
pollicization (with nerves and blood supply)
    82.61
Polya (gastrectomy) 43.7
Pomeroy (ligation and division of fallopian
    tubes) 66.32
Poncet
    lengthening of Achilles tendon 83.85
    urethrostomy, perineal 58.0
Porro (cesarean section) 74.99
posterior chamber (eye) NEC 14.9
Potts-Smith (descending aorta-left
    pulmonary artery anastomosis) 39.0
Printen and Mason (high gastric bypass)
    44.31
prostate NEC (see also Prostatectomy)
    60.69
    specified type 60.99
pterygium 11.39
    with corneal graft 11.32
Puestow (pancreaticojejunostomy) 52.96
pull-through NEC 48.49
pulmonary NEC 33.99
push-back (cleft palate repair) 27.62
Putti-Platt (capsulorrhaphy of shoulder for
    recurrent dislocation) 81.82
pyloric exclusion 44.39
pyriform sinus NEC 29.99
"rabbit ear" (anterior urethropexy) (Tudor)
    59.79
Ramadier (intrapetrosal drainage) 20.22
Ramstedt (pyloromyotomy) (with wedge
    resection) 43.3
Rankin
    exteriorization of intestine 46.03
    proctectomy (complete) 48.5
Rashkind (balloon septostomy) 35.41
Rastelli (creation of conduit between right
    ventricle and pulmonary artery)
    35.92
    in repair of
        pulmonary artery atresia 35.92
        transposition of great vessels 35.92
        truncus arteriosus 35.83
Raz-Pereyra procedure (bladder neck
    suspension) 59.79
rectal NEC 48.99
rectocele NEC 70.52
re-entry (aorta) 39.54
renal NEC 55.99
respiratory (tract) NEC 33.99
retina NEC 14.9
Ripstein (repair of rectal prolapse) 48.75
Rodney Smith (radical subtotal
    pancreatectomy) 52.53
Roux-en-Y
    bile duct 51.36
    cholecystojejunostomy 51.32
    esophagus (intrathoracic) 42.54
    pancreaticojejunostomy 52.96
Roux-Goldthwait (repair of patellar
    dislocation) 81.44
Roux-Herzen-Judine (jejunal loop
    interposition) 42.63

Ruiz-Mora (proximal phalangectomy for hammer toe) 77.99
Russe (bone graft of scaphoid) 78.04
Saemisch (corneal resection) 11.1
salivary gland or duct NEC 26.99
Salter (innominate osteotomy) 77.39
Sauer-Bacon (abdominoperineal resection) 48.5
Schanz (femoral osteotomy) 77.35
Schauta (-Amreich) (radical vaginal hysterectomy) 68.7
Schede (thoracoplasty) 33.34
Scheie
    cautery of sclera 12.62
    sclerostomy 12.62
Schlatter (total gastrectomy) 43.99
Schroeder (endocervical excision) 67.39
Schuchardt (nonobstetrical episiotomy) 71.09
Schwartze (simple mastoidectomy) 20.41
sclera NEC 12.89
Scott
    intestinal bypass for obesity 45.93
    jejunocolostomy (bypass) 45.93
scrotum NEC 61.99
Seddon-Brooks (transfer of pectoralis major tendon) 83.75
Semb (apicolysis of lung) 33.39
seminal vesicle NEC 60.79
Senning (correction of transposition of great vessels) 35.91
Sever (division of soft tissue of arm) 83.19
Sewell (heart) 36.2
sex transformation NEC 64.5
Sharrard (iliopsoas muscle transfer) 83.77
shelf (hip arthroplasty) 81.40
Shirodkar (encirclement suture, cervix) 67.5
sigmoid NEC 46.99
Silver (bunionectomy) 77.59
Sistrunk (excision of thyroglossal cyst) 06.7
Skene's gland NEC 71.8
skin NEC 86.99
skull NEC 02.99
sling
    eyelid
        fascia lata, palpebral 08.36
        frontalis fascial 08.32
        levator muscle 08.33
        orbicularis muscle 08.36
        palpebral ligament, fascia lata 08.36
        tarsus muscle 08.35
    fascial (fascia lata)
        eye 08.32
        for facial weakness (trigeminal nerve paralysis) 86.81
        palpebral ligament 08.36
        tongue (fascial) 25.59
    tongue (fascial) 25.59
    urethra (suprapubic) 59.4
        retropubic 59.5
    urethrovesical 59.5
Slocum (pes anserinus transfer) 81.47
Sluder (tonsillectomy) 28.2
Smith (open osteotomy of mandible) 76.62
Smith-Peterson (radiocarpal arthrodesis) 81.25
Smithwick (sympathectomy) 05.29
Soave (endorectal pull-through) 48.41
soft tissue NEC 83.99
    hand 82.99

Sonneberg (inferior maxillary neurectomy) 04.07
Sorondo-Ferre (hindquarter amputation) 84.19
Soutter (iliac crest fasciotomy) 83.14
Spalding-Richardson (uterine suspension) 69.22
spermatic cord NEC 63.99
sphincter of Oddi NEC 51.89
spinal (canal) (cord) (structures) NEC 03.99
Spinelli (correction of inverted uterus) 75.93
Spivack (permanent gastrostomy) 43.19
spleen NEC 41.99
S.P. Rogers (knee disarticulation) 84.16
Ssabanejew-Frank (permanent gastrostomy) 43.19
Stacke (simple mastoidectomy) 20.41
Stallard (conjunctivocystorhinostomy) 09.82
    with insertion of tube or stent 09.83
Stamm (-Kader) (temporary gastrostomy) 43.19
Steinberg 44.5
Steindler
    fascia stripping (for cavus deformity) 83.14
    flexorplasty (elbow) 83.77
    muscle transfer 83.77
sterilization NEC
    female (see also specific operation) 66.39
    male (see also Ligation, vas deferens) 63.70
Stewart (renal plication with pyeloplasty) 55.87
stomach NEC 44.99
Stone (anoplasty) 49.79
Strassman (metroplasty) 69.49
    metroplasty (Jones modification) 69.49
    uterus 68.22
Strayer (gastrocnemius recession) 83.72
stress incontinence — see Repair, stress incontinence
Stromeyer-Little (hepatotomy) 50.0
Strong (unbridling of celiac artery axis) 39.91
Sturmdorf (conization of cervix) 67.2
subcutaneous tissue NEC 86.99
sublingual gland or duct NEC 26.99
submaxillary gland or duct NEC 26.99
Summerskill (dacryocystorhinostomy by intubation) 09.81
Surmay (jejunostomy) 46.39
Swenson
    bladder reconstruction 57.87
    proctectomy 48.49
Swinney (urethral reconstruction) 58.46
Syme
    ankle amputation through malleoli of tibia and fibula 84.14
    urethrotomy, external 58.0
sympathetic nerve NEC 05.89
Taarnhoj (trigeminal nerve root decompression) 04.41
Tack (sacculotomy) 20.79
Talma-Morrison (omentopexy) 54.74
Tanner (devascularization of stomach) 44.99
TAPVC NEC 35.82
tarsus NEC 08.99
    muscle sling 08.35

tendon NEC 83.99
    extraocular NEC 15.9
    hand NEC 82.99
testis NEC 62.99
tetralogy of Fallot
    partial repair — see specific procedure
    total (one-stage) 35.81
Thal (repair of esophageal stricture) 42.85
thalamus (stereotactic) 01.41
Thiersch
    anus 49.79
    skin graft 86.69
        hand 86.62
Thompson
    cleft lip repair 27.54
    correction of lymphedema 40.9
    quadricepsplasty 83.86
    thumb apportion with bone graft 82.69
thoracic duct NEC 40.69
thorax NEC 34.99
Thorek (partial cholecystectomy) 51.21
three-snip, punctum 09.51
thymus NEC 07.99
thyroid gland NEC 06.98
TKP (thermokeratoplasty) 11.74
Tomkins (metroplasty) 69.49
tongue NEC 25.99
    flap, palate 27.62
    tie 25.91
tonsil NEC 28.99
Torek (-Bevan) (orchidopexy) (first stage) (second stage) 62.5
Torkildsen (ventriculocisternal shunt) 02.2
Torpin (cul-de-sac resection) 70.92
Toti (dacryocystorhinostomy) 09.81
Touchas 86.83
Touroff (ligation of subclavian artery) 38.85
trabeculae corneae cordis (heart) NEC 35.35
trachea NEC 31.99
Trauner (lingual sulcus extension) 24.91
truncus arteriosus NEC 35.83
Tsuge (macrodactyly repair) 82.83
Tudor "rabbit ear" (anterior urethropexy) 59.79
Tuffier
    apicolysis of lung 33.39
    vaginal hysterectomy 68.5
tunica vaginalis NEC 61.99
Turco (release of joint capsules in clubfoot) 80.48
Uchida (tubal ligation with or without fimbriectomy) 66.32
umbilicus NEC 54.99
urachus NEC 57.51
Urban (mastectomy) (unilateral) 85.47
    bilateral 85.48
ureter NEC 56.99
urethra NEC 58.99
urinary system NEC 59.99
uterus NEC 69.99
    supporting structures NEC 69.98
uvula NEC 27.79
vagina NEC 70.91
vascular NEC 39.99
vas deferens NEC 63.99
    ligation NEC 63.71
vein NEC 39.99
vena cava sieve 38.7
vertebra NEC 78.49
vesical (bladder) NEC 57.99
vessel NEC 39.99

cardiac NEC 36.99
Vicq d'Azyr (larynx) 31.1
Vidal (varicocele ligation) 63.1
Vineberg (implantation of mammary artery into ventricle) 36.2
vitreous NEC 14.79
vocal cord NEC 31.98
von Kraske (proctectomy) 48.64
Voss (hanging hip operation) 83.19
Vulpius (-Compere) (lengthening of gastrocnemius muscle) 83.85
vulva NEC 71.8
Ward-Mayo (vaginal hysterectomy) 68.5
Wardill (cleft palate) 27.62
Waters (extraperitoneal cesarean section) 74.2
Waterston (aorta-right pulmonary artery anastomosis) 39.0
Watkins (-Wertheim) (uterus interposition) 69.21
Watson-Jones
    hip arthrodesis 81.21
    reconstruction of lateral ligaments, ankle 81.49
    shoulder arthrodesis (extra-articular) 81.23
    tenoplasty 83.88
Weir
    appendicostomy 47.91
    correction of nostrils 21.86
Wertheim (radical hysterectomy) 68.6
West (dacryocystorhinostomy) 09.81
Wheeler
    entropion repair 08.44
    halving procedure (eyelid) 08.24
Whipple (radical pancreaticoduodenectomy) 52.7
    Child modification (radical subtotal pancreatectomy) 52.53
    Rodney-Smith modification (radical subtotal pancreatectomy) 52.53
White (lengthening of tendo calcaneus by incomplete tenotomy) 83.11
Whitehead
    glossectomy, radical 25.4
    hemorrhoidectomy 49.46
Whitman
    foot stabilization (talectomy) 77.98
    hip reconstruction 81.40
    repair of serratus anterior muscle 83.87
    trochanter wedge osteotomy 77.25
Wier (entropion repair) 08.44
Williams-Richardson (vaginal construction) 70.61
Wilms (thoracoplasty) 33.34
Wilson (angulation osteotomy for hallux valgus) 77.51
window
    antrum (nasal sinus) — see Antrotomy, maxillary
    aorticopulmonary 39.59
    bone cortex (see also Incision, bone) 77.10
        fascial 76.09
    nosoantral — see Antrotomy, maxillary
    pericardium 37.12
    pleural 34.09
Winiwarter (cholecystoenterostomy) 51.32
Witzel (temporary gastrostomy) 43.19
Woodward (release of high riding scapula) 81.83
Young
    epispadias repair 58.45
    tendon transfer (anterior tibialis) (repair of flat foot) 83.75
Yount (division of iliotibial band) 83.14
Zancolli
    capsuloplasty 81.72
    tendon transfer (biceps) 82.56
Ziegler (iridectomy) 12.14

Operculectomy 24.6
Ophthalmectomy 16.49
    with implant (into Tenon's capsule) 16.42
    with attachment of muscles 16.41
Ophthalmoscopy 16.21
Opponensplasty (hand) 82.56
Orbitomaxillectomy, radical 16.51
Orbitotomy (anterior) (frontal) (temporofrontal) (transfrontal) NEC 16.09
    with
        bone flap 16.01
        insertion of implant 16.02
    Kroenlein (lateral) 16.01
    lateral 16.01
Orchidectomy (with epididymectomy) (unilateral) 62.3
    bilateral (radical) 62.41
    remaining or solitary testis 62.42
Orchidopexy 62.5
Orchidoplasty 62.69
Orchidorrhaphy 62.61
Orchidotomy 62.0
Orchiectomy (with epididymectomy) (unilateral) 62.3
    bilateral (radical) 62.41
    remaining or solitary testis 62.42
Orchiopexy 62.5
Orchioplasty 62.69
Orthoroentgenography — see Radiography
Oscar Miller operation (midtarsal arthrodesis) 81.14
Osmond-Clark operation (soft tissue release with peroneus brevis tendon transfer) 83.75
Ossiculectomy NEC 19.3
    with
        stapedectomy (see also Stapedectomy) 19.19
        stapes mobilization 19.0
        tympanoplasty 19.53
        revision 19.6
Ossicultomy NEC 19.3
Ostectomy (partial), except facial — see also category 77.8
    facial NEC 76.39
        total 76.45
            with reconstruction 76.44
    first metatarsal head — see Bunionectomy
    for graft (autograft) (homograft) — see also category 77.7
        mandible 76.31
            total 76.42
                with reconstruction 76.41
    total, except facial — see also category 77.9
        facial NEC 76.45
            with reconstruction 76.44
        mandible 76.42
            with reconstruction 76.41
Osteoarthrotomy (see also Osteotomy) 77.30
Osteoclasis 78.70
    carpal, metacarpal 78.74
    clavicle 78.71
    ear 20.79
    femur 78.75
    fibula 78.77
    humerus 78.72
    patella 78.76
    pelvic 78.79
    phalanges (foot) (hand) 78.79
    radius 78.73
    scapula 78.71
    specified site NEC 78.79
    tarsal, metatarsal 78.78
    thorax (ribs) (sternum) 78.71
    tibia 78.77
    ulna 78.73
    vertebrae 78.79
Osteolysis — see category 78.4
Osteopathic manipulation (see also Manipulation, osteopathic) 93.67
Osteoplasty NEC — see category 78.4
    with bone graft — see Graft, bone
    for
        bone lengthening — see Lengthening, bone
        bone shortening — see Shortening, bone
        repair of malunion or nonunion of fracture — see Repair, fracture, malunion or nonunion
    carpal, metacarpal 78.44
    clavicle 78.41
    cranium NEC 02.06
        with
            flap (bone) 02.03
            graft (bone) 02.04
    facial bone NEC 76.69
    femur 78.45
    fibula 78.47
    humerus 78.42
    mandible, mandibular NEC 76.64
        body 76.63
        ramus (open) 76.62
            closed 76.61
    maxilla (segmental) 76.65
        total 76.66
    nasal bones 21.89
    patella 78.46
    pelvis 78.49
    phalanges (foot) (hand) 78.49
    radius 78.43
    scapula 78.41
    skull NEC 02.06
        with
            flap (bone) 02.03
            graft (bone) 02.04
    specified site NEC 78.49
    tarsal, metatarsal 78.48
    thorax (ribs) (sternum) 78.41
    tibia 78.47
    ulna 78.43
    vertebrae 78.49
Osteorrhaphy (see also Osteoplasty) 78.40
Osteosynthesis (fracture) — see Reduction, fracture
Osteotomy (adduction) (angulation) (block) (derotational) (displacement) (partial) (rotational) 77.30
    carpals, metacarpals 77.34
        wedge 77.24
    clavicle 77.31
        wedge 77.21
    facial bone 76.69
    femur 77.35
        wedge 77.25
    fibula 77.37

wedge 77.27
humerus 77.32
    wedge 77.22
mandible (segmental) (subapical) 76.64
    angle (open) 76.62
        closed 76.61
    body 76.63
    Gigli saw 76.61
    ramus (open) 76.62
        closed 76.61
maxilla (segmental) 76.65
    total 76.66
metatarsal 77.38
    wedge 77.28
        for hallux valgus repair 77.51
patella 77.36
    wedge 77.26
pelvic 77.39
    wedge 77.29
phalanges (foot) (hand) 77.39
    for repair of
        bunion — see Bunionectomy
        bunionette 77.54
        hallux valgus — see Bunionectomy
    wedge 77.29
        for repair of
            bunion — see Bunionectomy
            bunionette 77.54
            hallux valgus — see Bunionectomy

radius 77.33
    wedge 77.23
scapula 77.31
    wedge 77.21
specified site NEC 77.39
    wedge 77.29
tarsal 77.38
    wedge 77.28
thorax (ribs) (sternum) 77.31
    wedge 77.21
tibia 77.37
    wedge 77.27
toe 77.39
    for repair of
        bunion — see Bunionectomy
        bunionette 77.54
        hallux valgus — see Bunionectomy
    wedge 77.29
        for repair of
            bunion — see Bunionectomy
            bunionette 77.54
            hallux valgus — see Bunionectomy
ulna 77.33
    wedge 77.23
vertebrae 77.39
    wedge 77.29
Otonecrectomy (inner ear) 20.79
Otoplasty (external) 18.79
    auditory canal or meatus 18.6
    auricle 18.79
    cartilage 18.79
        reconstruction 18.71
    prominent or protruding 18.5
Otoscopy 18.11
Outfolding, sclera, for buckling (see also Buckling, scleral) 14.49
Outfracture, turbinates (nasal) 21.62
Output and clearance, circulatory 92.05
Overdistension, bladder (therapeutic) 96.25
Overlapping, sclera, for buckling (see also Buckling, scleral) 14.49
Oversewing
    pleural bleb 32.21
    ulcer crater (peptic) 44.40
        duodenum 44.42
        stomach 44.41
Oxford operation (for urinary incontinence) 59.4
Oxygen therapy (catalytic) (pump) 93.96
    hyperbaric 93.95
Oxygenation 93.96
    extracorporeal membrane (ECMO) 39.65
    hyperbaric 93.95
        wound 93.59

P

Pacemaker
    cardiac — *see also* Insertion, pacemaker, cardiac
        intraoperative (temporary) 39.64
        temporary (during and immediately following cardiac surgery) 39.64

Packing — *see also* Insertion, pack
    auditory canal 96.11
    nose, for epistaxis (anterior) 21.01
        posterior (and anterior) 21.02
    rectal 96.19
    sella turcica 07.79
    vaginal 96.14

Palatoplasty 27.69
    for cleft palate 27.62
        secondary or subsequent 27.63

Palatorrhaphy 27.61
    for cleft palate 27.62

Pallidectomy 01.42
Pallidoansotomy 01.42
Pallidotomy 01.42
Panas operation (linear proctotomy) 48.0
Pancoast operation (division of trigeminal nerve at foramen ovale) 04.02
Pancreatectomy (total) (with synchronous duodenectomy) 52.6
    partial NEC 52.59
        distal (tail) (with part of body) 52.52
        proximal (head) (with part of body) (with synchronous duodenectomy) 52.51
        radical 52.53
            subtotal 52.53
    radical 52.7
        subtotal 52.53

Pancreaticocystoduodenostomy 52.4
Pancreaticocystoenterostomy 52.4
Pancreaticocystogastrostomy 52.4
Pancreaticocystojejunostomy 52.4
Pancreaticoduodenectomy (total) 52.6
    partial NEC 52.59
        proximal 52.51
            radical subtotal 52.53
        radical (one-stage) (two-stage) 52.7
            subtotal 52.53

Pancreaticoduodenostomy 52.96
Pancreaticoenterostomy 52.96
Pancreaticogastrostomy 52.96
Pancreaticoileostomy 52.96
Pancreaticojejunostomy 52.96
Pancreatoduodenectomy (total) 52.6
    partial NEC 52.59
    radical (one-stage) (two-stage) 52.7
        subtotal 52.53

Pancreatogram 87.66
    endoscopic retrograde (ERP) 52.13

Pancreatolithotomy 52.09
    endoscopic 52.94

Pancreatotomy 52.09
Pancreolithotomy 52.09
    endoscopic 52.94

Panendoscopy 57.32
    specified site, other than bladder — *see* Endoscopy, by site

Panhysterectomy (abdominal) 68.4
    vaginal 68.5

Panniculectomy 86.83
Panniculotomy 86.83

Pantaloon operation (revision of gastric anastomosis) 44.5
Papillectomy, anal 49.39
    endoscopic 49.31
Papillotomy (pancreas) 51.82
    endoscopic 51.85
Paquin operation (ureteroneocystostomy) 56.74
Paracentesis
    abdominal (percutaneous) 54.91
    anterior chamber, eye 12.91
    bladder 57.11
    cornea 12.91
    eye (anterior chamber) 12.91
    thoracic, thoracis 34.91
    tympanum 20.09
        with intubation 20.01
Parasitology — *see* Examination, microscopic
Parathyroidectomy (partial) (subtotal) NEC 06.89
    complete 06.81
    ectopic 06.89
    global removal 06.81
    mediastinal 06.89
    total 06.81
Parenteral nutrition, total 99.15
    peripheral 99.15
Parotidectomy 26.30
    complete 26.32
    partial 26.31
    radical 26.32
Partsch operation (marsupialization of dental cyst) 24.4
Passage — *see* Insertion and Intubation
Passage of sounds, urethra 58.6
Patch
    blood, spinal (epidural) 03.95
    graft — *see* Graft
    spinal, blood (epidural) 03.95
    subdural, brain 02.12
Patellapexy 78.46
Patellaplasty NEC 78.46
Patellectomy 77.96
    partial 77.86
Pattee operation (auditory canal) 18.6
Pectenotomy (*see also* Sphincterotomy, anal) 49.59
Pedicle flap — *see* Graft, skin, pedicle
Peet operation (splanchnic resection) 05.29
PEG (percutaneous endoscopic gastrostomy) 43.11
PEJ (percutaneous endoscopic jejunostomy) 46.32
Pelvectomy, kidney (partial) 55.4
Pelvimetry 88.25
    gynecological 89.26
Pelviolithotomy 55.11
Pelvioplasty, kidney 55.87
Pelviostomy 55.12
    closure 55.82
Pelviotomy 77.39
    to assist delivery 73.94
Pelvi-ureteroplasty 55.87
Pemberton operation
    osteotomy of ilium 77.39
    rectum (mobilization and fixation for prolapse repair) 48.76

Penectomy 64.3
Pereyra operation (paraurethral suspension) 59.6
Perforation
    stapes footplate 19.0
Perfusion NEC 39.97
    carotid artery 39.97
    coronary artery 39.97
    for
        chemotherapy NEC 99.25
        hormone therapy NEC 99.24
    head 39.97
    hyperthermic (lymphatic), localized region or site 93.35
    intestine (large) (local) 46.96
        small 46.95
    kidney, local 55.95
    limb (lower) (upper) 39.97
    liver, localized 50.93
    neck 39.97
    subarachnoid (spinal cord) (refrigerated saline) 03.92
    total body 39.96
Pericardiectomy 37.31
Pericardiocentesis 37.0
Pericardiolysis 37.12
Pericardioplasty 37.4
Pericardiorrhaphy 37.4
Pericardiostomy (tube) 37.12
Pericardiotomy 37.12
Peridectomy 10.31
Perilimbal suction 89.11
Perimetry 95.05
Perineoplasty 71.79
Perineorrhaphy 71.71
    obstetrical laceration (current) 75.69
Perineotomy (nonobstetrical) 71.09
    to assist delivery — *see* Episiotomy
Periosteotomy (*see also* Incision, bone) 77.10
    facial bone 76.09
Perirectofistulectomy 48.93
Peritectomy 10.31
Peritomy 10.1
Peritoneocentesis 54.91
Peritoneoscopy 54.21
Peritoneotomy 54.19
Peritoneumectomy 54.4
Phacoemulsification (ultrasonic) (with aspiration) 13.41
Phacofragmentation (mechanical) (with aspiration) 13.43
    posterior route 13.42
    ultrasonic 13.41
Phalangectomy (partial) 77.89
    claw toe 77.57
    cockup toe 77.58
    hammer toe 77.56
    overlapping toe 77.58
    total 77.99
Phalangization (fifth metacarpal) 82.81
Pharyngeal flap operation (cleft palate repair) 27.62
    secondary or subsequent 27.63
Pharyngectomy (partial) 29.33
    with laryngectomy 30.3
Pharyngogram 87.09

contrast 87.06
Pharyngolaryngectomy 30.3
Pharyngoplasty (with silastic implant) 29.4
  for cleft palate 27.62
    secondary or subsequent 27.63
Pharyngorrhaphy 29.51
  for cleft palate 27.62
Pharyngoscopy 29.11
Pharyngotomy 29.0
Phenopeel (skin) 86.24
Phlebectomy 38.60
  with
    anastomosis 38.30
      abdominal 38.37
      head and neck NEC 38.32
      intracranial NEC 38.31
      lower limb 38.39
      thoracic NEC 38.35
      upper limb 38.33
    graft replacement 38.40
      abdominal 38.47
      head and neck NEC 38.42
      intracranial NEC 38.41
      lower limb 38.49
      thoracic NEC 38.45
      upper limb 38.43
  abdominal 38.67
  head and neck NEC 38.62
  intracranial NEC 38.61
  lower limb 38.69
  thoracic NEC 38.65
  upper limb 38.63
  varicose 38.50
    abdominal 38.57
    head and neck NEC 38.52
    intracranial NEC 38.51
    lower limb 38.59
    thoracic NEC 38.55
    upper limb 38.53
Phlebogoniostomy 12.52
Phlebography (contrast) (retrograde) 88.60
  by radioisotope — see Scan, radioisotope, by site
  adrenal 88.65
  femoral 88.66
  head 88.61
  hepatic 88.64
  impedance 88.68
  intra-abdominal NEC 88.65
  intrathoracic NEC 88.63
  lower extremity NEC 88.66
  neck 88.61
  portal system 88.64
  pulmonary 88.62
  specified site NEC 88.67
  vena cava (inferior) (superior) 88.51
Phleborrhaphy 39.32
▶**Phlebotomy** 38.99
Phonocardiogram, with ECG lead 89.55
Photochemotherapy NEC 99.83
  extracorporeal 99.88
Photocoagulation
  ciliary body 12.73
  eye, eyeball 16.99
  iris 12.41
  macular hole — see Photocoagulation, retina
  orbital lesion 16.92
  retina
    for
      destruction of lesion 14.25
      reattachment 14.55

      repair of tear or defect 14.35
    laser (beam)
      for
        destruction of lesion 14.24
        reattachment 14.54
        repair of tear or defect 14.34
    xenon arc
      for
        destruction of lesion 14.23
        reattachment 14.53
        repair of tear or defect 14.33
Photography 89.39
  fundus 95.11
Photopheresis, therapeutic 99.88
Phototherapy NEC 99.83
  newborn 99.83
  ultraviolet 99.82
Phrenemphraxis 04.03
  for collapse of lung 33.31
Phrenicectomy 04.03
  for collapse of lung 33.31
Phrenicoexeresis 04.03
  for collapse of lung 33.31
Phrenicotomy 04.03
  for collapse of lung 33.31
Phrenicotripsy 04.03
  for collapse of lung 33.31
Phrenoplasty 34.84
Physical medicine — see Therapy, physical
Physical therapy — see Therapy, physical
Physiotherapy, chest 93.99
Piercing ear, external (pinna) 18.01
Pigmenting, skin 86.02
Pilojection (aneurysm) (Gallagher) 39.52
Pinealectomy (complete) (total) 07.54
  partial 07.53
Pinealotomy (with drainage) 07.52
Pinning
  bone — see Fixation, bone, internal
  ear 18.5
Pinsker operation (obliteration of nasoseptal telangiectasia) 21.07
Piper operation (forceps) 72.6
Pirogoff operation (ankle amputation through malleoli of tibia and fibula) 84.14
Pituitectomy (complete) (total) (see also Hypophysectomy) 07.69
Placentogram, placentography 88.46
  with radioisotope (RISA) 92.17
Planing, skin 86.25
Plantation, tooth (bud) (germ) 23.5
  prosthetic 23.6
Plasma exchange 99.07
Plasmapheresis, therapeutic 99.71
Plastic repair — see Repair, by site
Plasty — see also Repair, by site
  bladder neck (V-Y) 57.85
  skin (without graft) 86.89
  subcutaneous tissue 86.89
Plateletpheresis, therapeutic 99.74
Play
  psychotherapy 94.36
  therapy 93.81
Pleating
  eye muscle 15.22
    multiple (two or more muscles) 15.4
  sclera, for buckling (see also Buckling, scleral) 14.49
Plethysmogram (carotid) 89.58

  air-filled (pneumatic) 89.58
  capacitance 89.58
  cerebral 89.58
  differential 89.58
  oculoplethysmogram 89.58
  photoelectric 89.58
  regional 89.58
  respiratory function measurement (body) 89.38
  segmental 89.58
  strain-gauge 89.58
  thoracic impedance 89.38
  venous occlusion 89.58
  water-filled 89.58
Pleurectomy NEC 34.59
Pleurocentesis 34.91
Pleurodesis 34.6
  chemical 34.92
    with cancer chemotherapy substance 34.92 [99.25]
    tetracycline 34.92 [99.21]
Pleurolysis (for collapse of lung) 33.39
Pleuropexy 34.99
Pleurosclerosis 34.6
  chemical 34.92
    with cancer chemotherapy substance 34.92 [99.25]
    tetracycline 34.92 [99.21]
Pleurotomy 34.09
Plexectomy
  choroid 02.14
  hypogastric 05.24
Plication
  annulus, heart valve 35.33
  bleb (emphysematous), lung 32.21
  broad ligament 69.22
  diaphragm (for hernia repair) (thoracic approach) (thoracoabdominal approach) 53.81
  eye muscle (oblique) (rectus) 15.22
    multiple (two or more muscles) 15.4
  fascia 83.89
    hand 82.89
  inferior vena cava 38.7
  intestine (jejunum) (Noble) 46.62
  Kelly (-Stoeckel) (urethrovesical junction) 59.3
  levator, for blepharoptosis 08.34
  ligament (see also Arthroplasty) 81.96
    broad 69.22
    round 69.22
    uterosacral 69.22
  mesentery 54.75
  round ligament 69.22
  sphincter, urinary bladder 57.85
  stomach 44.69
  superior vena cava 38.7
  tendon 83.85
    hand 82.55
  tricuspid valve (with repositioning) 35.14
  ureter 56.89
  urethra 58.49
  urethrovesical junction 59.3
  vein (peripheral) 39.59
  vena cava (inferior) (superior) 38.7
  ventricle (heart) 37.99
Plicotomy, tympanum 20.23
Plombage, lung 33.39
Pneumocentesis 33.93
Pneumocisternogram 87.02
Pneumoencephalogram 87.01

Pneumogram, pneumography
- extraperitoneal 88.15
- mediastinal 87.33
- orbit 87.14
- pelvic 88.13
- peritoneum NEC 88.13
- presacral 88.15
- retroperitoneum 88.15

Pneumogynecography 87.82
Pneumomediastinography 87.33
Pneumonectomy (complete) (extended) (radical) (standard) (total) (with mediastinaldissection) 32.5
- partial
  - complete excision, one lobe 32.4
  - resection (wedge), one lobe 32.3

Pneumonolysis (for collapse of lung) 33.39
Pneumonotomy (with exploration) 33.1
Pneumoperitoneum (surgically-induced) 54.96
- for collapse of lung 33.33
- pelvic 88.12

Pneumothorax (artificial) (surgical) 33.32
- intrapleural 33.32

Pneumoventriculogram 87.02
Politano-Leadbetter operation (ureteroneocystostomy) 56.74
Politerization, Eustachian tube 20.8
Pollicization (with carry over of nerves and blood supply) 82.61
Polya operation (gastrectomy) 43.7
Polypectomy — *see also* Excision, lesion, by site
- esophageal 42.32
  - endoscopic 42.33
- gastric (endoscopic) 43.41
- large intestine (colon) 45.42
- nasal 21.31

Polysomnogram 89.17
Pomeroy operation (ligation and division of fallopian tubes) 66.32
Poncet operation
- lengthening of Achilles tendon 83.85
- urethrostomy, perineal 58.0

Porro operation (cesarean section) 74.99
Positrocephalogram 92.11
Positron emission tomography (PET) — *see* Scan, radioisotope
Postmortem examination 89.8
Potts-Smith operation (descending aorta-left pulmonary artery anastomosis) 39.0
Poudrage
- intrapericardial 36.3
- pleural 34.6

PPN (peripheral parenteral nutrition) 99.15
Preparation (cutting), pedicle (flap) graft 86.71
Preputiotomy 64.91
Prescription for glasses 95.31
Pressure support
- ventilation [PSV] - *see* category 96.7

Printen and Mason operation (high gastric bypass) 44.31
Probing
- canaliculus, lacrimal (with irrigation) 09.42
- lacrimal
  - canaliculi 09.42
    - punctum (with irrigation) 09.41
  - nasolacrimal duct (with irrigation) 09.43
- with insertion of tube or stent 09.44
- salivary duct (for dilation of duct) (for removal of calculus) 26.91
  - with incision 26.0

Procedure — *see also* specific procedure
- diagnostic NEC
  - abdomen (region) 54.29
  - adenoid 28.19
  - adrenal gland 07.19
  - alveolus 24.19
  - amnion 75.35
  - anterior chamber, eye 12.29
  - anus 49.29
  - appendix 45.28
  - biliary tract 51.19
  - bladder 57.39
  - blood vessel (any site) 38.29
  - bone 78.80
    - carpal, metacarpal 78.84
    - clavicle 78.81
    - facial 76.19
    - femur 78.85
    - fibula 78.87
    - humerus 78.82
    - marrow 41.38
    - patella 78.86
    - pelvic 78.89
    - phalanges (foot) (hand) 78.89
    - radius 78.83
    - scapula 78.81
    - specified site NEC 78.89
    - tarsal, metatarsal 78.88
    - thorax (ribs) (sternum) 78.81
    - tibia 78.87
    - ulna 78.83
    - vertebrae 78.89
  - brain 01.18
  - breast 85.19
  - bronchus 33.29
  - buccal 27.24
  - bursa 83.29
  - canthus 08.19
  - cecum 45.28
  - cerebral meninges 01.18
  - cervix 67.19
  - chest wall 34.28
  - choroid 14.19
  - ciliary body 12.29
  - clitoris 71.19
  - colon 45.28
  - conjunctiva 10.29
  - cornea 11.29
  - cul-de-sac 70.29
  - dental 24.19
  - diaphragm 34.28
  - duodenum 45.19
  - ear
    - external 18.19
    - inner and middle 20.39
  - epididymis 63.09
  - esophagus 42.29
  - Eustachian tube 20.39
  - extraocular muscle or tendon 15.09
  - eye 16.29
    - interior chamber 12.29
    - posterior chamber 14.19
  - eyeball 16.29
  - eyelid 08.19
  - fallopian tube 66.19
  - fascia (any site) 83.29
  - fetus 75.25
  - gallbladder 51.19
  - ganglion (cranial) (peripheral) 04.19
    - sympathetic 05.19
  - gastric 44.19
  - globus pallidus 01.18
  - gum 24.19
  - heart 37.29
  - hepatic 50.19
  - hypophysis 07.19
  - ileum 45.19
  - intestine 45.29
    - large 45.28
    - small 45.19
  - iris 12.29
  - jejunum 45.19
  - joint (capsule) (ligament) (structure) NEC 81.98
    - facial 76.19
  - kidney 55.29
  - labia 71.19
  - lacrimal (system) 09.19
  - large intestine 45.28
  - larynx 31.48
  - ligament 81.98
    - uterine 68.19
  - liver 50.19
  - lung 33.29
  - lymphatic structure (channel) (gland) (node) (vessel) 40.19
  - mediastinum 34.29
  - meninges (cerebral) 01.18
    - spinal 03.39
  - mouth 27.29
  - muscle 83.29
    - extraocular (oblique) (rectus) 15.09
    - papillary (heart) 37.29
  - nail 86.19
  - nasopharynx 29.19
  - nerve (cranial) (peripheral) NEC 04.19
    - sympathetic 05.19
  - nipple 85.19
  - nose, nasal 21.29
    - sinus 22.19
  - ocular 16.29
    - muscle 15.09
  - omentum 54.29
  - ophthalmologic 16.29
  - oral (cavity) 27.29
  - orbit 16.29
  - orthodontic 24.19
  - ovary 65.19
  - palate 27.29
  - pancreas 52.19
  - papillary muscle (heart) 37.29
  - parathyroid gland 06.19
  - penis 64.19
  - perianal tissue 49.29
  - pericardium 37.29
  - periprostatic tissue 60.18
  - perirectal tissue 48.29
  - perirenal tissue 59.29
  - peritoneum 54.29
  - periurethral tissue 58.29
  - perivesical tissue 59.29
  - pharynx 29.19
  - pineal gland 07.19
  - pituitary gland 07.19
  - pleura 34.28
  - posterior chamber, eye 14.19
  - prostate 60.18
  - pulmonary 33.29
  - rectosigmoid 48.29
  - rectum 48.29
  - renal 55.29
  - respiratory 33.29
  - retina 14.19
  - retroperitoneum 59.29
  - salivary gland or duct 26.19
  - sclera 12.29
  - scrotum 61.19
  - seminal vesicle 60.19
  - sigmoid 45.28

sinus, nasal 22.19
skin 86.19
skull 01.19
soft tissue 83.29
spermatic cord 63.09
sphincter of Oddi 51.19
spine, spinal (canal) (cord) (meninges) (structure) 03.39
spleen 41.39
stomach 44.19
subcutaneous tissue 86.19
sympathetic nerve 05.19
tarsus 09.19
tendon NEC 83.29
   extraocular 15.09
testicle 62.19
thalamus 01.18
thoracic duct 40.19
thorax 34.28
thymus 07.19
thyroid gland 06.19
tongue 25.09
tonsils 28.19
tooth 24.19
trachea 31.49
tunica vaginalis 61.19
ureter 56.39
urethra 58.29
uterus and supporting structures 68.19
uvula 27.29
vagina 70.29
vas deferens 63.09
vesical 57.39
vessel (bloody) (any site) 38.2
vitreous 14.19
vulva 71.19
fistulizing, sclera NEC 12.69
miscellaneous (nonoperative) NEC 99.99
respiratory (nonoperative) NEC 93.99
surgical — see Operation

Proctectasis 96.22
Proctectomy (partial) (see also Resection, rectum) 48.69
  abdominoperineal 48.5
  complete (Miles) (Rankin) 48.5
  pull-through 48.49
Proctoclysis 96.37
Proctolysis 48.99
Proctopexy (Delorme) 48.76
  abdominal (Ripstein) 48.75
Proctoplasty 48.79
Proctorrhaphy 48.71
Proctoscopy 48.23
  with biopsy 48.24
  through stoma (artificial) 48.22
  transabdominal approach 48.21
Proctosigmoidectomy (see also Resection, rectum) 48.69
Proctosigmoidopexy 48.76
  with biopsy 48.24
  flexible 45.24
  through stoma (artificial) 48.22
  transabdominal approach 48.21
Proctostomy 48.1
Proctotomy (decompression) (linear) 48.0
Production — see also Formation
  atrial septal defect 35.42
  subcutaneous tunnel for esophageal anastomosis 42.86
    with anastomosis — see Anastomosis, esophagus, antesternal
Prognathic recession 76.64

Prophylaxis, dental (scaling) (polishing) 96.54
Prostatectomy (complete) (partial) NEC 60.69
  loop 60.2
  perineal 60.62
  radical (any approach) 60.5
  retropubic (punch) (transcapsular) 60.4
  suprapubic (punch) (transvesical) 60.3
  transcapsular NEC 60.69
    retropubic 60.4
  transurethral 60.2
  transvesical punch (suprapubic) 60.3
Prostatocystotomy 60.0
Prostatolithotomy 60.0
Prostatotomy (perineal) 60.0
Prostatovesiculectomy 60.5
Protection (of)
  individual from his surroundings 99.84
  surroundings from individual 99.84
Psychoanalysis 94.31
Psychodrama 94.43
Psychotherapy NEC 94.39
  biofeedback 94.39
  exploratory verbal 94.37
  group 94.44
    for psychosexual dysfunctions 94.41
  play 94.36
  psychosexual dysfunctions 94.34
  supportive verbal 94.38
PTCA (percutaneous transluminal coronary angioplasty) — see Angioplasty, balloon, coronary
Ptyalectasis 26.91
Ptyalithotomy 26.0
Ptyalolithotomy 26.0
Pubiotomy 77.39
  assisting delivery 73.94
Pubococcygeoplasty 59.71
Puestow operation (pancreaticojejunostomy) 52.96
Pull-through
  abdomino-anal 48.49
  abdominoperineal 48.49
    Duhamel type 48.65
  endorectal 48.41
Pulmowrap 93.99
Pulpectomy (see also Therapy, root canal) 23.70
Pulpotomy (see also Therapy, root canal) 23.70
Pump-oxygenator, for extracorporeal circulation 39.61
  percutaneous 39.66
Punch
  operation
    bladder neck, transurethral 57.49
    prostate — see Prostatectomy
  resection, vocal cords 30.22
Puncture
  antrum (nasal) (bilateral) (unilateral) 22.01
  artery NEC 38.98
    for
      arteriography (see also Arteriography) 88.40
      coronary arteriography (see also Arteriography, coronary) 88.57
  bladder, suprapubic (for drainage) NEC 57.18

    needle 57.11
    percutaneous (suprapubic) 57.17
  bursa 83.94
    hand 82.92
  cisternal 01.01
    with contrast media 87.02
  cranial 01.09
    with contrast media 87.02
  craniobuccal pouch 07.72
  craniopharyngioma 07.72
  fallopian tube 66.91
  fontanel, anterior 01.09
  heart 37.0
    for intracardiac injection 37.92
  hypophysis 07.72
  iris 12.12
  joint 81.91
  kidney (percutaneous) 55.92
  larynx 31.98
  lumbar (diagnostic) (removal of dye) 03.31
  lung (for aspiration) 33.93
  nasal sinus 22.01
  pericardium 37.0
  pituitary gland 07.72
  pleural cavity 34.91
  Rathke's pouch 07.72
  spinal 03.31
  spleen 41.1
    for biopsy 41.32
  sternal (for bone marrow biopsy) 41.31
    donor for bone marrow transplant 41.91
  vein NEC 38.99
    for
      phlebography (see also Phlebography) 88.60
    transfusion — see Transfusion
  ventricular shunt tubing 01.02
Pupillotomy 12.35
Push-back operation (cleft palate repair) 27.62
Putti-Platt operation (capsulorrhaphy of shoulder for recurrent dislocation) 81.82
Pyelogram (intravenous) 87.73
  infusion (continuous) (diuretic) 87.73
  percutaneous 87.75
  retrograde 87.74
Pyeloileostomy 56.71
Pyelolithotomy 55.11
Pyeloplasty 55.87
Pyelorrhaphy 55.81
Pyeloscopy 55.22
Pyelostolithotomy, percutaneous 55.03
Pyelostomy 55.12
  closure 55.82
Pyelotomy 55.11
Pyeloureteroplasty 55.87
Pylorectomy 43.6
Pyloroduodenotomy — see category 44.2
Pyloromyotomy (Ramstedt) (with wedge resection) 43.3
Pyloroplasty (Finney) (Heineke-Mikulicz) 44.29
  dilation, endoscopic 44.22
    by incision 44.21
  NEC 44.29
  revision 44.29
Pylorostomy — Gastrostomy

Q

Quadrant resection of breast 85.22
Quadricepsplasty (Thompson) 83.86
Quarantine 99.84
Quenuthoracoplasty 77.31
Quotient, respiratory 89.38

R

Rachicentesis 03.31
Rachitomy 03.09
Radiation therapy — *see also* Therapy, radiation
    teleradiotherapy — *see* Teleradiotherapy
Radical neck dissection — *see* Dissection, neck
Radicotomy 03.1
Radiculectomy 03.1
Radiculotomy 03.1
Radiography (diagnostic) NEC 88.39
    abdomen, abdominal (flat plate) NEC 88.19
        wall (soft tissue) NEC 88.09
    adenoid 87.09
    ankle (skeletal) 88.28
        soft tissue 88.37
    bone survey 88.31
    bronchus 87.49
    chest (routine) 87.44
        wall NEC 87.39
    clavicle 87.43
    contrast (air) (gas) (radio-opaque substance) NEC
        abdominal wall 88.03
        arteries (by fluoroscopy) — *see* Arteriography
        bile ducts NEC 87.54
        bladder NEC 87.77
        brain 87.02
        breast 87.35
        bronchus NEC (transcricoid) 87.32
            endotracheal 87.31
        epididymis 87.93
        esophagus 87.61
        fallopian tubes
            gas 87.82
            opaque dye 87.83
        fistula (sinus tract) — *see also* Radiography, contrast, by site
            abdominal wall 88.03
            chest wall 87.38
        gallbladder NEC 87.59
        intervertebral disc(s) 87.21
        joints 88.32
        larynx 87.07
        lymph — *see* Lymphangiogram
        mammary ducts 87.35
        mediastinum 87.33
        nasal sinuses 87.15
        nasolacrimal ducts 87.05
        nasopharynx 87.06
        orbit 87.14
        pancreas 87.66
        pelvis
            gas 88.12
            opaque dye 88.11
        peritoneum NEC 88.13
        retroperitoneum NEC 88.15
        seminal vesicles 87.91
        sinus tract — *see also* Radiography, contrast, by site
            abdominal wall 88.03
            chest wall 87.38
            nose 87.15
        skull 87.02
        spinal disc(s) 87.21
        trachea 87.32
        uterus
            gas 87.82
            opaque dye 87.83
        vas deferens 87.94
        veins (by fluoroscopy) — *see* Phlebography
        vena cava (inferior) (superior) 88.51
    dental NEC 87.12
    diaphragm 87.49
    digestive tract NEC 87.69
        barium swallow 87.61
        lower GI series 87.64
        small bowel series 87.63
        upper GI series 87.62
    elbow (skeletal) 88.22
        soft tissue 88.35
    epididymis NEC 87.95
    esophagus 87.69
        barium-swallow 87.61
    eye 95.14
    face, head, and neck 87.09
    facial bones 87.16
    fallopian tubes 87.85
    foot 88.28
    forearm (skeletal) 88.22
        soft tissue 88.35
    frontal area, facial 87.16
    genital organs
        female NEC 87.89
        male NEC 87.99
    hand (skeletal) 88.23
        soft tissue 88.35
    head NEC 87.09
    heart 87.49
    hip (skeletal) 88.26
        soft tissue 88.37
    intestine NEC 87.65
    kidney-ureter-bladder (KUB) 87.79
    knee (skeletal) 88.27
        soft tissue 88.37
    KUB (kidney-ureter-bladder) 87.79
    larynx 87.09
    lower leg (skeletal) 88.27
        soft tissue
    lower limb (skeletal) NEC 88.29
        soft tissue NEC 88.37
    lung 87.49
    mandible 87.16
    maxilla 87.16
    mediastinum 87.49
    nasal sinuses 87.16
    nasolacrimal duct 87.09
    nasopharynx 87.09
    neck NEC 87.09
    nose 87.16
    orbit 87.16
    pelvis (skeletal) 88.26
        pelvimetry 88.25
        soft tissue 88.19
    prostate NEC 87.92
    retroperitoneum NEC 88.16
    ribs 87.43
    root canal 87.12
    salivary gland 87.09
    seminal vesicles NEC 87.92
    shoulder (skeletal) 88.21
        soft tissue 88.35
    skeletal NEC 88.33
        series (whole or complete) 88.31
    skull (lateral, sagittal or tangential projection) NEC 87.17
    spine NEC 87.29
        cervical 87.22
        lumbosacral 87.24
        sacrococcygeal 87.24
        thoracic 87.23
    sternum 87.43
    supraorbital area 87.16
    symphysis menti 87.16
    teeth NEC 87.12
        full-mouth 87.11
    thigh (skeletal) 88.27
        soft tissue 88.37
    thyroid region 87.09
    tonsils and adenoids 87.09
    trachea 87.49
    ultrasonic — *see* Ultrasonography
    upper arm (skeletal) 88.21
        soft tissue 88.35
    upper limb (skeletal) NEC 88.24
        soft tissue NEC 88.35
    urinary system NEC 87.79
    uterus NEC 87.85
        gravid 87.81
    uvula 87.09
    vas deferens NEC 87.95
    wrist 88.23
    zygomaticomaxillary complex 87.16
Radioisotope
    scanning — *see* Scan, radioisotope
    therapy — *see* Therapy, radioisotope
Radiology
    diagnostic — *see* Radiography
    therapeutic — *see* Therapy, radiation
Raising, pedicle graft 86.71
Ramadier operation (intrapetrosal drainage) 20.22
Ramisection (sympathetic) 05.0
Ramstedt operation (pyeloromyotomy) (with wedge resection) 43.3
Range of motion testing 93.05
Rankin operation
    exteriorization of intestine 46.03
    proctectomy (complete) 48.5
Rashkind operation (balloon septostomy) 35.41
Rastelli operation (creation of conduit between right ventricle and pulmonary artery) 35.92
    in repair of
        pulmonary artery atresia 35.92
        transposition of great vessels 35.92
        truncus arteriosus 35.83
Raz-Pereyra procedure (Bladder neck suspension) 59.79
Readjustment — *see* Adjustment
Reamputation, stump 84.3
Reanastomosis — *see* Anastomosis
Reattachment
    amputated ear 18.72
    ankle 84.27
    arm (upper) NEC 84.24
    choroid and retina NEC 14.59
    by
        cryotherapy 14.52
        diathermy 14.51
        electrocoagulation 14.51
        photocoagulation 14.55
            laser 14.54
            xenon arc 14.53
    ear (amputated) 18.72
    extremity 84.29
        ankle 84.27

arm (upper) NEC 84.24
fingers, except thumb 84.22
   thumb 84.21
foot 84.26
forearm 84.23
hand 84.23
leg (lower) NEC 84.27
thigh 84.28
thumb 84.21
toe 84.25
wrist 84.23
finger 84.22
   thumb 84.21
foot 84.26
forearm 84.23
hand 84.23
joint capsule (*see also* Arthroplasty) 81.96
leg (lower) NEC 84.27
ligament — *see also* Arthroplasty
   uterosacral 69.22
muscle 83.74
   hand 82.54
   papillary (heart) 35.31
nerve (peripheral) 04.79
nose (amputated) 21.89
papillary muscle (heart) 35.31
penis (amputated) 64.45
retina (and choroid) NEC 14.59
   by
      cryotherapy 14.52
      diathermy 14.51
      electrocoagulation 14.51
      photocoagulation 14.55
         laser 14.54
         xenon arc 14.53
tendon (to tendon) 83.73
   hand 82.53
   to skeletal attachment 83.88
      hand 82.85
thigh 84.28
thumb 84.21
toe 84.25
tooth 23.5
uterosacral ligament(s) 69.22
vessels (peripheral) 39.59
   renal, aberrant 39.55
wrist 84.23

Recession
extraocular muscle 15.11
   multiple (two or more muscles) (with advancement of resection) 15.3
gastrocnemius tendon (Strayer operation) 83.72
levator palpebrae (superioris) muscle 08.38
prognathic jaw 76.64
tendon 83.72
   hand 82.52

Reclosure — *see also* Closure
disrupted abdominal wall (postoperative) 54.61

Reconstruction (plastic) — *see also* Construction and Repair, by site
alveolus, alveolar (process) (ridge) (with graft or implant) 24.5
artery (graft) — *see* Graft, artery
artificial stoma, intestine 46.40
auditory canal (external) 18.6
auricle (ear) 18.71
bladder 57.87
   with
      ileum 57.87 [45.51]
      sigmoid 57.87 [45.52]

bone, except facial (*see also* Osteoplasty) 78.40
   facial NEC 76.46
      with total ostectomy 76.44
   mandible 76.43
      with total mandibulectomy 76.41
breast, total 85.7
bronchus 33.48
canthus (lateral) 08.59
cardiac annulus 35.33
chest wall (mesh) (silastic) 34.79
cleft lip 27.54
conjunctival cul-de-sac 10.43
   with graft (buccal mucous membrane) (free) 10.42
cornea NEC 11.79
diaphragm 34.84
ear (external) (auricle) 18.71
   external auditory canal 18.6
   meatus (new) (osseous skin-lined) 18.6
   ossicles 19.3
   prominent or protruding 18.5
eyebrow 08.70
eyelid 08.70
   with graft or flap 08.69
      hair follicle 08.63
      mucous membrane 08.62
      skin 08.61
      tarsoconjunctival (one-stage) (two-stage) 08.64
   full-thickness 08.74
      involving lid margin 08.73
   partial-thickness 08.72
      involving lid margin 08.71
eye socket 16.64
   with graft 16.63
fallopian tube 66.79
foot and toes (with fixation device) 81.57
   with prosthetic implant 81.57
frontonasal duct 22.79
hip (total) (with prosthesis) 81.51
intraoral 27.59
joint — *see* Arthroplasty
lymphatic (by transplantation) 40.9
mandible 76.43
   with total mandibulectomy 76.41
mastoid cavity 19.9
mouth 27.59
nipple NEC 85.87
nose (total) (with arm flap) (with forehead flap) 21.83
ossicles (graft) (prosthesis) NEC 19.3
   with
      stapedectomy 19.19
      tympanoplasty 19.53
pelvic floor 71.79
penis (rib graft) (skin graft) (myocutaneous flap) 64.44
pharynx 29.4
scrotum (with pedicle flap) (with rotational flap) 61.49
skin (plastic) (without graft) NEC 86.89
   with graft — *see* Graft, skin
subcutaneous tissue (plastic) (without skin graft) NEC 86.89
   with graft — *see* Graft, skin
tendon pulley — (with graft) (with local tissue) 83.83
   for opponensplasty 82.71
      hand 82.71
thumb (osteoplastic) (with bone graft) (with skin graft) 82.69
trachea (with graft) 31.75
umbilicus 53.49

ureteropelvic junction 55.87
urethra 58.46
vagina 70.62
vas deferens, surgically divided 63.82

Recontour, gingiva 24.2
Recreational therapy 93.81
Rectectomy (*see also* Resection, rectum) 48.69
Rectopexy (Delorme) 48.76
   abdominal (Ripstein) 48.75
Rectoplasty 48.79
Rectorectostomy 48.74
Rectorrhaphy 48.71
Rectosigmoidectomy (*see also* Resection, rectum) 48.69
   transsacral 48.61
Rectosigmoidostomy 45.94
Rectostomy 48.1
   closure 48.72
Red cell survival studies 92.05
Reduction
adipose tissue 86.83
batwing arms 86.83
breast (bilateral) 85.32
   unilateral 85.31
bulbous tuberosities (mandible) (maxilla) (fibrous) (osseous) 24.31
buttocks 86.83
diastasis, ankle mortise (closed) 79.77
   open 79.87
dislocation (of joint) (manipulation) (with cast) (with splint) (with traction device) (closed) 79.70
   with fracture — *see* Reduction, fracture, by site
   ankle (closed) 79.77
      open 79.87
   elbow (closed) 79.72
      open 79.82
   finger (closed) 79.74
      open 79.84
   foot (closed) 79.78
      open 79.88
   hand (closed) 79.74
      open 79.84
   hip (closed) 79.75
      open 79.85
   knee (closed) 79.76
      open 79.86
   open (with external fixation) (with internal fixation) 79.80
   specified site NEC 79.89
   shoulder (closed) 79.71
      open 79.81
   specified site (closed) NEC 79.79
      open 79.89
   temporomandibular (closed) 76.93
      open 76.94
   toe (closed) 79.78
      open 79.88
   wrist (closed) 79.73
      open 79.83
elephantiasis, scrotum 61.3
epistaxis (*see also* Control, epistaxis) 21.00
fracture (bone) (with cast) (with splint) (with traction device) (closed) 79.00
   with internal fixation 79.10
   alveolar process (with stabilization of teeth)
      mandible (closed) 76.75
         open 76.77
      maxilla (closed) 76.73
         open 76.77

open 76.77
ankle — see Reduction, fracture, leg
arm (closed) NEC 79.02
    with external fixation 79.12
    open 79.22
        with internal fixation 79.32
blow-out — see Reduction, fracture, orbit
carpal, metacarpal (closed) 79.03
    with internal fixation 79.13
    open 79.23
        with internal fixation 79.33
epiphysis — see Reduction, separation
facial (bone) NEC 76.70
    closed 76.78
    open 76.79
femur (closed) 79.05
    with internal fixation 79.15
    open
        with internal fixation 79.35
fibula (closed) 79.07
    with internal fixation 79.16
    open 79.26
        with internal fixation 79.36
foot (closed) NEC 79.07
    with internal fixation 79.17
    open 79.27
        with internal fixation 79.37
hand (closed) NEC 79.03
    with internal fixation 79.13
    open 79.23
        with internal fixation 79.33
humerus (closed) 79.01
    with internal fixation 79.11
    open 79.21
        with internal fixation 79.31
jaw (lower) — see also Reduction, fracture, mandible
    upper — see Reduction, fracture, maxilla
larynx 31.64
leg (closed) NEC 79.06
    with internal fixation 79.16
    open 79.26
        with internal fixation 79.36
malar (closed) 76.71
    open 76.72
mandible (with dental wiring) (closed) 76.75
    open 76.76
maxilla (with dental wiring) (closed) 76.73
    open 76.74
nasal (closed) 21.71
    open 21.72
open 79.20
    with internal fixation 79.30
    specified site NEC 79.29
        with internal fixation 79.39
orbit (rim) (wall) (closed) 76.78
    open 76.79
patella (open) (with internal fixation) 79.36
phalanges
    foot (closed) 79.08
        with internal fixation 79.18
        open
            with internal fixation 79.38
    hand (closed) 79.04
        with internal fixation 79.14
        open 79.24
            with internal fixation 79.34
radius (closed) 79.02
    with internal fixation 79.12
    open 79.22
        with internal fixation 79.32
skull 02.02
specified site (closed) NEC 79.09
    with internal fixation 79.39
    open 79.29
        with internal fixation 79.39
spine 03.53
tarsal, metatarsal (closed) 79.07
    with internal fixation 79.17
    open 79.27
        with internal fixation 79.37
tibia (closed) 79.06
    with internal fixation 79.16
    open 79.26
        with internal fixation 79.36
ulna (closed) 79.02
    with internal fixation 79.12
    open 79.22
        with internal fixation 79.32
vertebra 03.53
zygoma, zygomatic arch (closed) 76.71
    open 76.72
fracture-dislocation — see Reduction, fracture
hemorrhoids (manual) 49.41
hernia — see also Repair, hernia
    manual 96.27
intussusception 46.80
    large intestine 46.82
        endoscopic (balloon) 46.85
    small intestine 46.81
malrotation, intestine (manual) (surgical) 46.80
    large 46.82
        endoscopic (balloon) 46.85
    small 46.81
mammoplasty (bilateral) 85.32
    unilateral 85.31
prolapse
    anus (operative) 49.94
    colostomy (manual) 96.28
    enterostomy (manual) 96.28
    ileostomy (manual) 96.28
    rectum (manual) 96.26
    uterus
        by pessary 96.18
        surgical 69.22
ptosis overcorrection 08.37
retroversion, uterus by pessary 96.18
separation, epiphysis (with internal fixation) (closed) 79.40
    femur (closed) 79.45
        open 79.55
    fibular (closed) 79.46
        open 79.56
    humerus (closed) 79.41
        open 79.51
    open 79.50
    specified site (closed) NEC — see also category 79.4
    open — see category 79.5
    tibia (closed) 79.46
        open 79.56
size
    abdominal wall (adipose) (pendulous) 86.83
    arms (adipose) (batwing) 86.83
    breast (bilateral) 85.32
        unilateral 85.31
    buttocks (adipose) 86.83
    finger (macrodactyly repair) 82.83
    skin 86.83
    subcutaneous tissue 86.83
    thighs (adipose) 86.83
torsion
    intestine (manual) (surgical) 46.80
        large 46.82
            endoscopic (balloon) 46.85
        small 46.81
    kidney pedicle 55.84
    omentum 54.74
    spermatic cord 63.52
        with orchiopexy 62.5
    testis 63.52
        with orchiopexy 62.5
    uterus NEC 69.98
        gravid 75.99
volvulus
    intestine 46.80
        large 46.82
            endoscopic (balloon) 46.85
        small 46.81
    stomach 44.92

Reefing, joint capsule (see also Arthroplasty) 81.96
Re-entry operation (aorta) 39.54
Re-establishment, continuity — see also Anastomosis
    bowel 46.50
    fallopian tube 66.79
    vas deferens 63.82
Referral (for)
    psychiatric aftercare (halfway house) (outpatient clinic) 94.52
    psychotherapy 94.51
    rehabilitation
        alcoholism 94.53
        drug addiction 94.54
        psychologic NEC 94.59
        vocational 94.55
Reformation
    cardiac pacemaker pocket, new site (skin) (subcutaneous) 37.79
    chamber of eye 12.99
Refracture
    bone (for faulty union) (see also Osteoclasis) 78.70
    nasal bones 21.88
Refusion, spine (any level) (any technique) 81.09
Regional blood flow study 92.05
Regulation, menstrual 69.6
Rehabilitation programs NEC 93.89
    alcohol 94.61
        with detoxification 94.63
        combined alcohol and drug 94.67
            with detoxification 94.69
    drug 94.64
        with detoxification 94.66
        combined drug and alcohol 94.67
            with detoxification 94.69
    sheltered employment 93.85
    vocational 93.85
Reimplantation
    adrenal tissue (heterotopic) (orthotopic) 07.45
    artery 39.59
        renal, aberrant 39.55
    bile ducts following excision of ampulla of Vater 51.62
    extremity — see Reattachment, extremity
    fallopian tube into uterus 66.74
    kidney 55.61
    lung 33.5
    ovary 65.72
    pancreatic tissue 52.81

parathyroid tissue (heterotopic)
  (orthotopic) 06.95
pulmonary artery for hemitruncus repair
  35.83
renal vessel, aberrant 39.55
testis in scrotum 62.5
thyroid tissue (heterotopic) (orthotopic)
  06.94
tooth 23.5
ureter into bladder 56.74
Reinforcement — *see also* Repair, by site
  sclera NEC 12.88
    with graft 12.87
Reinsertion — *see also* Insertion or Revision
  cystostomy tube 59.94
  fixation device (internal) (*see also* Fixation,
    bone, internal) 78.50
  heart valve (prosthetic) 35.95
  Holter (-Spitz) valve 02.42
  implant (expelled) (extruded)
    eyeball (with conjunctival graft) 16.62
    orbital 16.62
  nephrostomy tube 55.93
  pyelostomy tube 55.94
  ureteral stent (transurethral) 59.8
    with ureterotomy 59.8 [56.2]
  ureterostomy tube 59.93
  valve
    heart (prosthetic) 39.95
    ventricular (cerebral) 02.42
Relaxation — *see also* Release
  training 94.33
Release
  carpal tunnel (for nerve decompression)
    04.43
  celiac artery axis 39.91
  central slip, extensor tendon hand (mallet
    finger repair) 82.84
  chordee 62.42
  clubfoot NEC 83.84
  de Quervain's tenosynovitis 82.01
  Dupuytren's contracture (by palmar
    fasciectomy) 82.35
    by fasciotomy (subcutaneous) 82.12
      with excision 82.35
  Fowler (mallet finger repair) 82.84
  joint (capsule) (adherent) (constrictive)
    (*see also* Division, joint capsule)
    80.40
  laryngeal 31.92
  ligament (*see also* Division, ligament) 80.40
    median arcuate 39.91
  median arcuate ligament 39.91
  muscle (division) 83.19
    hand 82.19
  nerve (peripheral) NEC 04.49
    cranial NEC 04.42
    trigeminal 04.41
  pressure, intraocular 12.79
  scar tissue
    skin 86.64
    stoma — *see* Revision, stoma
  tarsal tunnel 04.44
  tendon 83.13
    hand 82.11
      extensor, central slip (repair mallet
        finger) 82.84
    sheath 83.01
      hand 82.01
  tenosynovitis 83.01
    abductor pollicis longus 82.01
    de Quervain's 82.01

external pollicis brevis 82.01
hand 82.01
torsion
  intestine 46.80
    large 46.82
      endoscopic (balloon) 46.85
    small 46.81
  kidney pedicle 55.84
  ovary 65.95
  testes 63.52
transverse carpal ligament (for nerve
  decompression) 04.43
trigger finger or thumb 82.01
urethral stricture 58.5
Volkmann's contracture
  excision of scar, muscle 83.32
  fasciotomy 83.14
  muscle transplantation 83.77
web contracture (skin) 86.84
Relief — *see* Release
Relocation — *see also* Revision
  cardiac pacemaker pocket, new site (skin)
    (subcutaneous) 37.79
Remobilization
  joint 93.16
  stapes 19.0
Removal — *see also* Excision
  Abrams bar (chest wall) 34.01
  Abscess — *see* Incision, by site
  adenoid tag(s) 28.6
  arch bars (orthodontic) 24.8
    immobilization device 97.33
  arterial graft or prosthesis 39.49
  arteriovenous shunt (device) 39.43
    with creation of new shunt 39.42
  Barton's tongs (skull) 02.95
    with synchronous replacement 02.94
  bladder sphincter, artificial 58.99
    with replacement 58.93
  blood clot — *see also* Incision, by site
    bladder (by incision) 57.19
      without incision 57.0
    kidney (without incision) 56.0
      by incision 55.01
    ureter (by catheter) (without incision)
      56.0
      by incision 56.2
  bone fragment (chip) (*see also* Incision,
    bone) 77.10
    joint (*see also* Arthrotomy) 80.10
    necrotic (*see also* Sequestrectomy,
      bone) 77.00
      joint (*see also* Arthrotomy) 80.10
    skull 01.25
      with debridement compound
        fracture 02.02
  bone growth stimulator — *see* category 78.6
  bony spicules, spinal canal 03.53
  brace 97.88
  breast implant 85.94
    tissue expander 85.96
  calcareous deposit
    bursa 83.03
      hand 82.03
    tendon, intratendinous 83.39
      hand 82.29
  calcification, heart valve leaflets — *see*
    Valvuloplasty, heart
  calculus
    bile duct (by incision) 51.49
      endoscopic 51.88
      percutaneous 51.98
    bladder (by incision) 57.19
      without incision 57.0

common duct (by incision) 51.41
  endoscopic 51.88
  percutaneous 51.96
gallbladder 51.04
kidney (by incision) 55.01
  without incision 56.0
  percutaneous 55.03
    with fragmentation
      (ultrasound) 55.04
  renal pelvis (by incision) 55.11
    percutaneous nephrostomy
      55.03
      with fragmentation 55.04
    transurethral 56.0
lacrimal
  canaliculi 09.42
    by incision 09.52
  gland 09.3
    by incision 09.0
  passage(s) 09.49
    by incision 09.59
  punctum 09.41
    by incision 09.51
  sac 09.49
    by incision 09.53
pancreatic duct (by incision) 52.09
  endoscopic 52.94
perirenal tissue 59.09
pharynx 29.39
prostate 60.0
salivary gland (by incision) 26.0
  by probe 26.91
ureter (by incision) 56.2
  without incision 56.0
urethra (by incision) 58.0
  without incision 58.6
caliper tongs (skull) 02.95
cannula
  for extracorporeal membrane
    oxygenation (ECMO) — omit
    code
cardiac pacemaker (device) (initial)
  (permanent) 37.89
  with replacement
    dual-chamber 37.87
    single-chamber device 37.85
    rate responsive 37.86
cardioverter/defibrillator pulse generator
  without replacement 37.99
cast 97.88
  with reapplication 97.13
    lower limb 97.12
    upper limb 97.11
catheter (indwelling) — *see also* Removal,
  tube
  bladder 97.64
  middle ear (tympanum) 20.1
  ureter 97.62
  urinary 96.64
  ventricular (cerebral) 02.43
    with synchronous replacement
      02.42
cerclage material, cervix 69.96
cerumen, ear 96.52
corneal epithelium 11.41
  for smear or culture 11.21
coronary artery obstruction (thrombus)
  36.09
  direct intracoronary artery
    infusion 36.04
  open chest approach 36.03
  percutaneous transluminal (balloon)
    (single vessel) 36.01
    with thrombolytic agent infusion 36.02
    multiple vessels 36.05
Crutchfield tongs (skull) 02.95

Removal — INDEX TO PROCEDURES — Removal

with synchronous replacement 02.94
cyst — *see also* Excision, lesion, by site
  dental 24.4
  lung 32.29
    endoscopic 32.28
cystic duct remnant 51.61
decidua (by)
  aspiration curettage 69.52
  curettage (D and C) 69.02
  manual 75.4
dental wiring (immobilization device) 97.33
  orthodontic 24.8
device (therapeutic) NEC 97.89
  abdomen NEC 97.86
  digestive system NEC 97.59
  drainage — *see* Removal, tube
  external fixation device 97.88
    mandibular NEC 97.36
    minifixator (bone) — *see* category 78.6
  for musculoskeletal immobilization NEC 97.88
  genital tract NEC 97.79
  head and neck NEC 97.39
  intrauterine contraceptive 97.71
  minifixator — *see* category 78.6
  thorax NEC 97.49
  trunk NEC 97.87
  urinary system NEC 96.69
diaphragm, vagina 97.73
drainage device — *see* Removal, tube
dye, spinal canal 03.31
ectopic fetus (from) 66.02
  abdominal cavity 74.3
  extraperitoneal (intraligamentous) 74.3
  fallopian tube (by salpingostomy) 66.02
    by salpingotomy 66.01
    with salpingectomy 66.62
  intraligamentous 74.3
  ovarian 74.3
  peritoneal (following uterine or tubal rupture) 74.3
  site NEC 74.3
  tubal (by salpingostomy) 66.02
    by salpingotomy 66.01
    with salpingectomy 66.62
electrodes
  bone growth stimulator — *see* category 78.6
  brain 01.22
    with synchronous replacement 02.93
    depth 01.22
      with synchronous replacement 02.93
    foramen ovale 01.22
      with synchronous replacement 02.93
    sphenoidal — omit code
      with synchronous replacement 02.96
  cardiac pacemaker (atrial) (transvenous) (ventricular) 37.77
    with replacement 37.76
  depth 01.22
    with synchronous replacement 02.93
  epicardial (myocardial) 37.77
    with replacement (by)
      atrial and/or ventricular lead(s) (electrode) 37.76
      epicardial lead 37.74
  epidural pegs 01.22
    with synchronous replacement 02.93
  foramen ovale 01.22
    with synchronous replacement 02.93
  intracranial 01.22
    with synchronous replacement 02.93
  peripheral nerve 04.93
    with synchronous replacement 04.92
  sphenoidal — omit code
    with synchronous replacement 02.96
  spinal
    with synchronous replacement 03.93
  temporary transvenous pacemaker system — omit code
electroencephalographic receiver (brain) (intracranial) 01.22
  with synchronous replacement 02.93
electronic
  stimulator
    bladder 57.98
    bone 78.6
    brain 01.22
      with synchronous replacement 02.93
      intracranial 01.22
        with synchronous replacement 02.93
    peripheral nerve 04.93
      with synchronous replacement 04.92
    skeletal muscle 83.93
      with synchronous replacement 83.92
    spinal 03.94
      with synchronous replacement 03.93
    ureter 56.94
electrostimulator — *see* Removal, electronic, stimulator, by site
embolus 38.00
  with endarterectomy — *see* Endarterectomy
  abdominal
    artery 38.06
    vein 38.07
  aorta (arch) (ascending) (descending) 38.04
  arteriovenous shunt or cannula 39.49
  bovine graft 39.49
  head and neck vessel NEC 38.02
  intracranial vessel NEC 38.01
  lower limb
    artery 38.08
    vein 38.09
  pulmonary (artery) (vein) 38.05
  thoracic vessel NEC 38.05
  upper limb (artery) (vein) 38.03
embryo — *see* Removal, ectopic fetus
encircling tube, eye (episcleral) 14.6
epithelial downgrowth, anterior chamber 12.93
external fixation device 97.88
  mandibular NEC 97.36
  minifixator (bone) — *see* category 78.6
extrauterine embryo — *see* Removal, ectopic fetus
eyeball 16.49
  with implant 16.42
    with attachment of muscle 16.41
fallopian tube — *see* Salpingectomy
feces (impacted) (by flushing) (manual) 96.38
fetus, ectopic — *see* Removal, ectopic fetus
fixation device
  external 97.88
    mandibular NEC 97.36
    minifixator (bone) — *see* category 78.6
  internal 78.60
    carpal, metacarpal 78.64
    clavicle 78.61
    facial (bone) 76.97
    femur 78.65
    fibula 78.67
    humerus 78.62
    patella 78.66
    pelvic 78.69
    phalanges (foot) (hand) 78.69
    radius 78.63
    scapula 78.61
    specified site NEC 78.69
    tarsal, metatarsal 78.68
    thorax (ribs) (sternum) 78.61
    tibia 78.67
    ulna 78.63
    vertebrae 78.69
foreign body NEC (*see also* Incision, by site) 98.20
  abdominal (cavity) 54.92
    wall 54.0
  adenoid 98.13
    by incision 28.91
  alveolus, alveolar bone 98.22
    by incision 24.0
  antecubital fossa 98.27
    by incision 86.05
  anterior chamber 12.00
    by incision 12.02
      with use of magnet 12.01
  anus (intraluminal) 98.05
    by incision 49.93
  artificial stoma (intraluminal) 98.18
  auditory canal, external 18.02
  axilla 98.27
    by incision 86.05
  bladder (without incision) 57.0
    by incision 57.19
  bone, except fixation device (*see also* Incision, bone) 77.10
    alveolus, alveolar 98.22
      by incision 24.0
  brain 01.39
    without incision into brain 01.24
  breast 85.0
  bronchus (intraluminal) 98.15
    by incision 33.0
  bursa 83.03
    hand 82.03
  canthus 98.22
    by incision 08.51
  cerebral meninges 01.31
  cervix (intraluminal) NEC 98.16
    penetrating 69.97
  choroid (by incision) 14.00
    with use of magnet 14.01
    without use of magnet 14.02
  ciliary body (by incision) 12.00
    with use of magnet 12.01
    without use of magnet 12.02
  conjunctiva (by magnet) 98.22
    by incision 10.0
  cornea 98.21
    by
      incision 11.1
      magnet 11.0
  duodenum 98.03

by incision 45.01
ear (intraluminal) 98.11
   by incision 18.09
epididymis 63.92
esophagus (intraluminal) 98.02
   by incision 42.09
extrapleural (by incision) 34.01
eye, eyeball (by magnet) 98.21
   anterior segment (by incision) 12.00
      with use of magnet 12.01
      without use of magnet 12.02
   posterior segment (by incision) 14.00
      with use of magnet 14.01
      without use of magnet 14.02
   superficial 98.21
eyelid 98.22
   by incision 08.09
fallopian tube
   by salpingostomy 66.02
   by salpingotomy 66.01
fascia 83.09
   hand 82.09
foot 98.28
gallbladder 51.04
groin region (abdominal wall) (inguinal) 54.0
gum 98.22
   by incision 24.0
hand 98.26
head and neck NEC 98.22
heart 37.11
internal fixation device — see Removal, fixation device, internal
intestine
   by incision 45.00
   large (intraluminal) 98.04
      by incision 45.03
   small (intraluminal) 98.03
      by incision 45.02
intraocular (by incision) 12.00
   with use of magnet 12.01
   without use of magnet 12.02
iris (by incision) 12.00
   with use of magnet 12.01
   without use of magnet 12.02
joint structures (see also Arthrotomy) 80.10
kidney (transurethral) (by endoscopy) 56.0
   by incision 55.01
   pelvis (transurethral) 56.0
      by incision 55.11
labia 98.23
   by incision 71.09
lacrimal
   canaliculi 09.42
      by incision 09.52
   gland 09.3
      by incision 09.0
   passage(s) 09.49
      by incision 09.59
   punctum 09.41
      by incision 09.51
   sac 09.49
      by incision 09.53
large intestine (intraluminal 98.04
   by incision 45.03
larynx (intraluminal) 98.14
   by incision 31.3
lens 13.00
   by incision 13.02
      with use of magnet 13.01
liver 50.0
lower limb, except foot 98.29
   foot 98.28

lung 33.1
mediastinum 34.1
meninges (cerebral) 01.31
   spinal 03.01
mouth (intraluminal) 98.01
   by incision 27.92
muscle 83.02
   hand 82.02
nasal sinus 22.50
   antrum 22.2
      with Caldwell-Luc approach 22.39
   ethmoid 22.51
   frontal 22.41
   maxillary 22.2
      with Caldwell-Luc approach 22.39
   sphenoid 22.52
nerve (cranial) (peripheral) NEC 04.04
   root 03.01
nose (intraluminal) 98.12
   by incision 21.1
oral cavity (intraluminal) 98.01
   by incision 27.92
orbit (by magnet) 98.21
   by incision 16.1
palate (penetrating) 98.22
   by incision 27.1
pancreas 52.09
penis 98.24
   by incision 64.92
pericardium 37.12
perineum (female) 98.23
   by incision 71.09
   male 98.25
      by incision 86.05
perirenal tissue 59.09
peritoneal cavity 54.91
perivesical tissue 59.19
pharynx (intraluminal) 98.13
   by pharyngotomy 29.0
pleura (by incision) 34.09
popliteal space 98.29
   by incision 86.05
rectum (intraluminal) 98.05
   by incision 48.0
renal pelvis (transurethral) 56.0
   by incision 56.1
retina (by incision) 14.00
   with use of magnet 14.01
   without use of magnet 14.02
retroperitoneum 54.92
sclera (by incision) 12.00
   with use of magnet 12.01
   without use of magnet 12.02
scrotum 98.24
   by incision 61.0
sinus (nasal) 22.50
   antrum 22.2
      with Caldwell-Luc approach 22.39
   ethmoid 22.51
   frontal 22.41
   maxillary 22.2
      with Caldwell-Luc approach 22.39
   sphenoid 22.52
skin NEC 98.20
   by incision 86.05
skull 01.24
   with incision into brain 01.39
small intestine (intraluminal) 98.03
   by incision 45.02
soft tissue NEC 83.09
   hand 82.09
spermatic cord 63.93
spinal (canal) (cord) (meninges) 03.01

stomach (intraluminal) 98.03
   bubble (balloon) 44.94
   by incision 43.0
subconjunctival (by magnet) 98.22
   by incision 10.0
subcutaneous tissue NEC 98.20
   by incision 86.05
supraclavicular fossa 98.27
   by incision 86.05
tendon (sheath) 83.01
   hand 82.01
testis 62.0
thorax (by incision) 34.09
thyroid (field) (gland) (by incision) 06.09
tonsil 98.13
   by incision 28.91
trachea (intraluminal) 98.15
   by incision 31.3
trunk NEC 98.25
tunica vaginalis 98.24
upper limb, except hand 98.27
   hand 98.26
ureter (transurethral) 56.0
   by incision 56.2
urethra (intraluminal) 98.19
   by incision 58.0
uterus (intraluminal) 98.16
vagina (intraluminal) 98.17
   by incision 70.14
vas deferens 63.6
vitreous (by incision) 14.00
   with use of magnet 14.01
   without use of magnet 14.02
vulva 98.23
   by incision 71.09
gallstones
   bile duct (by incision) NEC 51.49
      endoscopic 51.88
   common duct (by incision) 51.41
      endoscopic 51.88
      percutaneous 51.96
   duodenum 45.01
   gallbladder 51.04
   hepatic ducts 51.49
      endoscopic 51.88
   intestine 45.00
      large 45.03
      small NEC 45.02
   liver 50.0
Gardner Wells tongs (skull) 02.95
   with synchronous replacement 02.94
gastric bubble (balloon) 44.94
granulation tissue — see also Excision, lesion, by site
   with repair — see Repair, by site
   cranial 01.6
   skull 01.6
halo traction device (skull) 02.95
   with synchronous replacement 02.94
heart assist system 37.64
   with replacement 37.63
hematoma — see Drainage, by site
Hoffman minifixator device (bone) — see category 78.6
hydatidiform mole 68.0
impacted
   feces (rectum) (by flushing) (manual) 96.38
   tooth 23.19
      from nasal sinus (maxillary) 22.61
implant
   breast 85.94
   cochlear prosthetic device 20.99
   cornea 11.92
   lens (prosthetic) 13.8

Removal

middle ear NEC 20.99
ocular 16.71
    posterior segment 14.6
orbit 16.72
retina 14.6
tympanum 20.1
internal fixation device — see Removal, fixation device, internal
intrauterine contraceptive device (IUD) 97.71
joint (structure) 80.90
    ankle 80.97
    elbow 80.92
    foot and toe 80.98
    hand and finger 80.94
    hip 80.95
    knee 80.96
    other specified sites 80.99
    shoulder 80.91
    spine 80.99
    toe 80.98
    wrist 80.93
Kantrowitz heart pump 37.64
keel (tantalum plate), larynx 31.98
kidney — see also Nephrectomy
    mechanical 55.98
    transplanted or rejected 55.53
laminaria (tent), uterus 97.79
leads (cardiac) — see Removal, electrodes, cardiac pacemaker
lesion — see Excision, lesion, by site
ligamentum flavum (spine) — omit code
ligature
    fallopian tube 66.79
    ureter 56.86
    vas deferens 63.84
loose body
    bone — see Sequestrectomy, bone
    joint 80.10
    mesh (surgical) — see Removal, foreign body, by site
lymph node — see Excision, lymph, node
minifixator device (bone) — see category 78.6
    external fixation device 97.88
Mulligan hood, fallopian tube 66.94
    with synchronous replacement 66.93
muscle stimulator (skeletal) 83.93
    with replacement 83.92
myringotomy device or tube 20.1
nail (bed) (fold) 86.23
    internal fixation device — see Removal, fixation device, internal
necrosis
    skin 86.28
        excisional 86.22
neuropacemaker
    brain 01.22
        with synchronous replacement 02.93
    intracranial 01.22
        with synchronous replacement 02.93
    peripheral nerve 04.93
        with synchronous replacement 04.92
    spinal 03.94
        with synchronous replacement 03.93
neurostimulator
    brain 01.22
        with synchronous replacement 02.93
    intracranial 01.22

        with synchronous replacement 02.93
    peripheral nerve 04.93
        with synchronous replacement 04.92
    spinal 03.94
        with synchronous replacement 03.93
nonabsorbable surgical material NEC — see Removal, foreign body, by site
odontoma (tooth) 24.4
orbital implant 16.72
osteocartilagenous loose body, joint structures (see also Arthrotomy) 80.10
outer attic wall (middle ear) 20.59
ovo-testis (unilateral) 62.3
    bilateral 62.41
pacemaker
    brain (intracranial) 01.22
        with synchronous replacement 02.93
    cardiac (device) (initial) (permanent) 37.89
        with replacement
            dual-chamber device 37.87
            single-chamber device 37.85
                rate responsive 37.86
        electrodes (atrial) (tranvenous) (ventricular) 37.77
            with replacement 37.76
        epicardium (myocardium) 37.77
            with replacement (by)
                atrial and/or ventricular lead(s) (electrode) 37.76
                epicardial lead 37.74
        temporary transvenous pacemaker system — omit code
    intracranial 01.22
        with synchronous replacement 02.93
    neural
        brain 01.22
            with synchronous replacement 02.93
        peripheral nerve 04.93
            with synchronous replacement 04.92
        spine 03.94
            with synchronous replacement 03.93
    spinal 03.94
        with synchronous replacement 03.93
pack, packing
    dental 97.34
    intrauterine 97.72
    nasal 97.32
    rectum 97.59
    trunk NEC 97.85
    vagina 97.75
    vulva 97.75
pantopaque dye, spinal canal 03.31
patella (complete) 77.96
    partial 77.86
pectus deformity implant device 34.01
pelvic viscera, en masse (female) 68.8
    male 57.71
pessary, vagina NEC 97.74
pharynx (partial) 29.33
phlebolith — see Removal, embolus
placenta (by)
    aspiration curettage 69.52
    D and C 69.02

    manual 75.4
plaque, dental 96.54
plate, skull 02.07
    with synchronous replacement 02.05
polyp — see also Excision, lesion, by site
    esophageal 42.32
        endoscopic 42.33
    gastric (endoscopic) 43.41
    intestine 45.41
        endoscopic 45.42
    nasal 21.31
prosthesis
    bile duct 51.95
        nonoperative 97.55
    cochlear prosthetic device 20.99
    dental 97.35
    eye 97.31
    facial bone 76.99
    fallopian tube 66.94
        with synchronous replacement 66.93
    joint structure 80.00
        ankle 80.07
        elbow 80.02
        foot and toe 80.08
        hand and finger 80.04
        hip 80.05
        knee 80.06
        shoulder 80.01
        specified site NEC 80.09
        spine 80.09
        wrist 80.03
    lens 13.8
    penis (internal) without replacement 64.96
    Rosen (urethra) 59.99
    testicular, by incision 62.0
    urinary sphincter, artificial 58.99
        with replacement 58.93
pseudophakos 13.8
pterygium 11.39
    with corneal graft 11.32
pulse generator
    cardiac pacemaker 37.86
    cardioverter/defibrillator 37.99
pump assist device, heart 37.64
    with replacement 37.63
radioactive material — see Removal, foreign body, by site
redundant skin, eyelid 08.86
rejected organ
    kidney 55.53
    testis 62.42
reservoir, ventricular (Ommaya) (Rickham) 02.43
    with synchronous replacement 02.42
retained placenta (by)
    aspiration curettage 69.52
    D and C 69.02
    manual 75.4
retinal implant 14.6
rhinolith 21.31
rice bodies, tendon sheaths 83.01
    hand 82.01
Roger-Anderson minifixator device (bone) — see category 78.6
root, residual (tooth) (buried) (retained) 23.11
Rosen prosthesis (urethra) 59.99
Scribner shunt 39.43
scleral buckle or implant 14.6
secondary membranous cataract (with iridectomy) 13.65
secundines (by)
    aspiration curettage 69.52

D and C 69.02
    manual 75.4
sequestrum — *see* Sequestrectomy
seton, anus 49.93
Shepard's tube (ear) 20.1
Shirodkar suture, cervix 69.96
shunt
    arteriovenous 39.43
        with creation of new shunt 39.42
    lumbar-subarachnoid NEC 03.98
    pleurothecal 03.98
    salpingothecal 03.98
    spinal (thecal) NEC 03.98
    subarachnoid-peritoneal 03.98
    subarachnoid-ureteral 03.98
silastic tubes
    ear 20.1
    fallopian tubes 66.94
        with synchronous replacement 66.93
skin
    necrosis or slough 86.28
        excisional 86.22
        superficial layer (by dermabrasion) 86.25
skull tongs 02.95
    with synchronous replacement 02.94
splint 97.88
stent
    larynx 31.98
    ureteral 96.62
    urethral 96.65
stimoceiver (brain) (intracranial) 01.22
    with synchronous replacement 02.93
subdural
    grids 01.22
    strips 01.22
supernumerary digit(s) 86.26
suture(s) NEC 97.89
    abdominal wall 97.83
    by incision — *see* Incision, by site
    genital tract 97.79
    head and neck 97.38
    thorax 97.43
    trunk NEC 97.84
symblepharon — *see* Repair, symblepharon
temporary transvenous pacemaker system
    — omit code
testis (unilateral) 62.3
    bilateral 62.41
    remaining or solitary 62.42
thrombus 38.00
    with endarterectomy — *see* Endarterectomy
    abdominal
        artery 38.06
        vein 38.07
    aorta (arch) (ascending) (descending) 38.04
    arteriovenous shunt or cannula 39.49
    bovine graft 39.49
    coronary artery 36.09
    head and neck vessel NEC 38.02
    intracranial vessel NEC 38.01
    lower limb
        artery 38.08
        vein 38.09
    pulmonary (artery) (vein) 38.05
    thoracic vessel NEC 38.05
    upper limb (artery) (vein) 86.05
tissue expander (skin) NEC 86.05
    breast 85.96
toes, supernumerary 86.26
tongs, skull 02.95
    with synchronous replacement 02.94

tonsil tag 28.4
tooth (by forceps) (multiple) (single) NEC 23.09
    deciduous 23.01
    surgical NEC 23.19
        impacted 23.19
        residual root 23.11
        root apex 23.73
            with root canal therapy 23.72
trachoma follicles 10.33
T-tube (bile duct) 97.55
tube
    appendix 97.53
    bile duct (T-tube) NEC 97.55
    cholecystostomy 97.54
    cystostomy 97.63
    ear (button) 20.1
    gastrostomy 97.51
    large intestine 97.53
    liver 97.55
    mediastinum 97.42
    nephrostomy 97.61
    pancreas 97.56
    peritoneum 97.82
    pleural cavity 97.41
    pyelostomy 97.61
    retroperitoneum 97.81
    small intestine 97.52
    thoracotomy 97.41
    tracheostomy 97.37
    tympanostomy 20.1
    tympanum 20.1
    ureterostomy 97.62
ureteral splint (stent) 97.62
urethral sphincter, artificial 58.99
    with replacement 58.93
urinary sphincter, artificial 58.99
    with replacement 58.93
utricle 20.79
valve
    vas deferens 63.85
    ventricular (cerebral) 02.43
vascular graft or prosthesis 39.49
ventricular shunt or reservoir 02.43
    with synchronous replacement 02.42
Vinke tongs (skull) 02.95
    with synchronous replacement 02.94
vitreous (with replacement) 14.72
    anterior approach (partial) 14.71
    open sky approach 14.71
Wagner-Brooker minifixator device (bone)
    — *see* category 78.6
wiring, dental (immobilization device) 97.33
    orthodontic 24.8
Renipuncture (percutaneous) 55.92
Renogram 92.03
Renotransplantation NEC 55.69
Reopening — *see also* Incision, by site
    blepharorrhaphy 08.02
    canthorrhaphy 08.02
    cilia base 08.71
    craniotomy or craniectomy site 01.23
    fallopian tube (divided) 66.79
    iris in anterior chambers 12.97
    laminectomy or laminotomy site 03.02
    laparotomy site 54.12
    osteotomy site (*see also* Incision, bone) 77.10
        facial bone 76.09
    tarsorrhaphy 08.02
    thoracotomy site (for control of hemorrhage) (for examination) (for exploration) 34.03

thyroid field wound (for control of hemorrhage) (for examination) (for exploration) (forremoval of hematoma) 06.02
Repacking — *see* Replacement, pack, by site
Repair
    abdominal wall 54.72
    adrenal gland 07.44
    alveolus, alveolar (process) (ridge) (with graft) (with implant) 24.5
    anal sphincter 49.79
        laceration (by suture) 49.71
            obstetric (current) 76.62
            old 49.79
    aneurysm (false) (true) 39.52
        by or with
            clipping 39.51
            coagulation 39.52
            electrocoagulation 39.52
                excision or resection of vessel
                    — *see also*
                        Aneurysmectomy, by site
                with
                    anastomosis — *see*
                        aneurysmectomy,
                        with anastomosis, by
                        site
                    graft replacement — *see*
                        Aneurysmectomy,
                        with graft
                        replacement, by site
            filipuncture 39.52
            graft replacement — *see*
                Aneurysmectomy, with graft
                replacement, by site
            ligation 39.52
            methyl methacrylate 39.52
            occlusion 39.52
            suture 39.52
            trapping 39.52
            wiring 39.52
            wrapping (gauze) (methyl
                methacrylate) (plastic) 39.52
        coronary artery 36.91
        sinus of Valsalva 35.39
        thoracic aorta (dissecting), by
            fenestration 39.54
    anomalous pulmonary venous connection
        (total)
        one-stage 35.82
        partial — *see* specific procedure
        total 35.82
    anus 49.79
        laceration (by suture) 49.71
            obstetric (current) 76.62
            old 49.79
    aorta 39.31
    aorticopulmonary window 39.59
    arteriovenous fistula 39.53
        by or with
            clipping 39.53
            coagulation 39.53
            division 39.53
            excision or resection — *see also*
                Aneurysmectomy, by site
                with
                    anastomosis — *see*
                        Aneurysmectomy,
                        with anastomosis, by
                        site
                    graft replacement — *see*
                        Aneurysmectomy,
                        with graft
                        replacement, by site
            ligation 39.53

Repair   INDEX TO PROCEDURES   Repair

    coronary artery 36.99
    occlusion 39.53
    suture 39.53
artery NEC 39.59
  with
    patch graft 39.58
      with excision or resection of vessel — see Arteriectomy, with graft replacement, by site
      synthetic (Dacron) (Teflon) 39.57
      tissue (vein) (autogenous) (homograft) 39.56
    suture 39.31
  coronary NEC 36.99
    by angioplasty - see Angioplasty, coronary
    by atherectomy - see Angioplasty, coronary
artificial opening — see Repair, stoma
atrial septal defect 35.71
  with
    prosthesis (open heart technique) 35.51
      closed heart technique 35.52
    tissue graft 35.61
  combined with repair of valvular and ventricular septal defects — see Repair endocardialcushion defect
  in total repair of total anomalous pulmonary venous connection 35.82
atrioventricular canal defect (any type) 35.73
  with
    prosthesis 35.54
    tissue graft 35.63
bifid digit (finger) 82.89
bile duct NEC 51.79
  laceration (by suture) NEC 51.79
  common bile duct 51.71
bladder NEC 57.89
  exstrophy 57.86
  for stress incontinence — see Repair, stress incontinence
  laceration (by suture) 57.81
    obstetric (current) 76.61
    old 57.89
  neck 57.85
blepharophimosis 08.59
blepharoptosis 08.36
  by
    frontalis muscle technique (with)
      fascial sling 08.32
      suture 08.31
    levator muscle technique 08.34
      with resection or advancement 08.33
    orbicularis oculi muscle sling 08.36
    tarsal technique 08.35
blood vessel NEC 39.59
  with
    patch graft 39.58
      with excision or resection — see Angiectomy, with graft replacement
      synthetic (Dacron) (Teflon) 39.57
      tissue (vein) (autogenous) (homograft) 39.56
    resection — see Angiectomy
    suture 39.30
  coronary artery NEC 36.99
    by angioplasty - see Angioplasty, coronary
    by atherectomy - see Angioplasty, coronary
  peripheral vessel (angioplasty) (atherectomy) 39.59
bone NEC (see also Osteoplasty) — see category 78.4
  by synostosis technique — see Arthrodesis
  accessory sinus 22.79
  cranium NEC 02.06
    with
      flap (bone) 02.03
      graft (bone) 02.04
  for malunion, nonunion, or delayed union of fracture — see Repair, fracture, malunion ornonunion
  nasal 21.89
  skull NEC 02.06
    with
      flap (bone) 02.03
      graft (bone) 02.04
bottle, hydrocele of tunica vaginalis 61.2
brain (trauma) NEC 02.92
breast (plastic) (see also Mammoplasty) 85.89
broad ligament 69.29
bronchus NEC 33.48
  laceration (by suture) 33.41
bunionette (with osteotomy) 77.54
canaliculus, lacrimal 09.73
canthus (lateral) 08.59
cardiac pacemaker NEC 37.89
  electrode(s) (lead) NEC 37.75
cerebral meninges 02.12
cervix 67.69
  internal os 67.5
  laceration (by suture) 67.61
    obstetric (current) 75.51
    old 67.69
chest wall (mesh) (silastic) NEC 34.79
chordae tendineae 35.32
choroid NEC 14.9
  with retinal repair — see Repair, retina
cisternal chyli 40.69
claw toe 77.57
cleft
  hand 82.82
  laryngotracheal 31.69
  lip 27.54
  palate 27.62
    secondary or subsequent 27.63
coarctation of aorta — see Excision, coarctation of aorta
cochlear prosthetic device 20.99
  external components only 95.49
cockup toe 77.58
colostomy 46.43
conjunctiva NEC 10.49
  with scleral repair 12.81
  laceration 10.6
    with repair of sclera 12.81
  late effect of trachoma 10.49
cornea NEC 11.59
  with
    conjunctival flap 11.53
    transplant — see Keratoplasty
  postoperative dehiscence 11.52
coronary artery NEC 36.99
  by angioplasty - see Angioplasty, coronary
  by atherectomy - see Angioplasty, coronary
cranium NEC 02.06
  with
    flap (bone) 02.03
    graft (bone) 02.04
cusp, valve — see Repair, heart, valve
cystocele 70.51
  and rectocele 70.50
dental arch 24.8
diaphragm NEC 34.84
diastasis recti 83.65
diastematomyelia 03.59
ear (external) 18.79
  auditory canal or meatus 18.6
  auricle NEC 18.79
  cartilage NEC 18.79
  laceration (by suture) 18.4
  lop ear 18.79
  middle NEC 19.9
  prominent or protruding 18.5
ectropion 08.49
  by or with
    lid reconstruction 08.44
    suture (technique) 08.42
    thermocauterization 08.41
    wedge resection 08.43
encephalocele (cerebral) 02.12
endocardial cushion defect 35.73
  with
    prosthesis (grafted to septa) 35.54
    tissue graft 35.63
enterocele (female) 70.92
  male 53.9
enterostomy 46.40
entropion 08.49
  by or with
    lid reconstruction 08.44
    suture (technique) 08.42
    thermocauterization 08.41
    wedge resection 08.43
epicanthus (fold) 08.59
epididymis (and spermatic cord) NEC 63.59
  with vas deferens 63.89
epiglottis 31.69
episiotomy
  routine following delivery — see Episiotomy
  secondary 75.69
epispadias 58.45
esophagus, esophageal NEC 42.89
  fistula NEC 42.84
  stricture 42.85
exstrophy of bladder 57.86
eye, eyeball 16.89
  multiple structures 16.82
  rupture 16.82
  socket 16.64
    with graft 16.63
eyebrow 08.89
  linear 08.81
eyelid 08.89
  full-thickness 08.85
    involving lid margin 08.84
  laceration 08.81
    full-thickness 08.85
      involving lid margin 08.84
    partial-thickness 08.83
      involving lid margin 08.82
  linear 08.81
  partial-thickness 08.83
    involving lid margin 08.82
  retraction 08.38
fallopian tube (with prosthesis) 66.79
  by
    anastomosis 66.73
    reimplantation into
      ovary 66.72
      uterus 66.74
    suture 66.71

false aneurysm — *see* Repair, aneurysm
fascia 83.89
    by or with
        arthroplasty — *see* Arthroplasty
        graft (fascial) (muscle) 83.82
            hand 82.72
            tendon 83.81
                hand 82.79
        suture (direct) 83.65
            hand 82.46
    hand 82.89
        by
            graft NEC 82.79
                facial 82.72
                muscle 82.72
            suture (direct) 82.46
    joint — *see* Arthroplasty
filtering bleb (corneal) (scleral) (by excision) 12.82
    by
        corneal graft (*see also* Keratoplasty) 11.60
        scleroplasty 12.82
        suture 11.51
            with conjunctival flap 11.53
fistula — *see also* Closure, fistula
    anovaginal 70.73
    arteriovenous 39.53
        clipping 39.53
        coagulation 39.53
        division 39.53
        excision or resection — *see also* Aneurysmectomy, by site
        with
            anastomosis — *see* Aneurysmectomy, with anastomosis, by site
            graft replacement — *see* Aneurysmectomy, with graft replacement, by site
        ligation 39.53
    coronary artery 36.99
        occlusion 39.53
        suture 39.53
    cervicovesical 57.84
    cervix 67.62
    choledochoduodenal 51.72
    colovaginal 70.72
    enterovaginal 70.74
    enterovesical 57.83
    esophagocutaneous 42.84
    ileovesical 57.83
    intestinovaginal 70.74
    intestinovesical 57.83
    oroantral 22.71
    perirectal 48.93
    pleuropericardial 37.4
    rectovaginal 70.73
    rectovesical 57.83
    rectovesicovaginal 57.83
    scrotum 61.42
    sigmoidovaginal 70.74
    sinus
        nasal 22.71
        of Valsalva 35.39
    splencolic 41.95
    urethroperineovesical 57.84
    urethrovesical 57.84
    urethrovesicovaginal 57.84
    uterovesical 57.84
    vagina NEC 70.75
    vaginocutaneous 70.75
    vaginoenteric NEC 70.74
    vaginoileal 70.74
    vaginoperineal 70.75
    vagionvesical 57.84
    vesicocervicovaginal 57.84
    vesicocolic 57.83
    vesicocutaneous 57.84
    vesicoenteric 57.83
    vesicointestinal 57.83
    vesicometrorectal 57.83
    vesicoperineal 57.84
    vesicorectal 57.83
    vesicosigmoidal 57.83
    vesicosigmoidovaginal 57.83
    vesicourethral 57.84
    vesicourethrorectal 57.83
    vesicouterine 57.84
    vesicovaginal 57.84
    vulva 71.72
    vulvorectal 48.73
foramen ovale (patent) 35.71
    with
        prosthesis (open heart technique) 35.51
            closed heart technique 35.52
        tissue graft 35.61
fracture — *see also* Reduction, fracture
    larynx 31.64
    malunion or nonunion (delayed) NEC — *see* category 78.4
    with
        graft — *see* Graft, bone
        insertion (of)
            bone growth stimulator (invasive) — *see* category 78.9
            internal fixation device 78.5
        manipulation for realignment — *see* Reduction, fracture, by site, closed
        osteotomy
        with
            correction of alignment — *see* category 77.3
            with internal fixation device — *see* categories 77.3 [78.5]
            with intramedullary rod — *see* categories 77.3 [78.5]
        replacement arthroplasty — *see* Arthroplasty
        sequestrectomy — *see* category 77.0
        Sofield type procedure — *see* categories 77.3 [78.5]
        synostosis technique — *see* Arthrodesis
    vertebra 03.53
funnel chest (with implant) 34.74
gallbladder 51.91
gastroschisis 54.71
great vessels NEC 39.59
    laceration (by suture) 39.30
        artery 39.31
        vein 39.32
hallux valgus NEC 77.59
    resection of joint with prosthetic implant 77.59
hammer toe 77.56
hand 82.89
    with graft or implant 82.79
        fascia 82.72
        muscle 82.72
        tendon 82.79
heart 37.4
    assist system 37.63
    septum 35.70
        with
            prosthesis 35.50
            tissue graft 35.60
        atrial 35.71
            with
                prosthesis (open heart technique) 35.51
                    closed heart technique 35.52
                tissue graft 35.62
            combined with repair of valvular and ventricular septal defects — *see* Repair, endocardialcushion defect
            in total repair of
                tetralogy of Fallot 35.81
                total anomalous pulmonary venous connection 35.82
                truncus arteriosus 35.83
            combined with repair of valvular defect — *see* Repair, endocardial cushion defect
        ventricular 35.72
            with
                prosthesis 35.53
                tissue graft 35.62
            combined with repair of valvular and atrial septal defects — *see* Repair, endocardialcushion defect
            in total repair of
                tetralogy of Fallot 35.81
                total anomalous pulmonary venous connection 35.82
                truncus arteriosus 35.83
    valve (cusps) (open heart technique) 35.10
        with prosthesis or tissue graft 35.20
        aortic (without replacement) 35.11
            with
                prosthesis 35.22
                tissue graft 35.21
            combined with repair of atrial and ventricular septal defects — *see* Repair, endocardialcushion defect
        mitral (without replacement) 35.12
            with
                prosthesis 35.24
                tissue graft 35.23
        pulmonary (without replacement) 35.13
            with
                prosthesis 35.26
                    in total repair of tetralogy of Fallot 35.81
                tissue graft 35.25
        tricuspid (without replacement) 35.14

       with
           prosthesis 35.28
           tissue graft 35.27
hepatic duct 51.79
hernia NEC 53.9
    anterior abdominal wall NEC 53.59
       with prosthesis or graft 53.69
    colostomy 46.42
    crural 53.29
    cul-de-sac (Douglas') 70.92
    diaphragmatic
       abdominal approach 53.7
       thoracic, thoracoabdominal
          approach 53.80
    epigastric 53.59
       with prosthesis or graft 53.69
    esophageal hiatus
       abdominal approach 53.7
       thoracic, thoracoabdominal
          approach 53.80
    fascia 83.89
       hand 82.89
    femoral (unilateral) 53.29
       with prosthesis or graft 53.21
       bilateral 53.39
          with prosthesis or graft 53.31
    Ferguson 53.00
    Halsted 53.00
    Hill-Allison (hiatal hernia repair,
       transpleural approach) 53.80
    hypogastric 53.59
       with prosthesis or graft 53.69
    incisional 53.51
       with prosthesis or graft 53.61
    inguinal (unilateral) 53.05
       with prosthesis or graft 53.05
       bilateral 53.10
          with prosthesis or graft 53.17
          direct 53.11
             with prosthesis or graft
                53.14
          direct and indirect 53.13
             with prosthesis or graft
                53.16
          indirect 53.12
             with prosthesis or
                graft 53.15
       direct (unilateral) 53.01
          with prosthesis or graft 53.03
          and indirect (unilateral) 53.01
             with prosthesis or graft
                53.03
          bilateral 53.13
             with prosthesis or
                graft 53.16
          bilateral 53.11
             with prosthesis or graft
                53.14
       indirect (unilateral) 53.02
          with prosthesis or graft 53.04
          and direct (unilateral) 53.01
             with prosthesis or graft
                53.03
          bilateral 53.13
             with prosthesis or
                graft 53.16
          bilateral 53.12
             with prosthesis or graft
                53.15
    internal 53.9
    ischiatic 53.9
    ischiorectal 53.9
    lumbar 53.9
    manual 96.27
    obturator 53.9
    omental 53.9
    paraesophageal 53.7
    parahiatal 53.7
    paraileostomy 46.41
    parasternal 53.82
    parumbilical 53.49
       with prosthesis 53.41
    pericolostomy 46.42
    perineal (enterocele) 53.9
    preperitoneal 53.29
    pudendal 53.9
    retroperitoneal 53.9
    sciatic 53.9
    scrotal — *see* Repair, hernia, inguinal
    spigelian 53.59
       with prosthesis or graft 53.69
    umbilical 53.49
       with prosthesis 53.41
    uveal 12.39
    ventral 53.59
       incisional 53.51
       with prosthesis or graft 53.61
hydrocele
    round ligament 69.19
    spermatic cord 63.1
    tunica vaginalis 61.2
hymen 70.76
hypospadias 58.45
ileostomy 46.41
ingrown toenail 86.23
intestine, intestinal NEC 46.79
    fistula — *see* Closure, fistula, intestine
    laceration
       large intestine 46.75
       small intestine NEC 46.73
    stoma — *see* Repair, stoma
inverted uterus NEC 69.29
    manual
       nonobstetric 69.94
       obstetric 75.94
    obstetrical
       manual 75.94
       surgical 75.93
    vaginal approach 69.23
iris (rupture) NEC 12.39
jejunostomy 46.41
joint (capsule) (cartilage) NEC (*see also*
    Arthroplasty) 81.96
kidney NEC 55.89
knee (joint) NEC 81.47
    collateral ligaments 81.46
    cruciate ligaments 81.45
    five-in-one 81.42
    triad 81.43
labia — *see* Repair, vulva
laceration — *see* Suture, by site
lacrimal system NEC 09.99
    canaliculus 09.73
    punctum 09.72
       for eversion 09.71
laryngostomy 31.62
laryngotracheal cleft 31.69
larynx 31.69
    fracture 31.64
    laceration 31.61
leads (cardiac) NEC 37.75
ligament (*see also* Arthroplasty) 81.96
    broad 69.29
    collateral, knee NEC 81.46
    cruciate, knee NEC 81.45
    round 69.29
    uterine 69.29
lip NEC 27.59
    cleft 27.54
    laceration (by suture) 27.51
liver NEC 50.69
    laceration 50.61
lop ear 18.79
lung NEC 33.49
lymphatic (channel) (peripheral) NEC 40.9
    duct, left (thoracic) NEC 40.69
macrodactyly 82.83
mallet finer 82.84
mandibular ridge 76.64
mastoid (antrum) (cavity) 19.9
meninges (cerebral) NEC 02.12
    spinal NEC 03.59
       meningocele 03.51
       myelomeningocele 03.52
meningocele (spinal) 03.51
    cranial 02.12
mesentery 54.75
mouth NEC 27.59
    laceration NEC 27.52
muscle NEC 83.87
    by
       graft or implant (fascia) (muscle)
          83.82
          hand 82.72
          tendon 83.81
             hand 82.79
       suture (direct) 83.65
          hand 82.46
       transfer or transplantation (muscle)
          83.77
          hand 82.58
    hand 82.89
       by
          graft or implant NEC 82.79
             fascia 82.72
          suture (direct) 82.46
          transfer or transplantation
             (muscle) 82.58
musculotendinous cuff, shoulder 83.63
myelomeningocele 03.52
nasal
    septum (perforation) NEC 21.88
    sinus NEC 22.79
       fistula 22.71
nasolabial flaps (plastic) 21.86
nasopharyngeal atresia 29.4
nerve (cranial) (peripheral) NEC 04.79
    old injury 04.76
    revision 04.75
    sympathetic 05.81
nipple NEC 85.87
nose (external) (internal) (plastic) NEC (*see*
    also Rhinoplasty) 21.89
    laceration (by suture) 21.81
notched lip 27.59
omentum 54.74
omphalocele 53.49
    with prosthesis 53.41
orbit 16.89
    wound 16.81
ostium
    primum defect 35.73
       with
          prosthesis 35.54
          tissue graft 35.63
    secundum defect 35.71
       with
          prosthesis (open heart
             technique) 35.51
             closed heart technique
                35.52
          tissue graft 35.61
ovary 65.79
    with tube 65.73
overlapping toe 77.58
pacemaker

cardiac
    device (permanent) 37.89
    electrode(s) (lead) NEC 37.75
    pocket (skin) (subcutaneous) 37.79
palate NEC 27.69
    cleft 27.62
        secondary or subsequent 27.63
    laceration (by suture) 27.61
pancreas NEC 52.95
    Wirsung's duct 52.99
papillary muscle (heart) 35.31
patent ductus arteriosus 38.85
pectus deformity (chest) (carinatum)
    (excavatum) 34.74
pelvic floor NEC 70.79
    obstetric laceration (current) 75.69
    old 70.79
penis NEC 69.49
    for epispadias or hypospadias 58.45
    inflatable prosthesis 64.99
    laceration 64.41
pericardium 37.4
perineum (female) 71.79
    laceration (by suture) 71.71
        obstetric (current) 75.69
        old 71.79
    male NEC 86.89
        laceration (by suture) 86.59
peritoneum NEC 54.73
    by suture 54.64
pharynx NEC 29.59
    laceration (by suture) 29.51
    plastic 29.4
pleura NEC 34.93
postcataract wound dehiscence 11.52
    with conjunctival flap 11.53
pouch of Douglas 70.52
primum ostium defect 35.73
    with
        prosthesis 35.54
        tissue graft 35.63
prostate 60.93
ptosis, eyelid — see Repair, blepharoptosis
punctum, lacrimal NEC 09.72
    for correction of eversion 09.71
quadriceps (mechanism) 83.86
rectocele (posterior colporrhaphy) 70.52
    and cystocele 70.50
rectum NEC 48.79
    laceration (by suture) 48.71
    prolapse NEC 48.76
        abdominal approach 48.75
retina, retinal
    detachment 14.59
        by
            cryotherapy 14.52
            diathermy 14.51
            photocoagulation 14.55
                laser 14.54
                xenon arc 14.53
            scleral buckling (see also
                Buckling, scleral) 14.49
    tear or defect 14.39
        by
            cryotherapy 14.32
            diathermy 14.31
            photocoagulation 14.35
                laser 14.34
                xenon arc 14.33
retroperitoneal tissue 54.73
rotator cuff (suture) 83.63
round ligament 69.29
ruptured tendon NEC 83.88
    hand 82.86
salivary gland or duct NEC 26.49

sclera, scleral 12.89
    fistula 12.82
    staphyloma NEC 12.86
        with graft 12.85
scrotum 61.49
sinus
    nasal NEC 22.79
    of Valsalva (aneurysm) 35.39
skin (plastic) (without graft) 86.89
    laceration (by suture) 86.59
skull NEC 02.06
    with
        flap (bone) 02.03
        graft (bone) 02.04
spermatic cord NEC 63.59
    laceration (by suture) 63.51
sphincter ani 49.79
    laceration (by suture) 49.71
        obstetric (current) 75.62
        old 49.79
spina bifida NEC 03.59
    meningocele 03.51
    myelomeningocele 03.52
spinal (cord) (meninges) (structures) NEC
    03.59
    meningocele 03.51
    myelomeningocele 03.52
spleen 41.95
sternal defect 78.41
stoma
    bile duct 51.79
    bladder 57.22
    bronchus 33.42
    common duct 51.72
    esophagus 42.89
    gallbladder 51.99
    hepatic duct 51.79
    intestine 46.40
        large 46.43
        small 46.41
    kidney 55.89
    larynx 31.63
    rectum 48.79
    stomach 44.69
    thorax 34.79
    trachea 31.74
    ureter 56.62
    urethra 58.49
stomach NEC 44.69
    laceration (by suture) 44.61
stress incontinence (urinary) NEC 59.79
    by
        anterior urethropexy 59.79
        cystourethropexy (with levator
            muscle sling) 59.71
        paraurethral suspension (Pereyra)
            59.6
        periurethral suspension 59.6
        plication of urethrovesical junction
            59.3
        pubococcygeal sling 59.71
        retropubic urethral suspension 59.5
        suprapubic sling 59.4
        urethrovesical suspension 59.4
            gracilis muscle transplant 59.71
            levator muscle sling 59.71
subcutaneous tissue (plastic) (without skin
    graft) 86.89
    laceration (by suture) 86.59
supracristal defect (heart) 35.72
    with
        prosthesis 35.53
        tissue graft 35.62
symblepharon NEC 10.49

by division (with insertion of
    conformer) 10.5
with free graft 10.41
syndactyly 86.85
synovial membrane, joint — see
    Arthroplasty
telecanthus 08.59
tendon 83.88
    by or with
        arthroplasty — see Arthroplasty
        graft or implant (tendon) 83.81
            fascia 83.82
                hand 82.72
            hand 82.79
            muscle 83.82
                hand 82.72
        suture (direct) (immediate)
            (primary) (see also Suture,
            tendon) 83.64
            hand 82.45
        transfer or transplantation (tendon)
            83.75
            hand 82.56
    hand 82.86
        by
            graft or implant (tendon) 82.79
            suture (direct) (immediate)
                (primary) (see also
                Suture, tendon, hand)
                82.45
            transfer or transplantation
                (tendon) 82.56
    rotator cuff (direct suture) 83.63
    ruptured NEC 83.88
        hand 82.86
    sheath (direct suture) 83.61
        hand 82.41
testis NEC 62.69
tetralogy of Fallot
    partial — see specific procedure
    total (one-stage) 35.81
thoracic duct NEC 40.69
thoracostomy 34.72
thymus (gland) 07.93
tongue NEC 25.59
tooth NEC 23.2
    by
        crown (artificial) 23.41
        filling (amalgam) (plastic) (silicate)
            23.2
        inlay 23.3
total anomalous pulmonary venous
    connection
    partial — see specific procedure
    total (one-stage) 35.82
trachea NEC 31.79
    laceration (by suture) 31.71
tricuspid atresia 35.94
truncus arteriosus
    partial — see specific procedure
    total (one-stage) 35.83
tunica vaginalis 61.49
    laceration (by suture) 61.41
tympanum — see Tympanoplasty
ureter NEC 56.89
    laceration (by suture) 56.82
ureterocele 56.89
urethra NEC 58.49
    laceration (by suture) 58.41
        obstetric (current) 75.61
        old 58.49
    meatus 58.47
urethrocele (anterior colporrhaphy)
    (female) 70.51
    and rectocele 70.50

urinary sphincter, artificial (component) 58.99
urinary stress incontinence — *see* Repair, stress incontinence
uterus, uterine 69.49
    inversion — *see* Repair, inverted uterus
    laceration (by suture) 69.41
        obstetric (current) 75.50
        old 69.49
    ligaments 69.29
        by
            interposition 69.21
            plication 69.22
uvula 27.73
    with synchronous cleft palate repair 27.62
vagina, vaginal (cuff) (wall) NEC 70.79
    anterior 70.51
        with posterior repair 70.50
    cystocele 70.51
        and rectocele 70.50
    enterocele 70.92
    laceration (by suture) 70.71
        obstetric (current) 75.69
        old 70.79
    posterior 70.52
        with anterior repair 70.50
    rectocele 70.52
        and cystocele 70.50
    urethrocele 70.51
        and rectocele 70.50
varicocele 63.1
vas deferens 63.89
    by
        anastomosis 63.82
            to epididymis 63.83
        reconstruction 63.82
    laceration (by suture) 63.81
vein NEC 39.59
    with
        patch graft 39.58
            with excision or resection of vessel — *see* Phlebectomy, with graft replacement, by site
        synthetic (Dacron) (Teflon) 39.57
            tissue (vein) (autogenous) (homograft) 39.56
        suture 39.32
ventricular septal defect 35.72
    with
        prosthesis 35.53
            in total repair of tetralogy of Fallot 35.81
        tissue graft 35.62
    combined with repair of valvular and atrial septal defects — *see* Repair, endocardialcushion defect
    in total repair of
        tetralogy of Fallot 35.81
        truncus arteriosus 35.83
vertebral arch defect (spina bifida) 03.59
vulva NEC 71.79
    laceration (by suture) 71.71
        obstetrical (current) 75.69
        old 71.79
Wirsung's duct 52.99
wound (skin) (without graft) 86.59
    abdominal wall 54.63
        dehiscence 54.61
        postcataract dehiscence (corneal) 11.52

Replacement
    acetabulum (with prosthesis) 81.52
    ankle, total 81.56
    revision 81.59
    aortic valve (with prosthesis) 35.22
        with tissue graft 35.21
    artery — *see* Graft, artery
    bag — *see* Replacement, pack or bag
    Barton's tongs (skull) 02.94
    bladder
        with
            ileal loop 57.87 [45.51]
            sigmoid 57.87 [45.52]
            sphincter, artificial 58.93
    caliper tongs (skull) 02.94
    cannula
        arteriovenous shunt 39.94
        pancreatic duct 97.05
        vessel-to-vessel (arteriovenous) 39.94
    cardioverter/defibrillator (total system) 37.94
        leads only (electrodes) (sensing) (pacing) 37.97
        pulse generator only 37.98
    cast NEC 97.13
        lower limb 97.12
        upper limb 97.11
    catheter
        bladder (indwelling) 57.95
        cystostomy 59.94
        ventricular shunt (cerebral) 02.42
        wound 97.15
    Crutchfield tongs (skull) 02.94
    cystostomy tube (catheter) 59.94
    diaphragm, vagina 97.24
    drain — *see also* Replacement, tube
        vagina 97.26
        vulva 97.26
        wound musculoskeletal or skin 97.16
    ear (prosthetic) 18.71
    elbow (joint), total 81.84
    electrode(s) — *see* Implant, electrode or lead by site or name of device
        brain
            depth 02.93
            foramen ovale 02.93
            sphenoidal 02.96
        depth 02.93
        foramen ovale 02.93
        sphenoidal 02.96
    electroencephalographic receiver (brain) (intracranial) 02.93
    electronic
        cardioverter/defibrillator — *see* Replacement, cardioverter/defibrillator
        leads (electrode)(s) — *see* Replacement, pacemaker, electrode(s), cardiac
        stimulator — *see also* Implant, electronic stiumulator, by site
            bladder 57.97
            muscle (skeletal) 83.92
            ureter 56.93
    electrostimulator — *see* Implant, electronic stimulator by site
    enterostomy device (tube)
        large intestine 97.04
        small intestine 97.03
    epidural pegs 02.93
    femoral head, by prosthesis 81.52
        revision 81.53
    Gardner Wells tongs (skull) 02.94
    graft — *see* Graft
    holo traction device (skull) 02.94
    Harrington rod (with refusion of spine) 81.08
    heart
        artificial 37.63
        valve (with prosthesis) (with tissue graft) 35.20
            aortic (with prosthesis) 35.22
                with tissue graft 35.21
            mitral (with prosthesis) 35.24
                with tissue graft 35.23
            poppet (prosthetic) 35.95
            pulmonary (with prosthesis) 35.26
                with tissue graft 35.25
                in total repair of tetralogy of Fallot 35.81
            triscuspid (with prosthesis) 35.28
                with tissue graft 35.27
    hip (partial) (with fixation device) (with prosthesis) (with traction 81.52
        acetabulum 81.52
            revision 81.53
        femoral head 81.52
            revision 81.53
        total 81.51
            revision 81.53
    inverted uterus — *see* Repair, inverted uterus
    iris NEC 12.39
    kidney, mechanical 55.97
    knee (bicompartmental) (hemijoint) (partial) (total) (tricompartmental) (unicompartmental)81.54
        revision 81.55
    laryngeal stent 31.93
    leads (electrod)(s) — *see* Replacement, pacemaker, electrode(s), cardiac
    mechanical kidney 55.97
    mitral vale (with prosthesis) 35.24
        with tissue graft 35.23
    Mulligan hood, fallopian tube 66.93
    muscle stimulator (skeletal) 83.92
    nephrostomy tube 55.93
    neuropacemaker — *see* Implant, neuropacemaker, by site
    neurostimulator — *see also* Implant, neurostimulator, by site
        peripheral nerve 04.92
        skeletal muscle 83.92
    pacemaker
        brain 02.93
        cardiac device (initial) (permanent)
            dual-chamber device 37.87
            single-chamber device 37.85
                rate responsive 37.86
        electrode(s), cardiac (atrial) (transvenous) (ventricular) 37.76
            epicardium (myocardium) 37.74
        intracranial 02.93
        neural
            brain 02.93
            intracranial 02.93
            peripheral nerve 04.92
            spine 03.93
        spine 03.93
        temporary transvenous pacemaker system 37.78
    pack or bag
        nose 97.21
        teeth, tooth 97.22
        vagina 97.26
        vulva 96.26
        wound 97.16
    pessary, vagina NEC 97.25
    prosthesis
        acetabulum 81.53
        arm (bioelectric) (cineplastic) (kineplastic) 84.44

biliary tract 51.99
cochlear 20.96
channel (single) 20.97
    multiple 20.98
elbow 81.97
extremity (bioelectric) (cineplastic) (kineplastic) 84.40
    lower 84.48
    upper 84.44
fallopian tube (Mulligan hood) (stent) 66.93
femur 81.53
knee 81.55
leg (bioelectric) (cineplastic) (kineplastic) 84.48
penis (internal) (non-inflatable) 64.95
    inflatable (internal) 64.97
pulmonary valve (with prosthesis) 35.26
    with tissue graft 35.25
    in total repair of tetralogy of Fallot 35.81
pyelostomy tube 55.94
rectal tube 96.09
shoulder NEC 81.83
    partial 81.81
    total 81.80
skull
    plate 02.05
    tongs 02.94
specified appliance or device NEC 97.29
stent
    bile duct 97.05
    fallopian tube 66.93
    larynx 31.93
    pancreatic duct 97.05
    trachea 31.93
stimoceiver — see Implant, stimoceiver, by site
subdural
    grids 02.93
    strips 02.93
testis in scrotum 62.5
tongs, skull 02.94
tracheal stent 31.93
tricuspid valve (with prosthesis) 35.28
    with tissue graft 35.27
tube
    bile duct 97.05
    bladder 57.95
    cystostomy 59.94
    esophagostomy 97.01
    gastrostomy 97.02
    large intestine 97.04
    nasogastric 97.01
    nephrostomy 55.93
    pancreatic duct 97.05
    pyelostomy 55.94
    rectal 96.09
    small intestine 97.03
    tracheostomy 97.23
    ureterostomy 59.93
    ventricular (cerebral) 02.42
umbilical cord, prolapsed 73.92
ureter (with)
    bladder flap 56.74
    ileal segment implanted into bladder 56.89 [45.51]
ureterostomy tube 59.93
urethral sphincter, artificial 58.93
urinary sphincter, artificial 58.93
valve
    heart — see also Replacement, heart valve
    poppet (prosthesis) 35.95
ventricular (cerebral) 02.42
ventricular shunt (catheter) (valve) 02.42
Vinke tongs (skull) 02.94
vitreous (silicone) 14.75
    for retinal reattachment 14.59

Replant, replantation — *see also* Reattachment
extremity — *see* Reattachment, extremity
penis 64.45
scalp 86.51
tooth 23.5

Reposition
cardiac pacemaker
    electrode(s) (atrial) (transvenous) (ventricular) 37.75
    pocket 37.79
cardioverter/defibrillator
    lead(s) (sensing) (pacing) (epicardial patch) 37.99
    pulse generator 37.99
cilia base 08.71
iris 12.39
renal vessel, aberrant 39.55
thyroid tissue 06.94
tricuspid valve (with plication) 35.14

Resection — *see also* Excision, by site
abdominoendorectal (combined) 48.5
abdominoperineal (rectum) 48.5
    pull-through (Altmeier) (Swenson) NEC 48.49
        Duhamel type 48.65
alveolar process and palate (en bloc) 27.32
aneurysm — *see* Aneurysmectomy
aortic valve (for subvalvular stenosis) 35.11
artery — *see* Arteriectomy
bile duct NEC 51.69
    common duct NEC 51.63
bladder (partial) (segmental) (transvesical) (wedge) 57.6
    complete or total 57.79
    lesion NEC 57.59
        transurethral approach 57.49
    neck 57.59
        transurethral apporach 57.49
blood vessel — *see* Angiectomy
brain 01.59
    hemisphere 01.52
    lobe 01.53
breast — *see also* Mastectomy
    quadrant 85.22
    segmental 85.23
broad ligament 69.19
bronchus (sleeve) (wide sleeve) 32.1
    block (en bloc) (with radical dissection of brachial plexus, bronchus, lobe of lung, ribs,and sympathetic nerves) 32.6
bursa 83.5
    hand 82.31
cecum (and terminal ileum) 45.72
cerebral meninges 01.51
chest wall 34.4
clavicle 77.81
clitoris 71.4
colon (partial) (segmental) 45.79
    ascending (cecum and terminal ileum) 45.72
    cecum (and terminal ileum) 45.72
    complete 45.8
    descending (sigmoid) 45.76
    for interposition) 45.52
    Hartmann 45.75
    hepatic flexure 45.73
    left radical (hemicolon) 45.75
    multiple segmental 45.71
    right radical (hemicolon) (ileocolectomy) 45.73
    segmental NEC 45.79
        multiple 45.71
    sigmoid 45.76
    splenic flexure 45.75
    total 45.8
    transverse 45.74
conjunctiva, for pterygium 11.39
    corneal graft 11.32
cornual (fallopian tube) (unilateral) 66.69
    bilateral 66.63
diaphragm 34.81
endaural 20.79
endorectal (pull-through) (Soave) 48.41
    combined abdominal 48.5
esophagus (partial) (subtotal) (*see also* Esophagectomy) 42.41
    total 42.42
exteriorized intestine — *see* Resection, intestine, exteriorized
fascia 83.44
    for graft 83.43
        hand 82.34
    hand 82.35
        for graft 82.34
gallbladder (total) 51.22
gastric (partial) (sleeve) (subtotal) NEC (*see also* Gastrectomy) 43.89
    with anastomosis NEC 43.89
        esophagogastric 43.5
        gastroduodenal 43.6
        gastrogastric 43.89
        gastrojejunal 43.7
    complete or total NEC 43.99
        with intestinal interposition 43.91
    radical NEC 43.99
        with intestinal interposition 43.91
    wedge 43.42
        endoscopic 43.41
hallux valgus (joint) — *see also* Bunionectomy
    with prosthetic implant 77.59
hepatic
    duct 51.69
    flexure (colon) 45.73
infundibula, heart (right) 35.34
intestine (partial) NEC 45.79
    cecum (with terminal ileum) 45.72
    exteriorized (large intestine) 46.04
        small intestine 46.02
    for interposition 45.50
        large intestine 45.52
        small intestine 45.51
    hepatic flexure 45.73
    ileum 45.62
        with cecum 45.72
    large (partial) (segmental) NEC 45.79
        for interposition 45.52
        multiple segmental 45.71
        total 45.8
    left hemicolon 45.75
    multiple segmental (large intestine) 45.71
        small intestine 45.61
    right hemicolon 45.73
    segmental (large intestine) 45.79
        multiple 45.71
        small intestine 45.62
            multiplee 45.61
    sigmoid 45.76
    small (partial) (segmental) NEC 45.62
        for interposition 45.51

multiple segmental 45.61
total 45.63
total
    large intestine 45.8
    small intestine 45.63
joint structure NEC (*see also* Arthrectomy) 80.90
kidney (segmental) (wedge) 55.4
larynx — *see also* Laryngectomy
    submucous 30.29
lesion — *see* Excision, lesion, by site
levator palpebrae muscle 08.33
ligament (*see also* Arthrectomy) 80.90
    broad 69.19
    round 69.19
    uterine 69.19
lip (wedge) 27.43
liver (partial) (wedge) 50.22
    lobe (total) 50.3
    total 50.4
lung (wedge) NEC 32.29
    endoscopic 32.28
    segmental (any part) 32.3
meninges (cerebral) 01.51
    spinal 03.4
mesentery 54.4
muscle 83.45
    extraocular 15.13
        with
            advancement or recession of other eye muscle 15.3
            levator palpebrae 08.33
            Muller's, for blepharoptosis 08.35
            suture of original insertion 15.13
        orbicularis oculi 08.20
        tarsal, for blepharoptosis 08.35
    for graft 83.43
    hand 82.34
    hand 82.36
        for graft 82.34
    ocular — *see* Resection, muscle, extraocular
myocardium 37.33
nasal septum (submucous) 21.5
nerve (cranial) (peripheral) NEC 04.07
    phrenic 04.03
        for collapse of lung 33.31
    sympathetic 05.29
    vagus — *see* Vagotomy
nose (complete) (extended) (partial) (radical) 21.4
omentum 54.4
orbitomaxillary, radical 16.51
ovary — *see also* Oophorectomy wedge 65.22
palate (bony) (local) 27.31
    by wide excision 27.32
    soft 27.49
pancreas (total) (with synchronous duodenectomy) 52.6
    partial NEC 52.59
        distal (tail) (with part of body) 52.52
        proximal (head) (with part of body) (with synchronous duodenectomy) 52.51
        radical subtotal 52.53
    radical (one-stage) (two-stage) 52.7
    subtotal 52.53
pancreaticoduodenal (*see also* Pancreatectomy) 52.6
pelvic viscera (en masse) (female) 68.8
    male 57.71
penis 64.3
pericardium (partial) (for)
    chronic constrictive pericarditis 37.31
    drainage 37.12
    removal of adhesions 37.31
peritoneum 54.4
pharynx (partial) 29.33
phrenic nerve 04.03
    for collapse of lung 33.31
prostate — *see also* Prostatectomy
    transurethral (punch) 60.2
pterygium 11.39
radial head 77.83
rectosigmoid (*see also* Resection, rectum) 48.69
rectum (partial) NEC 48.69
    with
        pelvic exenteration 68.8
        transsacral sigmoidectomy 48.61
    abdominoendorectal (combined) 48.5
    abdominoperineal 48.5
        pull-through NEC 48.49
            Duhamel type 48.65
    anterior 48.63
        with colostomy (synchronous) 48.62
    Duhamel 48.65
    endorectal 48.41
        combined abdominal 48.5
    posterior 48.64
    pull-through NEC 48.49
        endorectal 48.41
    submucosal (Soave) 48.41
        combined abdominal 48.5
rib (transaxillary) 77.91
    as operative approach — omit code
    incidental to thoracic operation — omit code
right ventricle (heart), for infundibular stenosis 35.34
root (tooth) (apex) 23.73
    with root canal therapy 23.72
    residual or retained 23.11
round ligament 69.19
sclera 12.65
    with scleral buckling (*see also* Buckling, secleral) 14.49
    lamellar (for retinal reattachment) 14.49
        with implant 14.41
scrotum 61.3
soft tissue NEC 83.49
    hand 82.39
sphincter of Oddi 51.89
spinal cord (meninges) 03.4
splanchnic 05.29
splenic flexure (colon) 45.75
sternum 77.81
stomach (partial) (sleeve) (subtotal) NEC (*see also* Gastrectomy) 43.89
    with anastomosis NEC 43.89
        esophagogastric 43.5
        gastroduodenal 43.6
        gastrogasstric 43.89
        gastrojejunal 43.7
    complete or total NEC 43.99
        with intestinal interposition 43.91
    fundus 43.89
    radical NEC 43.99
        with intestinal interposition 43.91
    wedge 43.42
        endoscopic 43.41
submucous
    larynx 30.29
    nasal septum 21.5
vocal cords 30.22
synovial membrane (complete) (partial) (*see also* Synovectomy) 80.70
tarsolevator 08.33
tendon 83.42
    hand 82.33
thoracic structures (block) (en bloc) (radical) (brachial plexus, bronchus, lobes of lung, ribs, and sympathetic nerves) 32.6
thorax 34.4
tongue 25.2
    wedge 25.1
tooth root 23.73
    with root canal therapy 23.72
    apex (abscess) 23.73
        with root canal therapy 23.72
    residual or retained 23.11
trachea 31.5
transurethral
    bladder NEC 57.49
    prostate 60.2
transverse colon 45.74
turbinates — *see* Turbinectomy
ureter (partial) 56.41
    total 56.42
uterus — *see* Hysterectomy
vein — *see* Phlebectomy
ventricle (heart) (left) 35.34
vesical neck 57.59
    transurethral 57.49
vocal cords (punch) 30.22

▶ Respirator, volume-controlled (Bennett) (Byrd) - *see* Ventilation

Restoration
cardioesophageal angle 44.66
dental NEC 23.49
    by
        application of crown (artificial) 23.41
        insertion of bridge (fixed) 23.42
        removable 23.43
extremity — *see* Reattachment, extremtiy
eyebrow 08.70
    with graft 08.63
eye socket 16.64
    with graft 16.63
tooth NEC 23.2
    by
        crown (artificial) 23.41
        filling (amalgam) (plastic) (silicate) 23.2
        inlay 23.3

Resuscitation
artificial respiration 93.93
cardiac 99.60
    cardioversion 99.62
        atrial 99.61
    defibrillation 99.62
    external massage 99.63
        open chest 37.91
    intracardiac injection 37.92
cardiopulmonary 99.60
endotracheal intubation 96.04
manual 93.93
mouth-to-mouth 93.93
pulmonary 93.93

Resuture
abdominal wall 54.61
cardiac septum prosthesis 35.95
chest wall 34.71
heart valve prosthesis (poppet) 35.95

wound (skin and subcutaneous tissue) (without graft) NEC 86.59
Retinaculotomy NEC (*see also* Division, ligament) 80.40
   carpal tunnel (flexor) 04.43
Retraining
   cardiac 93.36
   vocational 93.85
Retrogasserian neurotomy 04.02
Revascularization
   cardiac (heart muscle) (myocardium) (direct) 36.10
     with
        bypass anastomosis
           aortocoronary (catheter stent) (homograft) (prosthesis) (saphenous vein graft) 36.10
              one coronary vessel 36.11
              two coronary vessels 36.12
              three coronary vessels 36.13
              four coronary vessels 36.14
           internal mammary-coronary artery (single vessel) 36.15
              double vessel 36.16
           specified type NEC 36.19
           thoracic artery-coronary artery (single vessel) 36.15
              double vessel 36.16
        implantation of artery into heart (muscle) (myocardium) (ventricle) 36.2
     indirect 36.2
     specified type NEC 36.3
Reversal, intestinal segment 45.50
   large 45.52
   small 45.51
Revision
   amputation stump 84.3
     current traumatic — *see* Amputation
   anastomosis
     biliary tract 51.94
     blood vessel 39.49
     gastric gastrointestinal (with jejunal interposition) 44.5
     intestine (large) 46.94
       small 46.93
     pleurothecal 03.97
     pyelointestinal 56.72
     salpingothecal 03.97
     subarachnoid-peritoneal 03.97
     subarachnoid-ureteral 03.97
     ureterointestinal 56.72
   ankle replacement (prosthesis) 81.59
   anterior segment (eye) wound (operative) NEC 12.83
   anteriovenous shunt (cannula) (for dialysis) 39.42
   arthroplasty — *see* Arthroplasty
   bone flap, skull 02.06
   breast implant 85.93
   bronchostomy 33.42
   cannula, vessel-to-vessel (arteriovenous) 39.94
   canthus, lateral 08.59
   cardiac pacemaker
     device (permanent) 37.89
       electrode(s) (atrial) (transvenous) (ventricular) 37.75
     pocket 37.79
   cholecystostomy 51.99
   cleft palate repair 27.63
   colostomy 46.43
   conduit, urinary 56.52
   cystostomy (stoma) 57.22
   elbow replacement (prosthesis) 81.97
   enterostomy (stoma) 46.40
     large intestine 46.43
     small intestine 46.41
   enucleation socket 16.64
     with graft 16.63
   esophagostomy 42.83
   exenteration cavity 16.66
     with secondary graft 16.65
   extraocular muscle surgery 15.6
   fenestration, inner ear 20.62
   filtering bleb 12.66
   fixation device (broken) (displaced) (*see also* Fixation, bone, internal) 78.50
   flap or pedicle graft (skin) 86.75
   foot replacement (prosthesis) 81.59
   gastric anastomosis (with jejunal interposition) 44.5
   gastroduodenostomy (with jejunal interposition) 44.5
   gastrointestinal anastomosis (with jejunal interposition) 44.5
   gastrojejunostomy 44.5
   gastrostomy 44.69
   hand replacement (prosthesis) 81.97
   heart procedure NEC 35.95
   hip replacement (acetabulum) (femoral head) (partial) (total) 81.53
   Holter (-Spitz) valve 02.42
   ileal conduit 56.52
   ileostomy 46.41
   jejunoileal bypass 46.93
   jejunostomy 46.41
   joint replacement
     acetabulum 81.53
     ankle 81.59
     elbow 81.97
     femoral head 81.53
     foot 81.59
     hand 81.97
     hip (partial) (total) 81.53
     knee 81.55
     lower extremity NEC 81.59
     toe 81.59
     upper extremity 81.97
     wrist 81.97
   knee replacement (prosthesis) 81.55
   laryngostomy 31.63
   lateral canthus 08.59
   mallet finger 82.84
   mastoid antrum 19.9
   mastoidectomy 20.92
   nephrostomy 55.89
   neuroplasty 04.75
   ocular implant 16.62
   orbital implant 16.62
   previous mastectomy site — *see* category 85.
   proctostomy 48.79
   prosthesis
     acetabulum
       hip 81.53
     ankle 81.59
     breast 85.93
     elbow 81.97
     femoral head 81.53
     foot 81.59
     hand 81.97
     heart valve (poppet) 35.95
     hip (partial) (total) 81.53
     knee 81.55
     lower extremity NEC 81.59
     shoulder 81.97
     toe 81.59
     upper extremity 81.97
     wrist 81.97
   pstosis overcorrection 08.37
   pyelostomy 55.12
   pyloroplasty 44.29
   rhinoplasty 21.84
   scar
     skin 86.84
       with excision 86.3
   scleral fistulization 12.66
   shoulder replacement (prosthesis) 81.97
   shunt
     arteriovenous (cannula) (for dialysis) 39.42
     lumbar-subarachnoid NEC 03.97
     peritoneojugular 54.99
     pleurothecal 03.97
     salpingothecal 03.97
     spinal (thecal) NEC 03.97
     subarachnoid-peritoneal 03.97
     subarachnoid-ureteral 03.97
     ventricular (cerebral) 02.42
   stapedectomy NEC 19.29
     with inus replacement (homograft) (prosthesis) 19.21
   stoma
     bile duct 51.79
     bladder (vesicostomy) 57.22
     bronchus 33.42
     common duct 51.72
     esophagus 42.89
     gallbladder 51.99
     hepatic duct 51.79
     intestine 46.60
       large 46.43
       small 46.41
     kidney 55.89
     larynx 31.63
     rectum 48.79
     stomach 44.69
     thorax 34.79
     trachea 31.74
     ureter 56.62
     urethra 58.49
   tack operation 20.79
   toe replacement (prosthesis) 81.59
   tracheostomy 31.74
   tympanoplasty 19.6
   uretero-ileostomy, cutaneous 56.52
   ureterostomy (cutaneous) (stoma) NEC 56.62
     ileal 56.52
   urethrostomy 58.49
   urinary conduit 56.52
   vascular procedure (previous) NEC 39.49
   ventricular shunt (cerebral) 02.42
   vesicostomy stoma 57.22
   wrist replacement (prosthesis) 81.97
Rhinectomy 21.4
Rhinocheiloplasty 27.59
   cleft lip 27.54
Rhinomanometry 89.12
Rhinoplasty (external) (internal) NEC 21.87
   augmentation (with graft) (with synthetic implant) 21.85
   limited 21.86
   revision 21.84
   tip 21.86
   twisted nose 21.84

Rhinorrhaphy (external) (internal) 21.81
    for epistaxis 21.09
Rhinoscopy 21.21
Rhinoseptoplasty 21.84
Rhinotomy 21.1
Rhizotomy (radiofrequency) (spinal) 03.1
    acoustic 04.01
    trigeminal 04.02
Rhytidectomy (facial) 86.82
    eyelid
        lower 08.86
        upper 08.87
Rhytidoplasty (facial) 86.82
Ripstein operation (repair of prolapsed rectum) 48.75
Rodney Smith operattion (radical subtotal pancreatectomy) 52.53
Roentgenography — *see* also Radiography, cardiac, negatvie contrast 88.58

Rollin gof conjunctiva 10.33
Root
    canal (tooth) (therapy) 23.70
        with
            apicoectomy 23.72
            irrigation 23.71
        resection (tooth) (apex) 23.73
            with root canal therapy 23.72
        residual or retained 23.11
Rotation of fetal head
    forceps (instrumental) (Kielland) (Scanzoni) (key-in-lock) 72.4
    manual 73.51
Routine
    chest x-ray 87.44
    psychiatric visit 94.12
Roux-en-Y operation
    bile duct 51.36
    cholecystojejunostomy 51.32

    esophagus (intrathoracic) 42.54
    pancreaticojejunostomy 52.96
Roux-Goldthwait operation (repair of recurrent patellar dislocation) 81.44
Roux-Herzen-Judine operation (jejunal loop interposition) 42.63
Rubin test (insufflation of fallopian tube) 66.8
Ruiz-Mora operation (proximal phalangectomy for hammer toe) 77.99
Rupture
    esophageal web 42.01
    joint adhesions, manual 93.26
    membranes, artificial 73.09
        for surgical induction of labor 73.01
    ovarian cyst, manual 65.93
Russe operation (bone graft of scaphoid) 78.04

S

Sacculotomy (tack) 20.79
Sacrectomy (partial) 77.89
   total 77.99
Saemisch operation (corneal section) 11.1
Salpingectomy (bilateral) (total)
      (transvaginal) 66.51
   with oophorectomy 65.61
   partial (unilateral) 66.69
      with removal of tubal pregnancy 66.62
      bilateral 66.63
         for sterilization 66.39
            by endoscopy 66.29
      remaining or solitary tube 66.52
         with ovary 65.62
   unilateral (total) 66.4
      with
         oophorectomy 65.4
         removal of tubal pregnancy 66.62
      partial 66.69
Salpingography 87.85
Salpingohysterostomy 66.74
Salpingo-oophorectomy (unilateral) 65.4
   bilateral (same operative episode) 65.61
   remaining or solitary tube and ovary 65.62
Salpingo-oophoroplasty 65.73
Salpingo-oophororrhaphy 65.79
Salpingo-oophorostomy 66.72
Salpingo-oophorotomy 65.0
Salpingoplasty 66.79
Salpingorrhaphy 66.71
Salpingosalpingostomy 66.73
Salpingostomy (for removal of non-ruptured
      ectopic pregnancy) 66.02
Salpingotomy 66.01
Salpingo-uterostomy 66.74
Salter operation (innominate osteotomy)
   77.39
**Sampling, blood for genetic
      determination of fetus** 75.33
Sandpapering (skin) 86.25
Saucerization
   bone (*see also* Excision, lesion, bone) 77.60
   rectum 48.99
Sauer-Bacon operation (abdominoperineal
      resection) 48.5
Scalenectomy 83.45
Scalenotomy 83.19
Scaling and polishing, dental 96.54
Scan, scanning
   C.A.T. (computerized axial tomography)
      88.38
      abdomen 88.01
      bone 88.38
         mineral density 88.98
      brain 87.03
      head 87.03
      kidney 87.71
      skeletal 88.38
         mineral density 88.98
      thorax 87.41
   computerized axial tomography (C.A.T.)
      (*see also* Scan, C.A.T.) 88.38
   C.T. - *see* Scan, C.A.T.
   gallium — *see* Scan, radioisotope
   liver 92.02
   positron emission tomography (PET) — *see*
      Scan, radioisotope
   radioisotope
      adrenal 92.09
      bone 92.14
         marrow 92.05
      bowel 92.04
      cardiac output 92.05
      cardiovascular 92.05
      cerebral 92.11
      circulation time 92.05
      eye 95.16
      gastrointestinal 92.04
      head NEC 92.12
      hematopoietic 92.05
      intestine 92.04
      iodine-131 92.01
      kidney 92.03
      liver 92.02
      lung 92.15
      lymphatic system 92.16
      myocardial infarction 92.05
      pancreatic 92.04
      parathyroid 92.13
      pituitary 92.11
      placenta 92.17
      protein-bound iodine 92.01
      pulmonary 92.15
      radio-iodine uptake 92.01
      renal 92.03
      specified site NEC 92.19
      spleen 92.05
      thyroid 92.01
      total body 92.18
      uterus 92.19
   renal 92.03
   thermal — *see* Thermography
Scapulectomy (partial) 77.81
   total 77.91
Scapulopexy 78.41
Scarification
   conjunctiva 10.33
   nasal veins (with packing) 21.03
   pericardium 36.3
   pleura 34.6
      chemical 34.92
         with cancer chemotherapy
            substance 34.92 [99.25]
            tetracycline 34.92 [99.21]
Schanz operation (femoral osteotomy)
   77.35
Schauta (-Amreich) **operation** (radical vaginal
      hysterectomy) 68.7
Schede operation (thoracoplasty) 33.34
Scheie operation
   cautery of sclera 12.62
   sclerostomy 12.62
Schlatter operation (total gastrectomy)
   43.99
Schroeder operation (endocervical
      excision) 67.39
Schuchardt operation (nonobstetrical
      episiotomy) 71.09
Schwartze operation (simple
      mastoidectomy) 20.41
Scintiphotography — *see* Scan, radioisotope
Scintiscan — *see* Scan, radioisotope
Sclerectomy (punch) (scissors) 12.65
   for retinal reattachment 14.49
   Holth's 12.65
   trephine 12.61
      with implant 14.41
Scleroplasty 12.89
Sclerosis — *see* Sclerotherapy
Sclerostomy (Scheie's) 12.62
Sclerotherapy
   esophageal varices (endoscopic) 42.33
   hemorrhoids 49.42
   pleura 34.92
      treatment of malignancy (cytoxic
         agent) 34.92 [99.25]
      with tetracycline 34.92 [99.21]
   varicose vein 39.92
   vein NEC 39.92
Sclerotomy (exploratory) 12.89
   anterior 12.89
      with
         iridectomy 12.65
         removal of vitreous 14.71
   posterior 12.89
      with
         iridectomy 12.65
         removal of vitreous 14.72
Scott operation
   intestinal bypass for obesity 45.93
   jejunocolostomy (bypass) 45.93
Scraping
   corneal epithelium 11.41
      for smear or culture 11.21
   trachoma follicles 10.33
Scrotectomy (partial) 61.3
Scrotoplasty 61.49
Scrotorrhaphy 61.41
Scrototomy 61.0
Scrub, posterior nasal (adhesions) 21.91
Sculpturing, heart valve — *see*
   Valvuloplasty, heart
Section — *see also* Division and Incision
   cesarean — *see* Cesarean section
   ganglion, sympathetic 05.0
   hypophyseal stalk (*see also*
      Hypophysectomy, partial) 07.63
   ligamentum flavum (spine) — omit code
   nerve (cranial) (peripheral) NEC 04.03
      acoustic 04.01
      spinal root (posterior) 03.1
      sympathetic 05.0
      trigeminal tract 04.02
   Saemisch (corneal) 11..1
   spinal ligament 80.49
      arcuate — omit code
      flavum — omit code
   tooth (impacted) 23.19
Seddon-Brooks operation (transfer of
      pectoralis major tendon) 83.75
Semb operation (apicolysis of lung) 33.39
Senning operation (correction of
      transposition of great vessels) 35.91
Separation
   twins (attached) (conjoined) (Siamese)
      84.93
      asymmetrical (unequal) 84.93
      symmetrical (equal) 84.92
Septectomy
   atrial (closed) 35.41
      open 35.42
      transvenous method (balloon) 35.41
   submucous (nasal) 21.5
Septoplasty NEC 21.88
   with submucous resection of septum 21.5
Septorhinoplasty 21.84

Septostomy (atrial) (balloon) 35.41
Septotomy, nasal 21.1
Sequestrectomy
    bone 77.00
        carpals, metacarpals 77.04
        clavicle 77.01
        facial 76.01
        femur 77.05
        fibula 77.07
        humerus 77.02
        nose 21.32
        patella 77.06
        pelvic 77.09
        phalanges (foot) (hand) 77.09
        radius 77.03
        scapula 77.01
        skull 01.25
        specified site NEC 77.09
        tarsals, metatarsals 77.08
        thorax (ribs) (sternum) 77.01
        tibia 77.07
        ulna 77.03
        vertebrae 77.09
    nose 21.32
    skull 01.24
Sesamoidectomy 77.98
Setback, ear 18.5
Sever operation (division of soft tissue of arm) 83.19
Severing of blepharorrhaphy 08.02
Sewell operation (heart) 36.2
Sharrard operation n(iliopsoas muscle transfer) 83.77
Shaving
    bone (see also Excision, lesion, bone) 77.60
    cornea (epithelium) 11.41
        for smear or culture 11.21
    patella 77.66
Shelf operation (hip arthroplasty) 81.40
Shirodkar operation (encirclement suture, cervix) 67.5
Shock therapy
    chemical 94.24
    electroconvulsive 94.27
    electrotonic 94.27
    insulin 94.24
    subconvulsive 94.26
Shortening
    bone (fusion) 78.20
        femur 78.25
        specified site NEC - see category 78.2
        tibia 78.27
        ulna 78.23
    endopelvic fascia 69.22
    extraocular muscle NEC 15.22
        multiple (two or more muscles) 15.4
    eyelid margin 08.71
    eye muscle NEC 15.22
        multiple (two or more muscles) (with lengthening) 15.4
    finger (macrodactyly repair) 82.83
    hell cord 83.85
    levator palpebrae muscle 08.33
    ligament — see also Arthroplasty
        round 69.22
        uterosacral 69.22
    muscle 83.85
        extraocular 15.22
            multiple (two or more muscles) 15.4
        hand 83.55
    sclera (for repair of retinal detachment) 14.59
        by scleral buckling (see also Buckling, scleral) 14.49
    tendon 83.85
        hand 82.55
    ureter (with reimplantation) 56.41
Shunt — see also Anastomosis and Bypass, vascular
    abdominovenous 54.94
    aorta-coronary sinus 36.3
    aorta (descending)-pulmonary (artery) 39.0
    aortocarotid 39.22
    aortoceliac 39.26
    aortofemoral 39.25
    aortoiliac 39.25
    aortoiliofemoral 39.25
    aortomesenteric 39.26
    aorto-myocardial (graft) 36.2
    aortorenal 39.24
    aortosubclavian 39.22
    apicoaortic 35.93
    arteriovenous NEC 39.29
        for renal dialysis (by)
            anastomosis 39.27
            external cannula 39.93
    ascending aorta to pulmonary artery (Waterston) 39.0
    axillary-femoral 39.29
    carotid-carotid 39.22
    carotid-subclavian 39.22
    caval-mesenteric 39.1
    corpora cavernosa-corpus spongiosum 64.98
    corpora-saphenous 64.98
    descending aorta to pulmonary artery (Potts-Smith) 39.0
    endolymphatic (-subarachnoid) 20.71
    endolymph-perilymph 20.71
    extracranial-intracranial (EC-IC) 39.28
    femoroperoneal 39.29
    femoropopliteal 39.29
    iliofemoral 39.25
    ilioiliac 39.25
    intestinal
        large-to-large 45.94
        small-to-large 45.93
        small-to-small 45.91
    left subclavian to descending aorta (Blalock-Park) 39.0
    left-to-right (systemic-pulmonary artery) 39.0
    left ventricle (heart) (apex) and aorta 35.93
    lienorenal 39.1
    lumbar-subarachnoid (with valve) NEC 03.79
    mesocaval 39.1
    peritoneal-jugular 54.94
    peritoneo-vascular 54.94
    peritoneovenous 54.94
    ▶ pleuroperitoneal 34.05
    pleurothecal (with valve) 03.79
    portacaval (double) 39.1
    portal-systemic 39.1
    portal vein to vena cava 39.1
    pulmonary-innominate 39.0
    pulmonary vein to atrium 35.82
    renoportal 39.1
    right atrium and pulmonary artery 35.94
    right ventricle and pulmonary artery (distal) 35.92
        in repair of
            pulmonary artery atresia 35.92
            transposition of great vessels 35.92
            truncus arteriosus 35.83
    salpingothecal (with valve) 03.79
    semicircular-subarachnoid 20.71
    spinal (thecal) (with valve) NEC 03.79
        subarachnoid-peritoneal 03.71
        subarachnoid-ureteral 03.72
    ▶ splenorenal (venous) 39.1
    ▶   arterial 39.26
    subarachnoid-peritoneal (with valve) 03.71
    subarachnoid-ureteral (with valve) 03.72
    subclavian-pulmonary 39.0
    subdural-peritoneal (with valve) 02.34
    superior mesenteric-caval 39.1
    systemic-pulmonary artery 39.0
    ▶ transjugular intrahepatic portosystemic (TIPS) 39.1
    vena cava to pulmonary artery (Green) 39.21
    ventricular (cerebral) (with valve) 02.2
        to
            abdominal cavity or organ 02.34
            bone marrow 02.39
            cervical subarachnoid space 02.2
            circulatory system 02.32
            cisterna magna 02.2
            extracranial site NEC 02.39
            gallbladder 02.34
            head or neck structure 02.31
            intracerebral site NEC 02.2
            lumbar site 02.39
            mastoid 02.31
            nasopharynx 02.31
            thoracic cavity 02.33
            ureter 02.35
            urinary system 02.35
            venous system 02.32
    ventriculoatrial (with valve) 02.32
    ventriculocaval (with valve) 02.32
    ventriculocisternal (with valve) 02.2
    ventriculolumbar (with valve) 02.39
    ventriculomastoid (with valve) 02.31
    ventriculonasopharyngeal 02.31
    ventriculopleural (with valve) 02.33
Sialoadenectomy (parotid) (sublingual) (submaxillary) 26.30
    complete 26.32
    partial 26.31
    radical 26.32
Sialoadenolithotomy 26.0
Sialoadenotomy 26.0
Sialodochoplasty NEC 26.49
Sialogram 87.09
Sialolithotomy 26.0
Sieve, vena cava 38.7
Sigmoid bladder 57.87 [45.52]
Sigmoidectomy 45.76
Sigmoidomyotomy 46.91
Sigmoidopexy (Moschowitz) 46.63
Sigmoidoproctectomy (see also Resection, rectum) 48.69
Sigmoidoproctostomy 45.94
Sigmoidorectostomy 45.94
Sigmoidorrhaphy 46.75
Sigmoidoscopy (rigid) 48.23
    with biopsy 45.25
    flexible 45.24
    through stoma (artificial) 45.22
    transabdominal 45.21
Sigmoidosigmoidostomy 45.94
    proximal to distal segment 45.76
Sigmoidostomy (see also Colostomy) 46.10
Sigmoidotomy 45.03

Sign language 93.75
Silver operation (bunionectomy) 77.59
Sinogram
    abdominal wall 88.03
    chest wall 87.38
    retroperitoneum 88.14
Sinusectomy (nasal) (complete) (partial) (with turbinectomy) 22.60
    antrum 22.62
        with Caldwell-Luc approach 22.61
    ethmoid 22.63
    frontal 22.42
    maxillary 22.62
        with Caldwell-Luc approach 22.61
    sphenoid 22.64
Sinusotomy (nasal) 22.50
    antrum (intranasal) 22.2
        with external approach (Caldwell-Luc) 22.39
            radical (with removal of membrane lining) 22.31
    ethmoid 22.51
    frontal 22.41
    maxillary (intranasal) 22.2
        external approach (Caldwell-Luc) 22.39
            radical (with removal of membrane lining) 22.31
    multiple 22.53
    perinasal 22.50
    sphenoid 22.52
Sistrunk operation (excision of thyroglossal cyst) 06.7
Size reduction
    abdominal wall (adipose) (pendulous) 86.83
    arms (adipose) (batwing) 86.83
    breast (bilateral) 85.32
        unilateral 85.31
    buttocks (adipose) 86.83
    skin 86.83
    subcutaneous tissue 86.83
    thighs (adipose) 86.83
Skeletal series (x-ray) 88.31
Sling — *see also* Operation, sling
    fascial (fascia lata)
        for facial weakness (trigeminal nerve paralysis) 86.81
        mouth 86.81
        orbicularis (mouth) 86.81
        tongue 25.59
    levator muscle (urethrocystopexy) 59.71
    pubococcygeal 59.71
    rectum (puborectalis) 48.76
    tongue (fascial) 25.59
Slitting
    canaliculus for
        passage of tube 09.42
        removal of streptothrix 09.42
    lens 13.2
    prepuce (dorsal) (lateral) 64.91
Slocum operation (pes anserinus transfer) 81.47
Sluder operation (tonsillectomy) 28.2
Small bowel series (x-ray) 87.63
Smith operation (open osteotomy of mandible) 76.62
Smith-Peterson operation n(radiocarpal arthrodesis) 81.25
Smithwick operation (sympathectomy) 05.29
Snaring, polyp, colon (endoscopic) 45.42
Snip, punctum (with dilation) 09.51

Soave operation (endorectal pull-through) 48.41
Somatotherapy, psychiatric NEC 94.29
Sonneberg operation (inferior maxillary neurectomy) 04.07
Sorondo-Ferre operation (hindquarter amputation) 84.19
Soutter operation (iliac crest fasciotomy) 83.14
SP Rogers operation (knee disarticulation) 84.16
Spaulding-Richardson operation (uterine suspension) 69.22
Spectrophotometry NEC 89.39
    blood 89.39
    placenta 89.29
    urine 89.29
Speech therapy NEC 93.75
Spermatocelectomy 63.2
Spermatocystectomy 60.73
Spermatocystotomy 60.72
Sphenoidectomy 22.64
Sphenoidotomy 22.52
Sphincterectomy, anal 49.6
Sphincteroplasty
    anal 49.79
        obstetrical laceration (current) 75.62
            old 49.79
    bladder neck 57.85
    pancreas 51.83
    sphincter of Oddi 51.83
Sphincterorrhaphy, anal 49.71
    obstetrical laceration (current) 75.62
    old 49.79
Sphincterotomy
    anal (external) (internal) 49.59
        left lateral 49.51
        posterior 49.52
    bladder (neck) (transurethral) 57.91
    choledochal 51.82
        endoscopic 51.85
    iris 12.12
    pancreatic 51.82
        endoscopic 51.85
    sphincter of Oddi 51.82
        endoscopic 51.85
    transduodenal ampullary 51.82
        endoscopic 51.85
Spinal anesthesia — omit code
Spinelli operation (correction of inverted uterus) 75.93
Spirometry (incentive) (respiratory) 89.37
Spivack operation (permanent gastrostomy) 43.19
Splanchnicectomy 05.29
Splanchnicotomy 05.0
Splenectomy (complete) (total) 41.5
    partial 41.43
Splenogram 88.64
    radioisotope 92.05
Splenolysis 54.5
Splenopexy 41.95
Splenoplasty 41.95
Splenoportogram (by splenic arteriography) 88.64
Splenorrhaphy 41.95
Splenotomy 41.2
Splinting
    dental (for immobilization) 93.55
        orthodontic 24.7
    musculoskeletal 93.54

    ureteral 56.2
Splitting — *see also* Division
    canaliculus 09.52
    lacrimal papilla 09.51
    spinal cord tracts 03.29
        percutaneous 03.21
    tendon sheath 83.01
        hand 82.01
Spondylosyndesis (*see also* Fusion, spinal) 81.00
Ssabanejew-Frank operation (permanent gastrostomy) 43.19
Stab, intercostal 34.09
Stabilization, joint — *see also* Arthrodesis
    patella (for recurrent dislocation) 81.44
Stacke operation (simple mastoidectomy) 20.41
Stallard operation (conjunctivocystorhinostomy) 09.82
    with insertion of tube or stent 09.83
Stamm (-Kader) operation (temporary gastrostomy) 43.19
Stapedectomy 19.19
    with incus replacement (homograft) (prosthesis) 19.11
    revision 19.29
        with incus replacement 19.21
Stapediolysis 19.0
Stapling
    artery 39.31
    blebs, lung (emphysematous) 32.21
    diaphysis (*see also* Stapling, epiphyseal plate) 78.20
    epiphyseal plate 78.20
        femur 78.25
        fibula 78.27
        humerus 78.22
        radius 78.23
        specified site NEC 78.29
        tibia 78.27
        ulna 78.23
    gastric varices 44.91
    graft — *see* Graft
    vein 39.32
Steinberg operation 44.5
Steindler operation
    fascia stripping (for cavus deformity) 83.14
    flexorplasty (elbow) 83.77
    muscle transfer 83.77
Sterilization
    female (*see also* specific operation) 66.39
    male NEC (*see also* Ligation, vas deferens) 63.70
Sternotomy 77.31
    as operative approach — omit code
    for bone marrow biopsy 41.31
Stewart operation (renal plication with pyeloplasty) 55.87
Stimulation (electronic) — *see also* Implant, electronic stimulator
    bone growth (percutaneous) — *see* category 78.9
        transcutaneous (surface) 99.86
    cardiac (external) 99.62
        internal 37.91
    carotid sinus 99.64
    electrophysiologic, cardiac 37.26
    nerve, peripheral or spinal cord, transcutaneous 93.39
Stitch, Kelly-Stoeckel (urethra) 59.3
Stomatoplasty 27.59

Stomatorrhaphy 27.52
Stone operation (anoplasty) 49.79
Strassman operation (metroplasty) 69.49
Strayer operation (gastrocnemius recession) 83.72
Stretching
   eyelid (with elongation) 08.71
   fascia 93.28
   foreskin 99.95
   iris 12.63
   muscle 93.27
   nerve (cranial) (peripheral) 04.91
   tendon 93.27
Stripping
   bone (*see also* Incision, bone) 77.10
   carotid sinus 39.8
   cranial suture 02.01
   fascia 83.14
      hand 82.12
   membrane for surgical induction of labor 73.1
   meninges (cerebral) 01.51
      spinal 03.4
   saphenous vein, varicose 38.59
   subdural membrane (cerebral) 01.51
      spinal 03.4
   varicose veins (lower limb) 38.59
      upper limb 38.53
   vocal cords 30.09
Stromeyer-Little operation (hepatotomy) 50.0
Strong operation (unbridling of celiac artery axis) 39.91
Stryker frame 93.59
Study
   bone mineral density 88.98
   bundle of His 37.29
   color vision 95.06
   conduction, nerve (median) 89.15
   dark adaptation, eye 95.07
   electrophysiologic stimulation and recording, cardiac 37.26
   function — *see also* Function, study
      radioisotope — *see* Scan, radioisotope
   lacrimal flow (radiographic) 87.05
   ocular motility 95.15
   pulmonary function — (*see* categories 89.37–89.38)
   radiographic — *see* Radiography
   radio-iodinated triolein 92.04
   renal clearance 92.03
   spirometer 89.37
   tracer — *see also* Scan, radioisotope
      eye (P32) 95.16
   ultrasonic — *see* Ultrasonography
   visual field 95.05
   xenon flow NEC 92.19
      cardiovascular 92.05
      pulmonary 92.15
Sturmdorf operation (conization of cervix) 67.2
Submucous resection
   larynx 30.29
   nasal septum 21.5
Summerskill operation (dacryocystorhinostomy by intubation) 09.81
Surmay operation (jejunostomy) 46.39
Suspension
   balanced, for traction 93.45
   bladder NEC 57.89
   diverticulum pharynx 29.59
   kidney 55.7
   Olshausen (uterus) 69.22
   ovary 65.79
   paraurethral (Pereyra) 59.6
   periurethral 59.6
   urethra (retropubic) (sling) 59.5
   urethrovesical
      Goebel-Frangenheim-Stoeckel 59.4
      gracilis muscle transplant 59.71
      levator muscle sling 59.71
      Marshall-Marchetti (-Krantz) 59.5
      Millin-Read 59.4
      suprapubic 59.4
   uterus (abdominal or vaginal approach) 69.22
   vagina 70.77
Suture (laceration)
   abdominal wall 54.63
      secondary 54.61
   adenoid fossa 28.7
   adrenal (gland) 07.44
   aneurysm (cerebral) (peripheral) 39.52
   anus 49.71
      obstetric laceration (current) 75.62
      old 49.79
   aorta 39.31
   aponeurosis (*see also* Suture, tendon) 83.64
   arteriovenous fistula 39.53
   artery 39.31
   bile duct 51.79
   bladder 57.81
      obstetric laceration (current) 75.61
   blood vessel NEC 39.30
      artery 39.31
      vein 39.32
   breast (skin) 85.81
   bronchus 33.41
   bursa 83.99
      hand 82.99
   canaliculus 09.73
   cecum 46.75
   cerebral meninges 02.11
   cervix (traumatic laceration) 67.61
      internal os, encirclement 67.5
      obstetric laceration (current) 75.51
      old 67.69
   chest wall 34.71
   cleft palate 27.62
   clitoris 71.4
   colon 46.75
   common duct 51.71
   conjunctiva 10.6
   cornea 11.51
      with conjunctival flap 11.53
   corneoscleral 11.51
      with conjunctival flap 11.53
   diaphragm 34.82
   duodenum 46.71
      ulcer (bleeding) (perforated) 44.42
         endoscopic 44.43
   dura mater (cerebral) 02.11
      spinal 03.59
   ear, external 18.4
   enterocele 70.92
   entropion 08.42
   epididymis (and)
      spermatic cord 63.51
      vas deferens 63.81
   episiotomy — *see* Episiotomy
   esophagus 42.82
   eyeball 16.89
   eyebrow 08.81
   eyelid 08.81
      with entropion or ectropion repair 08.42
   fallopian tube 66.71
   fascia 83.65
      hand 82.46
      to skeletal attachment 83.89
         hand 82.89
   gallbladder 51.91
   ganglion, sympathetic 05.81
   gingiva 24.32
   great vessel 39.30
      artery 39.31
      vein 39.32
   gum 24.32
   heart 37.4
   hepatic duct 51.79
   hymen 70.76
   ileum 46.73
   intestine 46.79
      large 46.75
      small 46.73
   jejunum 46.73
   joint capsule 81.96
      with arthroplasty — *see* Arthroplasty
      ankle 81.94
      foot 81.94
      lower extremity NEC 81.95
      upper extremity 81.93
   kidney 55.81
   labia 71.71
   laceration — *see* Suture, by site
   larynx 31.61
   ligament 81.96
      with arthroplasty — *see* Arthroplasty
      ankle 81.94
      broad 69.29
      Cooper's 54.64
      foot and toes 81.94
      gastrocolic 54.73
      knee 81.95
      lower extremity NEC 81.95
      sacrouterine 69.29
      upper extremity 81.93
      uterine 69.29
   ligation — *see* Ligation
   lip 27.51
   liver 50.61
   lung 33.43
   meninges (cerebral) 02.11
      spine 03.59
   mesentery 54.75
   mouth 27.52
   muscle 83.65
      hand 82.46
      ocular (oblique) (rectus) 15.7
   nerve (cranial) (peripheral) 04.3
      sympathetic 05.81
   nose (external) (internal) 21.81
      for epistaxis 21.09
   obstetric laceration NEC 75.69
      bladder 75.61
      cervix 75.51
      corpus uteri 75.52
      pelvic floor 75.69
      perineum 75.69
      rectum 75.62
      sphincter ani 75.62
      urethra 75.61
      uterus 75.50
      vagina 75.69
      vulva 75.69
   omentum 54.64
   ovary 65.71

palate 27.61
    cleft 27.62
palpebral fissure 08.59
pancreas 52.95
pelvic floor 71.71
    obstetric laceration (current) 75.69
penis 64.41
peptic ulcer (bleeding) (perforated) 44.40
pericardium 37.4
perineum (female) 71.71
    after delivery 75.69
        episiotomy repair — see Episiotomy
    male 86.59
periosteum 78.10
    carpal, metacarpal 78.24
    femur 78.25
    fibula 78.27
    humerus 78.22
    pelvic 78.29
    phalanges (foot) (hand) 78.29
    radius 78.23
    specified site NEC 78.29
    tarsal, metatarsal 78.28
    tibia 78.27
    ulna 78.23
    vertebrae 78.29
peritoneum 54.64
periurethral tissue to symphysis pubis 59.5
pharynx 29.51
pleura 34.93
rectum 48.71
    obstetric laceration (current) 75.62
retina (for reattachment) 14.59
sacrouterine ligament 69.29
salivary gland 26.41
scalp 86.59
    replantation 86.51
sclera (with repair of conjunctiva) 12.81
scrotum (skin) 61.41
secondary
    abdominal wall 54.61
    episiotomy 75.69
    peritoneum 54.64
sigmoid 46.75
skin (mucous membrane) (without graft) 86.59
    with graft — see Graft, skin
    breast 85.81
    ear 18.4
    eyebrow 08.81
    eyelid 08.81
    nose 21.81
    penis 64.41
    scalp 86.59
        replantation 86.51
    scrotum 61.41
    vulva 71.71
specified site NEC — see Repair, by site
spermatic cord 63.51
sphincter ani 49.71
    obstetric laceration (current) 75.62
    old 49.79

spinal meninges 03.59
spleen 41.95
stomach 44.61
    ulcer (bleeding) (perforated) 44.41
        endoscopic 44.43
subcutaneous tissue (without skin graft) 86.59
    with graft — see Graft, skin
tendon (direct) (immediate) (primary) 83.64
    delayed (secondary) 83.62
        hand NEC 82.43
            flexors 82.42
    hand NEC 82.45
        delayed (secondary) 82.43
        flexors 82.44
            delayed (secondary) 82.42
    ocular 15.7
    rotator cuff 83.63
    sheath 83.61
        hand 82.41
    supraspinatus (rotator cuff repair) 83.63
    to skeletal attachment 83.88
        hand 82.85
Tenon's capsule 15.7
testis 62.61
thymus 07.93
thyroid gland 06.93
tongue 25.51
tonsillar fossa 28.7
trachea 31.71
tunica vaginalis 61.41
ulcer (bleeding) (perforated) (peptic) 44.40
    duodenum 44.42
        endoscopic 44.43
    gastric 44.41
        endoscopic 44.43
    intestine 46.79
    skin 86.59
    stomach 44.41
        endoscopic 44.43
ureter 56.82
urethra 58.41
    obstetric laceration (current) 75.61
uterosacral ligament 69.29
uterus 69.41
    obstetric laceration (current) 75.50
    old 69.49
uvula 27.73
vagina 70.71
    obstetric laceration (current) 75.69
    old 70.79
vas deferens 63.81
vein 39.32
vulva 71.71
    obstetric laceration (current) 75.69
    old 71.79
Suture-ligation — see also Ligation
    blood vessel — see Ligation, blood vessel
Sweep, anterior iris 12.97

Swenson operation
    bladder reconstruction 57.87
    proctectomy 48.49
Swinney operation (urethral reconstruction) 58.46
Switch, switching
    coronary arteries 35.84
    great arteries, total 35.84
Syme operation
    ankle amputation through malleoli of tibia and fibula 84.14
    urethrotomy, external 58.0
Sympathectomy NEC 05.29
    cervical 05.22
    cervicothoracic 05.22
    lumbar 05.23
    periarterial 39.7
    presacral 05.24
    renal 05.29
    thoracolumbar 05.23
    tympanum 20.91
Sympatheticotripsy 05.0
Symphysiotomy 77.39
    assisting delivery (obstetrical) 73.94
    kidney (horseshoe) 55.85
Symphysis, pleural 34.6
Synchondrotomy (see also Division, cartilage) 80.40
Syndactylization 86.89
Syndesmotomy (see also Division, ligament) 80.40
Synechiotomy
    endometrium 68.21
    iris (posterior) 12.33
        anterior 12.32
Synovectomy (joint) (complete) (partial) 80.70
    ankle 80.77
    elbow 80.72
    foot and toe 80.78
    hand and finger 80.74
    hip 80.75
    knee 80.76
    shoulder 80.71
    specified site NEC 80.79
    spine 80.79
    tendon sheath 83.42
        hand 82.33
    wrist 80.73
Syringing
    lacrimal duct or sac 09.43
    nasolacrimal duct 09.43
    with
        dilation 09.43
        insertion of tube or stent 09.44

T

Taarnhoj operation (trigeminal nerve root decompression) 04.41
Tack operation (sacculotomy) 20.79
Take-down
  anastomosis
    arterial 39.49
    blood vessel 39.49
    gastric, gastrointestinal 44.5
    intestine 46.93
    stomach 44.5
    vascular 39.49
    ventricular 02.43
  arterial bypass 39.49
  arteriovenous shunt 39.43
    with creation of new shunt 39.42
  cecostomy 46.52
  colostomy 46.52
  duodenostomy 46.51
  enterostomy 46.50
  esophagostomy 42.83
  gastroduodenostomy 44.5
  gastrojejunostomy 44.5
  ileostomy 46.51
  intestinal stoma 46.50
    large 46.52
    small 46.51
  jejunoileal bypass 46.93
  jejunostomy 46.51
  laryngostomy 31.62
  sigmoidostomy 46.52
  stoma
    bile duct 51.79
    bladder 57.82
    bronchus 33.42
    common duct 51.72
    esophagus 42.83
    gallbladder 51.92
    hepatic duct 51.79
    intestine 46.50
      large 46.52
      small 46.51
    kidney 55.82
    larynx 31.62
    rectum 48.72
    stomach 44.62
    thorax 34.72
    trachea 31.72
    ureter 56.83
    urethra 58.42
  systemic-pulmonary artery anastomosis 39.49
    in total repair of tetralogy of Fallot 35.81
  tracheostomy 31.72
  vascular anastomosis or bypass 39.49
  ventricular shunt (cerebral) 02.43
Talectomy 77.98
Talma-Morison operation (omentopexy) 54.74
Tamponade
  esophageal 96.06
  intrauterine (nonobstetric) 69.91
    after delivery or abortion 75.8
    antepartum 73.1
  vagina 96.14
    after delivery or abortion 75.8
    antepartum 73.1
Tanner operation (devascularization of stomach) 44.99
Tap
  abdomen 54.91
  chest 34.91
  cisternal 01.01
  cranial 01.09
  joint 81.91
  lumbar (diagnostic) (removal of dye) 03.31
  perilymphatic 20.79
  spinal (diagnostic) 03.31
  subdural (through fontanel) 01.09
  thorax 34.91
Tarsectomy 08.20
  de Grandmont 08.35
Tarsoplasty (*see also* Reconstruction, eyelid) 08.70
Tarsorrhaphy (lateral) 08.52
  division or severing 08.02
Tattooing
  cornea 11.91
  skin 86.02
Tautening, eyelid for entropion 08.42
Telemetry (cardiac) 89.54
Teleradiotherapy
  beat particles 92.25
  Betatron 92.24
  cobalt-60 92.23
  electrons 92.25
  iodine-125 92.23
  linear accelerator 92.24
  neutrons 92.26
  particulate radiation NEC 92.26
  photons 92.24
  protons 92.26
  radioactive cesium 92.23
  radioisotopes NEC 92.23
Temperature gradient study (*see also* Thermography) 88.89
Temperment assessment 94.02
Tendinoplasty — *see* Repair, tendon
Tendinosuture (immediate) (primary) (*see also* Suture, tendon) 83.64
  hand (*see also* Suture, tendon, hand) 82.45
Tendolysis 83.91
  hand 82.91
Tendoplasty — *see* Repair, tendon
Tenectomy 83.39
  eye 15.13
    levator palpebrae 08.33
    multiple (two or more tendons) 15.3
  hand 82.29
  levator palpebrae 08.33
  tendon sheath 83.31
    hand 82.21
Tenodesis (tendon fixation to skeletal attachment) 83.88
  Fowler 82.85
  hand 82.85
Tenolysis 83.91
  hand 82.91
Tenomyoplasty (*see also* Repair, tendon) 83.88
  hand (*see also* Repair, tendon, hand) 82.86
Tenomyotomy — *see* Tenonectomy
Tenonectomy 83.42
  for graft 83.41
    hand 82.32
  hand 82.33
    for graft 82.32
Tenontomyoplasty — *see* Repair, tendon
Tenontoplasty — *see* Repair, tendon
Tenoplasty (*see also* Repair, tendon) 83.88
  hand (*see also* Repair, tendon, hand) 82.86
Tenorrhaphy (*see also* Suture, tendon) 83.64
  hand (*see also* Suture, tendon, hand) 82.45
  to skeletal attachment 83.88
    hand 82.85
Tenosuspension 83.88
  hand 82.86
Tenosuture (*see also* Suture, tendon) 83.64
  hand (*see also* Suture, tendon, hand) 82.45
  to skeletal attachment 83.88
    hand 82.85
Tenosynovectomy 83.42
  hand 82.33
Tenotomy 83.13
  Achilles tendon 83.11
  adductor (hip) (subcutaneous) 83.12
  eye 15.12
    levator palpebrae 08.38
    multiple (two or more tendons) 15.4
  hand 82.11
  levator palpebrae 08.38
  pectoralis minor tendon (decompression thoracic outlet) 83.13
  stapedius 19.0
  tensor tympani 19.0
Tenovaginotomy — *see* Tenotomy
Tensing, orbicularis oculi 08.59
Termination of pregnancy
  by
    aspiration curettage 69.51
    dilation and curettage 69.01
    hysterectomy — *see* Hysterectomy
    hysterotomy 74.91
    intra-amniotic injection (saline) 75.0
Test, testing (for)
  auditory function NEC 95.46
  Bender Visual-Motor Gestalt 94.02
  Benton Visual Retention 94.02
  cardiac (vascular)
    function NEC 89.59
    stress 89.44
      bicycle ergometer 89.43
      Masters' two-step 89.42
      treadmill 89.41
  Denver developmental (screening) 94.02
  fetus, fetal
    nonstress (fetal activity acceleration determinations) 75.35
    oxytocin challenge (contraction stress) 75.35
    sensitivity (to oxytocin) — omit code
  14 C-Urea breath 89.39
  function
    cardiac NEC 89.59
    hearing NEC 95.46
    muscle (by)
      electromyography 93.08
      manual 93.04
    neurologic NEC 89.15
    vestibular 95.46
      clinical 95.44
  glaucoma NEC 95.26
  hearing 95.47
    clinical NEC 95.42
  intelligence 94.01

Thal operation

internal jugular-subclavian venous reflux 89.62
intracarotid amobarbital (Wada) 89.10
Master's two-step stress (cardiac) 89.42
muscle function (by)
    electromyography 93.08
    manual 93.04
neurologic function NEC 89.15
nocturnal penile tumescence 89.29
provocative, for glaucoma 95.26
psychologic NEC 94.08
psychometric 94.01
radio-cobalt B12 Shilling 92.04
range of motion 93.05
rotation (Barany chair) (hearing) 95.45
sleep disorder function — (see categories 89.17–89.18)
Stanford-Binet 94.01
tuning fork (hearing) 95.42
Thallium stress (transesophageal pacing) 89.44
► Urea breath, (14 C) 89.39
vestibular function NEC 95.46
    thermal 95.44
Wada (hemispheric function) 89.10
whispered speech (hearing) 95.42

Thal operation (repair of esophageal stricture) 42.85
Thalamectomy 01.41
Thalamotomy 01.41
Theleplasty 85.87
Therapy
    Antabuse 94.25
    art 93.89
    aversion 94.33
    behavior 94.33
    Bennett respirator — see category 96.7
    blind rehabilitation NEC 93.78
    Byrd respirator — see category 96.7
    carbon dioxide 94.25
    cobalt-60 92.23
    conditioning, psychiatric 94.33
    continuous positive airway pressure (CPAP) 93.90
    croupette, croup tent 93.94
    daily living activities 93.83
        for the blind 93.78
    dance 93.89
    desensitization 94.33
    detoxification 94.25
    diversional 93.81
    domestic tasks 93.83
        for the blind 93.78
    educational (bed-bound children) (handicapped) 93.82
    electroconvulsive (ECT) 94.27
    electroshock (EST) 94.27
        subconvulsive 94.26
    electrotonic (ETT) 94.27
    encounter group 94.44
    extinction 94.33
    family 94.42
    fog (inhalation) 93.94
    gamma ray 92.23
    group NEC 94.44
        for psychosexual dysfunctions 94.41
    hearing NEC 95.49
    heat NEC 93.35
        for cancer treatment 99.85
    helium 93.98
    hot pack(s) 93.35
    hyperbaric oxygen 93.95
        wound 93.59
    hyperthermia NEC 93.35
        for cancer treatment 99.85
    individual, psychiatric NEC 94.39
        for psychosexual dysfunction 94.34
    industrial 93.89
    infrared irradiation 93.35
    inhalation NEC 93.96
    insulin shock 94.24
    intermittent positive pressure breathing (IPPB) 93.91
    IPPB (intermittent positive pressure breathing) 93.91
    lithium 94.22
    manipulative, osteopathic (see also Manipulation, osteopathic) 93.67
    manual arts 93.81
    methadone 94.25
    mist (inhalation) 93.94
    music 93.84
    nebulizer 93.94
    neuroleptic 94.23
    occupational 93.83
    oxygen 93.96
        catalytic 93.96
        hyperbaric 93.95
            wound 93.59
        wound (hyperbaric) 93.59
    paraffin bath 93.35
    physical NEC 93.39
        combined (without mention of components) 93.38
        diagnostic NEC 93.09
    play 93.81
        psychotherapeutic 94.36
    positive and expiratory pressure - see category 96.7
    psychiatric NEC 94.39
        drug NEC 94.25
        lithium 94.22
    radiation 92.29
        contact (150 KVP or less) 92.21
        deep (200–300 KVP) 92.22
        high voltage (200–300 KVP) 92.22
        low voltage (150 KVP or less) 92.21
        megavoltage 92.24
        orthovoltage 92.22
        particle source NEC 92.26
        photon 92.24
        radioisotope (teleradiotherapy) 92.23
        retinal lesion 14.26
        superficial (150 KVP or less) 92.21
        supervoltage 92.24
    radioisotope, radioisotopic NEC 92.29
        implantation or insertion 92.27
        injection or instillation 92.28
        teleradiotherapy 92.23
    radium (radon) 92.23
    recreational 93.81
    rehabilitation NEC 93.89
    respiratory NEC 93.99
►   bi-level airway pressure 93.90
        continuous positive airway pressure [CPAP]
        endotracheal respiratory assistance - see category 96.7
        intermittent mandatory ventilation [IMV] - see category 96.7
        intermittent positive pressure breathing [IPPB] 93.91
        negative pressure (continuous) [CNP] 93.99
        other continuous (unspecified duration) 96.70
            for less than 96 consecutive hours 96.71
            for 96 consecutive hours or more 96.72
        positive and expiratory pressure [PEEP] - see category 96.7
        pressure support ventilation [PSV] - see category 96.7
    root canal 23.70
        with
            apicoectomy 23.72
            irrigation 23.71
    shock
        chemical 94.24
        electric 94.27
            subconvulsive 94.26
        insulin 94.24
    speech 93.75
        for correction of defect 93.74
    ultrasound 93.35
        hyperthermia for cancer treatment 99.85
    ultraviolet light 99.82

Thermocautery — see Cauterization
Thermography 88.89
    blood vessel 88.86
    bone 88.83
    breast 88.85
    cerebral 88.81
    eye 88.82
    lymph gland 88.89
    muscle 88.84
    ocular 88.82
    osteoarticular 88.83
    specified site NEC 88.89
    vein, deep 88.86
Thermokeratoplasty 11.74
Thermosclerectomy 12.62
Thermotherapy (hot packs) (paraffin bath) NEC 93.35
Thiersch operation
    anus 49.79
    skin graft 86.69
        hand 86.62
Thompson operation
    cleft lip repair 27.54
    correction of lymphedema 40.9
    quadricepsplasty 83.86
    thumb apposition with bone graft 82.69
Thoracectomy 34.09
    for lung collapse 33.34
Thoracentesis 34.91
Thoracocentesis 34.91
Thoracolysis (for collapse of lung) 33.39
Thoracoplasty (anterior) (extrapleural) (paravertebral) (posterolateral) (complete) (partial) 33.34
Thoracoscopy, transpleural (for exploration) 34.21
    for lung collapse 33.32
Thoracotomy (with drainage) 34.09
    as operative approach — omit code
    exploratory 34.02
Three-snip operation, punctum 09.51
Thrombectomy 38.00
    with endarterectomy — see Endarterectomy
    abdominal
        artery 38.06
        vein 38.07
    aorta (arch) (ascending) (descending) 38.04
    bovine graft 39.49

Thromboendarterectomy — continued
- coronary artery 36.09
- head and neck vessel NEC 38.02
- intracranial vessel NEC 38.01
- lower limb
  - artery 38.08
  - vein 38.09
- pulmonary vessel 38.05
- thoracic vessel NEC 38.05
- upper limb (artery) (vein) 38.03

Thromboendarterectomy 38.10
- abdominal 38.16
- aorta (arch) (ascending) (descending) 38.14
- coronary artery 36.09
  - open chest approach 36.03
- head and neck NEC 38.12
- intracranial NEC 38.11
- lower limb 38.15
- thoracic NEC 38.15
- upper limb 38.13

Thymectomy 07.80
- partial 07.81
- total 07.82

Thymopexy 07.99
Thyrochondrotomy 31.3
Thyrocricoidectomy 30.29
Thyrocricotomy (for assistance in breathing) 31.1
Thyroidectomy NEC 06.39
- by mediastinotomy (see also Thyroidectomy, substernal) 06.50
- with laryngectomy — see Laryngectomy
- complete or total 06.4
  - substernal (by mediastinotomy) (transsternal route) 06.52
  - transoral route (lingual) 06.6
- lingual (complete) (partial) (subtotal) (total) 06.6
- partial or subtotal NEC 06.39
  - with complete removal of remaining lobe 06.2
  - submental route (lingual) 06.6
  - substernal (by mediastinotomy) (transsternal route) 06.51
- remaining tissue 06.4
- submental route (lingual) 06.6
- substernal (by mediastinotomy) (transsternal route) 06.50
  - complete or total 06.52
  - partial or subtotal 06.51
- transoral route (lingual) 06.6
- transsternal route (see also Thyroidectomy, substernal) 06.50
- unilateral (with removal of isthmus) (with removal of portion of other lobe) 06.2

Thyroidorrhaphy 06.93
Thyroidotomy (field) (gland) NEC 06.09
- postoperative 06.02

Thyrotomy 31.3
- with tantalum plate 31.69

Toilette
- skin — see Debridement, skin or subcutaneous tissue
- tracheostomy 96.55

Token economy (behavior therapy) 94.33
Tomkins operation (metroplasty) 69.49
Tomography — see also Radiography
- abdomen NEC 88.02
- cardiac 87.42
- computerized axial NEC 88.38
  - abdomen 88.01
- bone 88.38
  - quantitative 88.98
- brain 87.03
- head 87.03
- kidney 87.71
- skeletal 88.38
  - quantitative 88.98
- thorax 87.41
- head NEC 87.04
- kidney NEC 87.72
- lung 87.42
- thorax NEC 87.42

Tongue tie operation 25.91
Tonography 95.26
Tonometry 89.11
Tonsillectomy 28.2
- with adenoidectomy 28.3

Tonsillotomy 28.0
Topectomy 01.32
Torek (-Bevan) operation (orchidopexy) (first stage) (second stage) 62.5
Torkildsen operation (ventriculocisternal shunt) 02.2
Torpin operation (cul-de-sac resection) 70.92
Toti operation (dacryocystorhinostomy) 09.81
Touchas operation 86.63
Touroff operation (ligation of subclavian artery) 38.85
Toxicology — see Examination, microscopic
TPN (total parenteral nutrition) 99.15
Trabeculectomy ab externo 12.64
Trabeculodialysis 12.59
Trabeculotomy ab externo 12.54
Trachelectomy 67.4
Trachelopexy 69.22
Tracheloplasty 67.69
Trachelorrhaphy (Emmet) (suture) 67.61
- obstetrical 75.51

Trachelotomy 69.95
- obstetrical 73.93

Tracheocricotomy (for assistance in breathing) 31.1
Tracheofissure 31.1
Tracheography 87.32
Tracheolaryngotomy (emergency) 31.1
- permanent opening 31.29

Tracheoplasty 31.79
- with artificial larynx 31.75

Tracheorrhaphy 31.71
Tracheoscopy NEC 31.42
- through tracheotomy (stoma) 31.41

Tracheostomy (emergency) (temporary) (for assistance in breathing) 31.1
- mediastinal 31.21
- permanent NEC 31.29
- revision 31.74

Tracheotomy (emergency) (temporary) (for assistance in breathing) 31.1
- permanent 31.29

Tracing, carotid pulse with ECG lead 89.56
Traction
- with reduction of fracture or dislocation — see Reduction, fracture and Reduction, dislocation
- adhesive tape (skin) 93.46
- boot 93.46
- Bryant's (skeletal) 93.44
- Buck's 93.46
- caliper tongs 93.41
  - with synchronous insertion of device 02.94
- Cortel's (spinal) 93.42
- Crutchfield tongs 93.41
  - with synchronous insertion of device 02.94
- Dunlop's (skeletal) 93.44
- gallows 93.46
- Gardner Wells 93.41
  - with synchronous insertion of device 02.94
- halo device, skull 93.41
  - with synchronous insertion of device 02.94
- Lyman Smith (skeletal) 93.44
- manual, intermittent 93.21
- mechanical, intermittent 93.21
- Russell's (skeletal) 93.44
- skeletal NEC 93.44
  - intermittent 93.43
- skin, limbs NEC 93.46
- spinal NEC 93.42
  - with skull device (halo) (caliper) (Crutchfield) (Gardner Wells) (Vinke) (tongs) 93.41
    - with synchronous insertion of device 02.94
- Thomas' splint 93.45
- Vinke tongs 93.41
  - with synchronous insertion of device 02.94

Tractotomy
- brain 01.32
- medulla oblongata 01.32
- mesencephalon 01.32
- percutaneous 03.21
- spinal cord (one-stage) (two-stage) 03.29
- trigeminal (percutaneous) (radiofrequency) 04.02

Training (for) (in)
- ADL (activities of daily living) 93.83
  - for the blind 93.78
- ambulation 93.22
- braille 93.77
- crutch walking 93.24
- dyslexia 93.71
- dysphasia 93.72
- esophageal speech (postlaryngectomy) 93.73
- gait 93.22
- joint movements 93.14
- lip reading 93.75
- Moon (blind reading) 93.77
- orthoptic 95.35
- prenatal (natural childbirth) 93.37
- prosthetic or orthotic device usage 93.24
- relaxation 94.33
- speech NEC 93.75
  - esophageal 93.73
  - for correction of defect 93.74
- use of lead dog for the blind 93.76
- vocational 93.85

Transactional analysis
- group 94.44
- individual 94.39

Transection — see also Division
- artery (with ligation) (see also Division, artery) 38.80
  - renal, aberrant (with reimplantation) 39.55

bone (see also Osteotomy) 77.30
fallopian tube (bilateral) (remaining)
    (solitary) 66.39
    by endoscopy 66.22
    unilateral 66.92
isthmus, thyroid 06.91
muscle 83.19
    eye 15.13
        multiple (two or more muscles) 15.3
    hand 82.19
nerve (cranial) (peripheral) NEC 04.03
    acoustic 04.01
    root (spinal) 03.1
    sympathetic 05.0
    tracts in spinal cord 03.29
    trigeminal 04.02
    vagus (transabdominal) (see also Vagotomy) 44.00
pylorus (with wedge resection) 43.3
renal vessel, aberrant (with reimplantation) 39.55
spinal
    cord tracts 03.29
    nerve root 03.1
tendon 83.13
    hand 82.11
uvula 27.71
vas deferens 63.71
vein (with ligation) (see also Division, vein) 38.80
    renal, aberrant (with reimplantation) 39.55
    varicose (lower limb) 38.59

Transfer, transference
bone shaft, fibula into tibia 78.47
digital (to replace absent thumb) 82.69
    finger (to thumb) (same hand) 82.61
    to
        finger, except thumb 82.81
        opposite hand (with amputation) 82.69 [84.01]
    toe (to thumb) (with amputation) 82.69 [84.11]
        to finger, except thumb 82.81 [84.11]
fat pad NEC 86.89
    with skin graft — see Graft, skin, full-thickness
finger (to replace absent thumb) (same hand) 82.61
    to
        finger, except thumb 82.81
        opposite hand (with amputation) 82.69 [84.01]
muscle origin 83.77
    hand 82.58
nerve (cranial) (peripheral) (radial anterior) (ulnar) 04.6
pedicle graft 86.74
pes anserinus (tendon) (repair of knee) 81.47
tarsoconjunctival flap, from opposing lid 08.64
tendon 83.75
    hand 82.56
    pes anserinus (repair of knee) 81.47
toe-to-thumb (free) (pedicle) (with amputation) 82.69 [84.11]

Transfixion — see also Fixation
iris (bombe) 12.11

Transfusion (of) 99.03
antihemophilic factor 99.06
antivenin 99.16
blood (whole) 99.03
    expander 99.08
    surrogate 99.09
bone marrow 41.00
    allogenic 41.03
        with purging 41.02
    allograft 41.03
        with purging 41.02
    autograft 41.01
    autologous 41.01
coagulation factors 99.06
Dextran 99.08
exchange 99.01
    intraperitoneal 75.2
    in utero (with hysterotomy) 75.2
exsanguination 99.01
gamma globulin 99.14
granulocytes 99.09
intrauterine 75.2
packed cells 99.04
plasma 99.07
platelets 99.05
replacement, total 99.01
serum NEC 99.07
substitution 99.01
thrombocytes 99.05

Transillumination
nasal sinuses 89.35
skull (newborn) 89.16

Translumbar aortogram 88.42

Transplant, transplantation
artery 39.59
    renal, aberrant 39.55
autotransplant — see Reimplantation
blood vessel 39.59
    renal, aberrant 39.55
bone (see also Graft, bone) 78.00
    marrow 41.00
        allogeneic 41.03
            with purging 41.02
        allograft 41.03
            with purging 41.02
        autograft 41.01
        autologous 41.01
        stem cell (autologous) (hematopoietic) 41.04
combined heart-lung 33.6
conjunctiva, for pterygium 11.39
corneal (see also Keratoplasty) 11.60
dura 02.12
fascia 83.82
    hand 82.72
finger (replacing absent thumb) (same hand) 82.61
    to
        finger, except thumb 82.81
        opposite hand (with amputation) 82.69 [84.01]
gracilis muscle (for) 83.77
    anal incontinence 49.74
    urethrovesical suspension 59.71
hair follicles
    eyebrow 08.63
    eyelid 08.63
    scalp 86.64
heart (orthotopic) 37.5
    combined with lung 33.6
ileal stoma to new site 46.23
kidney NEC 55.69
liver 50.59
    auxiliary (permanent) (temporary) (recipient's liver in situ) 50.51
lung 33.5
    combined with heart 33.6
lymphatic structure(s) (peripheral) 40.9
mammary artery to myocardium or ventricular wall 36.2
muscle 83.77
    gracilis (for) 83.77
        anal incontinence 49.74
        urethrovesical suspension 59.71
    hand 82.58
    temporalis 83.77
        with orbital exenteration 16.59
nerve (cranial) (peripheral) 04.6
ovary 65.92
pancreas 52.80
    heterotransplant 52.83
    homotransplant 52.82
    reimplantation 52.81
pes anserinus (tendon) (repair of knee) 81.47
renal NEC 55.69
    vessel, aberrant 39.55
salivary duct opening 26.49
skin — see Graft, skin
spermatic cord 63.53
spleen 41.94
▸ stem cells (autologous) (hematopoietic) 41.04
tendon 83.75
    hand 82.56
    pes anserinus (repair of knee) 81.47
    superior rectus (blepharoptosis) 08.36
testis to scrotum 62.5
thymus 07.94
thyroid tissue 06.94
toe (replacing absent thumb) (with amputation) 82.69 [84.11]
    to finger, except thumb 82.81 [84.11]
tooth 23.5
ureter to
    bladder 56.74
    ileum (external diversion) 56.51
        internal diversion only 56.71
    intestine 56.71
    skin 56.61
vein (peripheral) 39.59
    renal, aberrant 39.55
vitreous 14.72
    anterior approach 14.71

Transposition
extraocular muscles 15.5
eyelash flaps 08.63
eye muscle (oblique) (rectus) 15.5
finger (replacing absent thumb) (same hand) 82.61
    to
        finger, except thumb 82.81
        opposite hand (with amputation) 82.69 [84.01]
interatrial venous return 35.91
jejunal (Henley) 43.81
joint capsule (see also Arthroplasty) 81.96
muscle NEC 83.79
    extraocular 15.5
    hand 82.59
nerve (cranial) (peripheral) (radial anterior) (ulnar) 04.6
nipple 85.86
pterygium 11.31
tendon NEC 83.76
    hand 82.57
vocal cords 31.69

Transureteroureterostomy 56.75

Transversostomy (see also Colostomy) 46.10
Trapping, aneurysm (cerebral) 39.52
Trauner operation (lingual sulcus extension) 24.91
Trephination, trephining
    accessory sinus — see Sinusotomy
    corneoscleral 12.89
    cranium 01.24
    nasal sinus — see Sinusotomy
    sclera (with iridectomy) 12.61
Trial (failed) forceps 73.3
Trigonectomy 57.6
Trimming, amputation stump 84.3
Triple arthrodesis 81.12
Trochanterplasty 81.40
Tsuge operation (macrodactyly repair) 82.83
Tuck, tucking — see also Plication
    eye muscle 15.22
        multiple (two or more muscles) 15.4
    levator palpebrae, for blepharoptosis 08.34

Tudor 'rabbit ear' operation (anterior urethropexy) 59.79
Tuffler operation
    apicolysis of lung 33.39
    vaginal hysterectomy 68.5
Tunnel, subcutaneous (antethoracic) 42.86
    with esophageal anastomosis 42.68
Turbinectomy (complete) (partial) NEC 21.69
    by
        cryosurgery 21.61
        diathermy 21.61
    with sinusectomy — see Sinusectomy
Turco operation (release of joint capsules in clubfoot) 80.48
Tylectomy (breast) (partial) 85.21
Tympanectomy 20.59
    with tympanoplasty — see Tympanoplasty
Tympanogram 95.41
Tympanomastoidectomy 20.42

Tympanoplasty (type I) (with graft) 19.4
    with
        air pocket over round window 19.54
        fenestra in semicircular canal 19.55
        graft against
            incus or malleus 19.52
            mobile and intact stapes 19.53
        incudostapediopexy 19.52
    epitympanic, type I 19.4
    revision 19.6
    type
        II (graft against incus or malleus) 19.52
        III (graft against mobile and intact stapes) 19.53
        IV (air pocket over round window) 19.54
        V (fenestra in semicircular canal) 19.55
Tympanosympathectomy 20.91
Tympanotomy 20.09
    with intubation 20.01

U

Uchida operation (tubal ligation with or without fimbriectomy) 66.32
UFR (uroflowmetry) 89.24
Ultrasonography
    abdomen 88.76
    aortic arch 88.73
    biliary tract 88.74
    breast 88.73
    deep vein thrombosis 88.77
    digestive system 88.74
    eye 95.13
    head and neck 88.71
    heart 88.72
    intestine 88.74
    lung 88.73
    midline shift, brain 88.71
    multiple sites 88.79
    peripheral vascular system 88.77
    retroperitoneum 88.76
    thorax NEC 88.73
    total body 88.79
    urinary system 88.75
    uterus 88.79
        gravid 88.78
Ultrasound
    diagnostic — *see* Ultrasonography
    fragmentation (of)
        cataract (with aspiration) 13.41
        urinary calculus, stones 59.95
    inner ear 20.79
    therapy 93.35
Umbilectomy 54.3
Unbridling
    blood vessel, peripheral 39.91
    celiac artery axis 39.91
Uncovering — *see* Incision, by site
Undercutting
    hair follicle 86.09
    perianal tissue 49.02
Unroofing — *see also* Incision, by site
    external
        auditory canal 18.02
        ear NEC 18.09
    kidney cyst 55.39

UPP (urethral pressure profile) 89.25
Upper GI series (x-ray) 87.62
Uranoplasty (for cleft palate repair) 27.62
Uranorrhaphy (for cleft palate repair) 27.62
Uranostaphylorrhaphy 27.62
Urban operation (mastectomy) (unilateral) 85.47
    bilateral 85.48
Ureterectomy 56.40
    with nephrectomy 55.51
    partial 56.41
    total 56.42
Ureterocecostomy 56.71
Ureterocelectomy 56.41
Ureterocolostomy 56.71
Ureterocystostomy 56.74
Ureteroenterostomy 56.71
Ureteroileostomy (internal diversion) 56.71
    external diversion 56.51
Ureterolithotomy 56.2
Ureterolysis 59.02
    with freeing or repositioning of ureter 59.01
Ureteroneocystostomy 56.74
Ureteropexy 56.85
Ureteroplasty 56.89
Ureteroplication 56.89
Ureteroproctostomy 56.71
Ureteropyelography (intravenous) (diuretic infusion) 87.73
    percutaneous 87.75
    retrograde 87.74
Ureteropyeloplasty 55.87
Ureteropyelostomy 55.86
Ureterorrhaphy 56.82
Ureteroscopy 56.31
    with biopsy 56.33
Ureterosigmoidostomy 56.71
Ureterostomy (cutaneous) (external) (tube) 56.61
    closure 56.83
    ileal 56.51

Ureterotomy 56.2
Ureteroureterostomy (crossed) 56.75
    lumbar 56.41
    resection with end-to-end anastomosis 56.41
    spatulated 56.41
Urethral catheterization, indwelling 57.94
Urethral pressure profile (UPP) 89.25
    Urethrectomy (complete) (partial) (radical) 58.3
    with
        complete cystectomy 57.79
        pelvic exenteration 68.8
        radical cystectomy 57.71
Urethrocystography (retrograde) (voiding) 87.76
Urethrocystopexy (by) 59.79
    levator muscle sling 59.71
    retropubic suspension 59.5
    suprapubic suspension 59.4
Urethrolithotomy 58.0
Urethrolysis 58.5
Urethropexy 58.49
    anterior 59.79
Urethroplasty 58.49
    augmentation (Polytef injection) 59.79
Urethrorrhaphy 58.41
Urethroscopy 58.22
    for control of hemorrhage of prostate 60.94
    perineal 58.21
Urethrostomy (perineal) 58.0
Urethrotomy (external) 58.0
    internal (endoscopic) 58.5
Uroflowmetry (UFR) 89.24
Urography (antegrade) (excretory) (intravenous) 87.73
    retrograde 87.74
Uteropexy (abdominal approach) (vaginal approach) 69.22
Uvulectomy 27.72
Uvulotomy 27.71

V

Vaccination (prophylactic) (against) 99.59
    anthrax 99.55
    brucellosis 99.55
    cholera 99.31
    common cold 99.51
    disease NEC 99.55
        arthropod-borne viral NEC 99.54
    encephalitis, arthropod-borne viral 99.53
    German measles 99.47
    hydrophobia 99.44
    infectious parotitis 99.46
    influenza 99.52
    measles 99.45
    mumps 99.46
    paratyphoid fever 99.32
    pertussis 99.37
    plague 99.34
    poliomyelitis 99.41
    rabies 99.44
    Rocky Mountain spotted fever 99.55
    rubella 99.47
    rubeola 99.45
    smallpox 99.42
    Staphylococcus 99.55
    Streptococcus 99.55
    tuberculosis 99.33
    tularemia 99.35
    typhoid 99.32
    typhus 99.55
    undulant fever 99.55
    yellow fever 99.43
Vacuum extraction, fetal head 72.79
    with episiotomy 72.71
Vagectomy (subdiaphragmatic) (*see also* Vagotomy) 44.00
Vaginal douche 96.44
Vaginectomy 70.4
Vaginofixation 70.77
Vaginoperineotomy 70.14
Vaginoplasty 70.79
Vaginorrhaphy 70.71
    obstetrical 75.69
Vaginoscopy 70.21
Vaginotomy 70.14
    for
        culdocentesis 70.0
        pelvic abscess 70.12
Vagotomy (gastric) 44.00
    parietal cell 44.02
    selective NEC 44.03
        highly 44.02
        Holle's 44.02
        proximal 44.02
    truncal 44.01
Valvotomy — *see* Valvulotomy
Valvulectomy, heart — *see* Valvuloplasty, heart
Valvuloplasty
    heart (open heart technique) (without valve replacement) 35.10
        with prosthesis or tissue graft — *see* Replacement, heart, valve, by site
        aortic valve 35.11
            percutaneous (balloon) 35.96
            combined with repair of atrial and ventricular septal defects — *see* Repair, endocardialcushion defect
        mitral valve 35.12
            percutaneous (balloon) 35.96
        pulmonary valve 35.13
            in total repair of tetralogy of Fallot 35.81
            percutaneous (balloon) 35.96
        tricuspid valve 35.14
Valvulotomy
    heart (closed heart technique) (transatrial) (transventricular) 35.00
        aortic valve 35.01
        mitral valve 35.02
        open heart technique — *see* Valvuloplasty, heart
        pulmonary valve 35.03
            in total repair of tetralogy of Fallot 35.81
        tricuspid valve 35.04
Varicocelectomy, spermatic cord 63.1
Varicotomy, peripheral vessels (lower limb) 38.59
    upper limb 38.53
Vascularization — *see* Revascularization
Vasectomy (complete) (partial) 63.73
Vasogram 87.94
Vasoligation 63.71
    gastric 38.86
Vasorrhaphy 63.81
Vasostomy 63.6
Vasotomy 63.6
Vasotripsy 63.71
Vasovasostomy 63.82
Vectorcardiogram (VCG) (with ECG) 89.53
Venectomy — *see* Phlebectomy
Venipuncture NEC 38.99
    for injection of contrast material — *see* Phlebography
Venography — *see* Phlebography
Venorrhaphy 39.32
Venotomy 38.00
    abdominal 38.07
    head and neck NEC 38.02
    intracranial NEC 38.01
    lower limb 38.09
    thoracic NEC 38.05
    upper limb 38.03
Venotripsy 39.98
Venovenostomy 39.29
Ventilation
- bi-level airway pressure 93.90
- continuous positive airway pressure [CPAP] 93.90
- endotracheal respiratory assistance - *see* category 96.7
- intermittent positive airway pressure breathing [IPPB] 93.91
- mechanical
-     endotracheal respiratory assistance — *see* category 96.7
-     intermittent mandatory ventilation [IMV] — *see* category 96.7
-     other continuous (unspecified duration) 96.70
-         for less than 96 consecutive hours 96.71
-         for 96 consecutive hours or more 96.72
-     positive and expiratory pressure [PEEP] — *see* category 96.7
-     pressure support ventilation [PSV] — *see* category 96.7
- negative pressure (continuous) [CNP] 93.99

Ventriculocholecystostomy 02.34
Ventriculocisternostomy 02.2
Ventriculocordectomy 30.29
Ventriculogram, Ventriculography (cerebral) 87.02
    cardiac
        left ventricle (outflow tract) 88.53
            combined with right heart 88.54
        right ventricle (outflow tract) 88.52
            combined with left heart 88.54
    radionuclide cardiac 92.05
Ventriculomyocardiotomy 37.11
Ventriculoperitoneostomy 02.34
Ventriculopuncture 01.09
    through previously implanted catheter or reservoir (Ommaya) (Rickham) 01.02
Ventriculoseptopexy (*see also* Repair, ventricular septal defect) 35.72
Ventriculoseptoplasty (*see also* Repair, ventricular septal defect) 35.72
Ventriculostomy 02.2
Ventriculotomy
    cerebral 02.2
    heart 37.1
Ventriculoureterostomy 02.35
Ventriculovenostomy 02.32
Ventrofixation, uterus 69.22
Ventrohysteropexy 69.22
Ventrosuspension, uterus 69.22
VEP (visual evoked potential) 95.23
Version, obstetrical (bimanual) (cephalic) (combined) (internal) (podalic) 73.21
    with extraction 73.22
    Braxton Hicks 73.21
        with extraction 73.22
    external (bipolar) 73.91
    Potter's (podalic) 73.21
        with extraction 73.22
    Wigand's (external) 73.91
    Wright's (cephalic) 73.21
        with extraction 73.22
Vesicolithotomy (suprapubic) 57.19
Vesicostomy 57.21
Vesicourethroplasty 57.85
Vesiculectomy 60.73
    with radical prostatectomy 60.5
Vesiculogram, seminal 87.92
    contrast 87.91
Vesicultomy 60.72
Vestibuloplasty (buccolabial) (lingual) 24.91
Vestibulotomy 20.79
Vicq D'azyr operation (larynx) 31.1
Vidal operation (varicocele ligation) 63.1
Vidlanectomy 05.21
Villusectomy (*see also* Synovectomy) 80.70
Vision check 95.09
Visual evoked potential (VEP) 95.23
Vitrectomy (mechanical) (posterior approach) 14.74
    with scleral buckling 14.49
    anterior approach 14.73
Vocational

assessment 93.85
retraining 93.85
schooling 93.82
Voice training (postlaryngectomy) 93.73
von Kraske operation (proctectomy) 48.64
Voss operation (hanging hip operation) 83.19

Vulpius (-Compere) operation (lengthening of gastrocnemius muscle) 83.85
Vulvectomy (bilateral) (simple) 71.62
   partial (unilateral) 71.61
   radical (complete) 71.5
   unilateral 71.61
VY operation (repair)
   bladder 57.89

   neck 57.85
ectropion 08.44
lip 27.59
skin (without graft) 86.89
subcutaneous tissue (without skin graft) 86.89
tongue 25.59

W

Wads test (hemispheric function) 89.10
Ward-Mayo operation (vaginal hysterectomy) 68.5
Washing — *see* Lavage and Irrigation
Waterston operation (aorta-right pulmonary artery anastomosis) 39.0
Watkins (-Wertheim) **operation** (uterus interposition) 69.21
Watson-Jones operation
   hip arthrodesis 81.21
   reconstruction of lateral ligaments, ankle 81.49
   shoulder arthrodesis (extra-articular) 81.23
   tenoplasty 83.88
Webbing (syndactylization) 86.89
Weir operation
   appendicostomy 47.91
   correction of nostrils 21.86
Wertheim operation (radical hysterectomy) 68.6
West operation (dacryocystorhinostomy) 09.81
Wheeler operation
   entropion repair 08.44
   halving procedure (eyelid) 08.24
Whipple operation (radical pancreaticoduodenectomy) 52.7
   Child modification (radical subtotal pancreatectomy) 52.53
   Rodney Smith modification (radical subtotal pancreatectomy) 52.53
White operation (lengthening of tendo calcaneus by incomplete tenotomy) 83.11
Whitehead operation
   glossectomy, radical 25.4
   hemorrhoidectomy 49.46
Whitman operation
   foot stabilization (talectomy) 77.98
   hip reconstruction 81.40
   repair of serratus anterior muscle 83.87
   talectomy 77.98
   trochanter wedge osteotomy 77.25
Wier operation (entropion repair) 08.44
Williams-Richardson operation (vaginal construction) 70.61
Wilms operation (thoracoplasty) 33.34
Wilson operation (angulation osteotomy for hallux valgus) 77.51
Window operation
   antrum (nasal sinus) — *see* Antrotomy, maxillary
   aorticopulmonary 39.59
   bone cortex (*see also* Incision, bone) 77.10
      facial 76.09
   nasoantral — *see* Antrotomy, maxillary
   pericardium 37.12
   pleura 34.09
Winiwarter operation (cholecystoenterostomy) 51.32
Wiring
   aneurysm 39.52
   dental (for immobilization) 93.55
      with fracture-reduction — *see* Reduction, fracture
   orthodontic 24.7
Wirsungojejunostomy 52.96
Witzel operation (temporary gastrostomy) 43.19
Woodward operation (release of high riding scapula) 81.83
Wrapping, aneurysm (gauze) (methyl methacrylate) (plastic) 39.52

X

Xenograft 86.65
Xerography, breast 87.36
Xeromammography 87.36
Xiphoidectomy 77.81
X-ray
   chest (routine) 87.44
      wall NEC 87.39
   contrast — *see* Radiography, contrast
   diagnostic — *see* Radiography
   injection of radio-opaque substance — *see* Radiography, contrast
   skeletal series, whole or complete 88.31
   therapeutic — *see* Therapy, radiation

Y

Young operation
   epispadias repair 58.45
   tendon transfer (anterior tibialis) (repair of flat foot) 83.75
Yount operation (division of iliotibial band) 83.14

Z

Zancolli operation
   capsuloplasty 81.72
   tendon transfer (biceps) 82.56
Ziegler operation (iridectomy) 12.14
Zonulolysis (with lens extraction) (*see also* Extraction, cataract, intracapsular) 13.19
Z-plasty
   epicanthus 08.59
   eyelid (*see also* Reconstruction, eyelid) 08.70
   hypopharynx 29.4
   skin (scar) (web contracture) 86.84
      with excision of lesion 86.3